Ta₁

Pocketbook

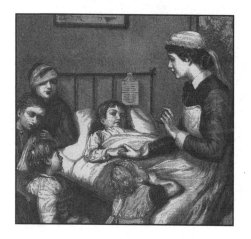

Todd J. Flosi, MD, FAAP
Director, Inpatient Pediatrics
Ventura County Medical Center
Clinical Instructor, Department of Family Medicine
UCLA School of Medicine
Los Angeles, California

Stephanie L. D'Augustine, MD, FAAP
General Pediatrics
Ventura County Health Care Agency
Ventura, California

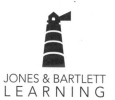

JONES & BARTLETT
L E A R N I N G

World Headquarters
Jones & Bartlett Learning
5 Wall Street
Burlington, MA 01803
978-443-5000
info@jblearning.com
www.jblearning.com

Jones & Bartlett Learning books and products are available through most bookstores and online booksellers. To contact Jones & Bartlett Learning directly, call 800-832-0034, fax 978-443-8000, or visit our website, www.jblearning.com.

Substantial discounts on bulk quantities of Jones & Bartlett Learning publications are available to corporations, professional associations, and other qualified organizations. For details and specific discount information, contact the special sales department at Jones & Bartlett Learning via the above contact information or send an email to specialsales@jblearning.com.

Production Credits
Executive Acquisitions Editor: Nancy Anastasi Duffy
Production Assistant: Alex Schab
Digital Marketing Manager: Jennifer Sharp
Manufacturing and Inventory Control Supervisor: Amy Bacus
Composition: diacriTech
Cover Design: Kristin E. Parker
Manager of Photo Research, Rights & Permissions: Lauren Miller
Cover Image: Courtesy of The National Library of Medicine
Printing and Binding: Edwards Brothers Malloy
Cover Printing: Edwards Brothers Malloy

ISBN: 978-1-4496-3638-8

6048

Printed in the United States of America
18 17 16 15 14   10 9 8 7 6 5 4 3 2 1

Tarascon Pediatric Inpatient Pocketbook

Table of Contents

Editorial Board

Abbreviations

↑	increased
↑↑	greatly increased
↓	decreased
→	leading to
>	greater than
≥	greater than or equal to
<	less than
≤	less than or equal to
~	approximately
+/−	with or without *or* plus or minus
17-OHP	17-hydroxyprogesterone
2hPG	2 hours post-CHO load
AA	amino acids
AAN	American Academy of Neurology
AAP	American Academy of Pediatrics
ABCs	airway, breathing, circulation
ABG	arterial blood gas
ABPA	allergic bronchopulmonary aspergillosis
ABPM	ambulatory blood pressure monitoring
Abs	antibodies
abx	antibiotics
AC	activated charcoal
ACE	angiotensin-converting enzyme
ACEi	angiotensin-converting enzyme inhibitor
ACS	acute chest/coronary syndrome
ACTH	adrenocorticotropic hormone
ADEM	acute disseminated encephalomyelitis
ADH	antidiuretic hormone
AF	atrial fibrillation
AG	anion gap
AGA	appropriate for gestational age
AGE	acute gastroenteritis
AHO	acute hematogenous osteomyelitis
AIDP	autoimmune demyelinating polyneuropathy
AIS	arterial ischemic stroke
AKIN	Acute Kidney Injury Network
ALL	acute lymphoblastic leukemia
ALT	alanine aminotransferase
ALTE	apparent life-threatening event
AM	morning
AML	acute myeloid leukemia
AMS	altered mental status
ANC	absolute neutrophil count
anti-DS DNA	anti-double-stranded DNA
anti-FXa	anti-factor Xa assay
aPTT	activated partial thromboplastin time
AR	aortic regurgitation
ARA	arachidonic acid
ARDS	acute respiratory distress syndrome
ARF	acute renal failure
AS	aortic stenosis
ASAP	as soon as possible
ASD	atrial septal defect
ASDOS	atrial septal defect occlusion system
ASIS	anterior superior iliac spine
ASO	antistreptolysin O antibody
AST	aspartate transaminase
ATA	antithyroglobulin antibodies
ATG	antithymocyte globulin
ATN	acute tubular necrosis
AV	aortic valve
AVM	arteriovenous malformation
AVN	avascular necrosis
BAL	bronchoalveolar lavage *or* Dimercaprol
BG	blood glucose
bid	twice per day
BiPAP	bilevel positive airway pressure
BMT	bone marrow transplant
BP	blood pressure
BPD	bronchopulmonary dysplasia
bpm	beats per minute
BRAT	bananas, rice, applesauce, toast
BRBPR	bright red blood per rectum
BSA	body surface area
BUN	blood urea nitrogen
BVM	bag-valve mask
BW	body weight
Ca	calcium
CAH	congenital adrenal hyperplasia
CaSR	calcium-sensing receptor
CBC	complete blood count
CBCd	complete blood count with differential
cc	cubic centimeter
CcO$_2$	capillary oxygen content
CCAM	congenital cystic adenomatoid malformation
CCHD	congenital coronary heart disease
CDC	Centers for Disease Control and Prevention
CDPH	California Department of Public Health
CF	cystic fibrosis
CFRD	cystic fibrosis-related diabetes
CFTR	cystic fibrosis transmembrane conductance regulator
CGD	chronic granulomatous disease
CHD	congenital heart disease
CHF	congestive heart failure
CHO	carbohydrate
CIDP	chronic inflammatory demyelinating polyneuropathy
CK	creatine kinase

cm	centimeter	EGD	esophagoscopy
CMAP	compound muscle action potential	EMG	electromyography
CMV	cytomegalovirus	ENT	ear, nose, and throat
CN	cranial nerve	EOD	early onset disease
CNS	central nervous system	ERCP	endoscopic retrograde
CO	carbon monoxide		cholangiopancreatography
CO_2	carbon dioxide	ESR	erythrocyte sedimentation rate
coarct	coarctation of the aorta	ESRD	end-stage renal disease
COC	combined oral contraceptive	ESWL	extracorporeal shock wave
CP	cerebral palsy		lithotripsy
CPAP	continuous positive airway pressure	ETOH	alcohol
CPK	creatine phosphokinase	ETT	endotracheal tube
Cr	creatinine		
CrCl	creatinine clearance	FB	foreign body
CRP	C-reactive protein	FBG	fasting blood glucose
CRRT	continuous renal replacement	FDA	Food and Drug Administration
	therapy	FDG-PET	18-fluorodeoxyglucose positron
CSF	cerebrospinal fluid		emission tomography
CT	computed tomography	Fe	iron
Cu	copper	FE	fractional excretion
CVA	cerebrovascular accident	FENa	fractional excretion of sodium
CVC	central venous catheter	FEV_1	forced expiratory volume in
CVL	central venous line		1 second
CvO_2	venous oxygen content	FFP	fresh frozen plasma
CVST	cerebral sinovenous thrombosis	FHH	familial hypocalciuric
CXR	chest radiograph		hypercalcemia
		FHx	family history
$D_{25}W$	dextrose 25% in water	FiO_2	fraction of inspired oxygen
DAT	direct antiglobulin (Coombs) test	fL	femtoliters
DDAVP	1-desamino-8-D-arginine	Fr	French (catheter)
	vasopressin	FSGN	focal segmental glomerulosclerosis
DDH	developmental dysplasia of the hip	FSH	follicle-stimulating hormone
DIC	disseminated intravascular	FT4	free thyroxine
	coagulation	FTT	failure to thrive
DIP	desquamative interstitial	FVIII	factor VIII
	pneumonitis		
DFA	direct fluorescence antibody	g	gram
DHA	docosahexaenoic acid	G6PD	glucose-6-phosphate
div	divided		dehydrogenase
DKA	diabetic ketoacidosis	GA	gestational age
dL	deciliter	GBS	Guillain-Barré syndrome *or* Group B
DMPA	depot medroxyprogesterone acetate		streptococcus
DNase	antideoxyribonuclease	GC	*Neisseria gonorrhoeae*
DNSI	deep neck space infection	GCS	Glasgow Coma Scale
DOC	deoxycorticosterone	GER	gastroesophageal reflux
DOL	day of life	GERD	gastroesophageal reflux disease
DPB	diastolic blood pressure	GFR	glomerular filtration rate
DTR	deep tendon reflex	GH	growth hormone
DUOX2	dual oxidase 2	GI	gastrointestinal
DWI	diffusion-weighted imaging	GNR	gram-negative rod
DXA	dual-energy X-ray absorptiometry	gtt	drop
		GVHD	graft-versus-host disease
EBV	Epstein-Barr Virus		
ECG	electrocardiogram	h	hour
ECMO	extracorporeal membrane	H_2O	water
	oxygenation	Hb	hemoglobin
ED	emergency department	HbA1c	hemoglobin A1c
EDTA	ethylenediaminetetraacetic acid	HbCO	carboxyhemoglobin
EEG	electroencephalogram	HBIG	hepatitis B immunoglobulin
eFe	elemental iron	HbS	sickle hemoglobin
EGA	estimated gestational age		

HCl	hydrogen chloride	LH	luteinizing hormone
HCO₃	bicarbonate	LMA	laryngeal mask airway
HCT	hematocrit	LMWH	low molecular weight heparin
HFFI	high-frequency flow interrupter	LOC	level of consciousness
HFJV	high-frequency jet ventilator	LOD	late-onset disease
HFOV	high-frequency oscillator ventilator	LP	lumbar puncture
Hib	*Haemophilus influenzae* type b	LR	lactated Ringer's
HIV	human immunodeficiency virus	LV	left atrium
HLHS	hypoplastic left heart syndrome		
HOB	head of bed	m	meter
HPLC	high-performance liquid chromatography	MAP	mean airway pressure
		MAS	McCune–Albright syndrome *or* macrophage activating syndrome
HPT	hypothalamic-pituitary-thyroid		
HPV	human papillomavirus	MCAD	medium-chain acyl-CoA dehydrogenase deficiency
hr	hour		
HR	heart rate	mcg	microgram
HSP	Henoch-Schönlein purpura	MCHC	mean corpuscular hemoglobin concentration
HSV	herpes simplex		
HTLV	human T-lymphotropic virus	mcL	microliter
HTN	hypertension	MCT	medium chain triglyceride
HUS	hemolytic uremic syndrome	MCV	mean corpuscular volume
Hz	hertz	MDI	metered-dose inhaler
		MELAS	mitochondrial encephalopathy, lactic acidosis, and stroke-like episode
IAP	intrapartum antibiotic prophylaxis		
IBD	irritable bowel disorder		
iCa	ionized calcium	MEN	multiple endocrine neoplasia
ICP	intracranial pressure	mEq	milliequivalent
ICS	intercostal space	mg	milligram
IDM	infant of diabetic mother	Mg	magnesium
I:E	inspiratory to expiratory ratio	MH	microscopic hematuria
IgA	immunoglobulin A	MHC	minor histocompatibility complex
IgE	immunoglobulin E	MIC	minimum inhibitory concentration
IL-1	interleukin-1	min	minute
IM	intramuscular	mL	milliliter
IN	intranasal	mmad	massive macronodular adrenal hyperplasia
INR	international normalized ratio		
IO	intraosseous	mmHg	millimeters of mercury
iPTH	intact parathyroid hormone	mmol	millimole
IU	international unit	MMR	measles, mumps, rubella
IUD	intrauterine device	Mn	manganese
IUGR	intrauterine growth restriction	Mo	molybdenum
IV	intravenous	mOsm	milliosmole
IVC	inferior vena cava	MPGN	membranoproliferative glomerulonephritis
IVF	intravenous fluids		
IVIG	intravenous immunoglobulin	MRA	magnetic resonance angiography
		MRCP	magnetic resonance cholangiopancreatography
J	joule		
JIA	juvenile idiopathic arthritis	MRI	magnetic resonance imaging
		MRSA	methicillin-resistant *Staphylococcus aureus*
K	potassium		
KCl	potassium chloride	ms	millisecond
kg	kilogram	MTHFR	methylenetetrahydrofolate reductase
KI	potassium iodide		
		MV	mitral valve
		MVI	multivitamin for infusion
L	left *or* liter		
LA	left atrium	N/A	not applicable
LDH	lactate dehydrogenase	Na	sodium
LFT	liver function test	NAAT	nucleic acid amplification test
LGA	large for gestational age	NaCl	sodium chloride
LGI	lower gastrointestinal tract	NaHCO3	sodium bicarbonate

NAS	neonatal abstinence syndrome	PID	pelvic inflammatory disease
NCCAH	non-classical congenital adrenal hyperplasia	PIG	pulmonary interstitial glycogenesis
		PKD	polycystic kidney disease *or* pyruvate kinase deficiency
NEC	necrotizing enterocolitis		
NEHI	neuroendocrine cell hyperplasia in infancy	PM	afternoon/night
		PMN	polymorphonuclear
NF	neurofibromatosis	PO	orally
ng	nanogram	PPHN	persistent pulmonary hypertension of the newborn
NG	nasogastric		
NGAL	neutrophil gelatinase-associated lipocalin	PPI	proton pump inhibitor
		PPNAD	primary pigmented adrenocortical nodular disease
NGT	nasogastric tube		
NHL	non-Hodgkin's lymphoma	PPV	positive predictive value *or* positive pressure ventilation
NIPPV	nasal intermittent positive pressure ventilation		
		PR	rectally
nmol	nanomole	PRA	plasma renin activity
NMJ	neuromuscular junction	PRBC	packed red blood cells
NPH	isophane insulin	prn	as needed
NPO	nothing per orem (nothing by mouth)	PS	pulmonic stenosis
		PSGN	post-strep glomerulonephritis
NPV	negative predictive value	pSLE	pediatric systemic lupus erythematosus
NS	normal saline		
NSAID	nonsteroidal anti-inflammatory drug	PT	prothrombin time
		PTH	parathyroid hormone
		PTLD	post-transplant lymphoproliferative disease
O₂	oxygen		
oCRH	ovine corticotropin-releasing hormone	PTU	propylthiouracil
		PTSD	posttraumatic stress disorder
OFC	occipital–frontal circumference	PTT	partial thromboplastin time
OG	orogastric		
OGT	orogastric tube	q	every
OGTT	oral glucose tolerance test	qd	daily
OR	operating room	qid	four times per day
ORS	oral rehydration solution	qod	every other day
OT	occupational therapy	QTc	corrected QT interval
OTC	over the counter		
oz	ounce	R	right
		RBC	red blood cells
PA	pulmonary artery	RDA	recommended dietary allowance
PaO₂	partial pressure of oxygen	RDS	respiratory distress syndrome
PCO₂	partial pressure of carbon dioxide	RDW	red cell distribution width
PCN	penicillin	retic	reticulocyte count
PCOS	polycystic ovarian syndrome	RF	rheumatoid factor
PCP	*Pneumocystis* pneumonia	RIDT	rapid influenza diagnostic test
PCR	polymerase chain reaction	RLQ	right lower quadrant
PDA	patent ductus arteriosus	RNP	ribonucleoprotein
PE	physical exam *or* pulmonary embolism	RR	respiratory rate
		RSI	rapid-sequence intubation
PEEP	positive end-expiratory pressure	RSV	respiratory syncytial virus
PEF	peak expiratory flow	RTA	renal tubular acidosis
PFO	patent foramen ovale	RT-PCR	reverse transcriptase polymerase chain reaction
PFT	pulmonary function test		
PGE1	prostaglandin E1	RUQ	right upper quadrant
PHACE	*p*osterior fossa, *h*emangioma, *a*rterial lesions, *c*ardiac, and *e*ye anomalies	RUS	renal ultrasound
		RV	right ventricular
		RVH	right ventricular hypertrophy
Phos	phosphorous	Rx	treatment
PI	primary immunodeficiency		
PICC	peripherally inserted central catheter	SBP	systolic blood pressure
		SCD	sickle cell disease
PICU	pediatric intensive care unit		

SES	socioeconomic status	tPA	tissue plasminogen activator
sg	specific gravity	TPN	total parenteral nutrition
SGA	small for gestational age	TSB	total serum bilirubin
SIADH	syndrome of inappropriate anti-diuretic hormone	TSH	thyroid-stimulating hormone
		TSHR	thyroid-stimulating hormone receptor
SIDS	sudden infant death syndrome		
SIMV	synchronized intermittent mandatory ventilation	TSS	trans-sphenoidal surgery
		TTKG	transtubular potassium gradient
SJS	Stevens-Johnson syndrome	TTP	thrombotic thrombocytopenic purpura
SLE	systemic lupus erythematosus		
SMX	sulfamethoxazole	TV	tidal volume
sol	solution		
SpO$_2$	oxygen saturation	U	unit
SQ	subcutaneously	UAC	umbilical artery catheter
SSKI	saturated solution of potassium iodide	UCa	urine calcium
		UCr	urine creatinine
SSRI	selective serotonin reuptake inhibitor	UFC	urinary free cortisol
		UGI	upper gastrointestinal tract
STI	sexually transmitted infection	UH	unfractionated heparin
SVC	superior vena cava	UNICEF	United Nations Children's Fund
SvO$_2$	venous oxygen saturation	UOP	urine output
SVT	supraventricular tachycardia	UP	urine protein
sx	symptoms	US	ultrasound
		USPSTF	US Preventive Services Task Force
T1DM	type 1 diabetes mellitus	UTI	urinary tract infection
T3	triiodothyronine	UVC	umbilical venous catheter
T4	thyroxine		
TA	tricuspid atresia		
TAC	tacrolimus	VATS	video-assisted thoracoscopic surgery
TAPVR	total anomalous pulmonary venous return		
		VCUG	voiding cystourethrogram
TB	tuberculosis	VF	ventricular fibrillation
tbili	total bilirubin	VKA	vitamin K antagonist
TBSA	total body surface area	VKDB	vitamin K deficiency bleeding
TCA	tricyclic antidepressant	VOC	vaso-occlusive crisis
TcB	transcutaneous bilirubin monitor	VOD	veno-occlusive disease
TCD	transcranial Doppler	VP	ventriculoperitoneal
TDD	total daily dose	V/Q	ventilation/perfusion
TEF	tracheoesophageal fistula	VSD	ventricular septal defect
TEN	toxic epidermal necrolysis	VT	ventricular tachycardia
TG	triglycerides	VTE	venous thrombotic event
TGA	transposition of the great arteries	VUR	vesicoureteral reflux
THAM	tris-hydroxymethyl aminomethane	vWD	von Willebrand's disease
TIA	transient ischemic attack	VZV	varicella zoster virus
TIBC	total iron-binding capacity	WAGR	Wilm's tumor, aniridia, genitourinary anomalies, mental retardation
tid	three times per day		
TLS	tumor lysis syndrome		
TMP	trimethoprim	WBC	white blood cells
TNF	tumor necrosis factor	WBI	whole-bowel irrigation
TOF	tetralogy of Fallot	WHO	World Health Organization
TOGV	transposition of the great vessels	WPW	Wolff-Parkinson-White
TORCH	toxoplasma, "other" (such as syphilis), rubella, cytomegalovirus, hepatitis, HIV	yo	years old
		Zn	zinc

ARRHYTHMIAS AND ECG EVALUATION

Table 1.1 Normal ECG Values

Age	P-R interval[a]	QRS interval[a]	QRS axis (mean)	QTc[b]
0–7 days	0.08–0.12	0.04–0.08	80–160 (125)	0.34–0.54
1–4 weeks	0.08–0.12	0.04–0.07	60–160 (110)	0.30–0.50
1–3 months	0.08–0.12	0.04–0.08	40–120 (80)	0.32–0.47
3–6 months	0.08–0.12	0.04–0.08	20–80 (65)	0.35–0.46
6–12 months	0.09–0.13	0.04–0.08	0–100 (65)	0.31–0.49
1–3 years	0.10–0.14	0.04–0.08	20–100 (55)	0.34–0.49
3–8 years	0.11–0.16	0.05–0.09	40–80 (60)	< 0.45
8–16 years	0.12–0.17	0.05–0.09	20–80 (65)	< 0.45

[a] seconds [b] QTc = QT interval/(square root of RR interval)

Table 1.2 ECG Diagnosis of Chamber Enlargement (hypertrophy)

Right Ventricular Hypertrophy/RVH	Biventricular Hypertrophy
• R in V1 > 20 mm (> 25 mm < 1 months old) • S in V6 > 6 mm (> 12 mm < 1 months old) • Upright T in V3R, R in V1 after 5 days old • QR pattern in V3R, V1 **Left Ventricular Hypertrophy/LVH** • R in V6 > 25 mm (> 21 mm < 1 year) • S in V1 > 30 mm (> 20 mm < 1 year) • R in V6 + S in V1 > 60 mm (use V5 if R in V5 > R in V6) • Abnormal R/S ratio • S in V1 > 2 X R in V5	• RVH and (S in V1 or R in V6) exceeding mean for age • LVH and (R in V1 or S in V6) exceeding mean for age **Right Atrial Hypertrophy** • Peak P value > 3 mm (< 6 months), > 2.5 mm (≥ 6 months) **Left Atrial Hypertrophy** • P in II > 0.09 seconds • P in V1 with late negative defl ection > 0.04 seconds and > 1 mm deep

Table 1.3 ECG Findings in Medical Disorders

Disorder	Typical ECG Findings (not necessarily most common)
Calcium	↑ Ca: short QT, AV block, ↓ HR. ↓ Ca: long QT, ↑ HR
CNS bleed	Diffuse deep T inversion, prominent U, QT > 60% of normal
Digoxin effect	Downward curve of ST segment, flat/inverted Ts, short QT
Hyperkalemia	Peaked Ts, wide then flat Ps, wide QRS and QT, sine wave
Hypokalemia	Flat T waves, U waves, ST depression
Thyroid	*Hypo:* ↓ HR, ↓ voltage, ST ↓, flat/↓ T waves; *Hyper:* ↑ HR
Kawasaki disease	Prolonged P-R, nonspecific ST-T changes
Lyme disease	AV block, pericarditis, intraventricular conduction delays
Myocarditis	Diffuse nonspecific ST-T Δ, AV block, ventricular ectopy
Pericarditis	Flat/concave ST ↓, PR segment depression, ↓ voltage

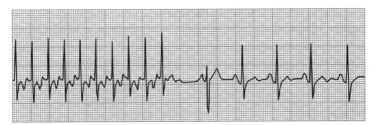

Figure 1.1 Supraventricular Tachycardia

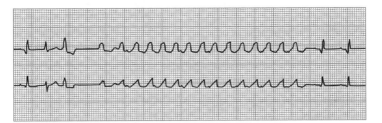

Figure 1.2 Ventricular Tachycardia

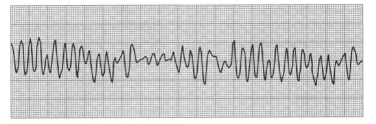

Figure 1.3 Ventricular Fibrillation

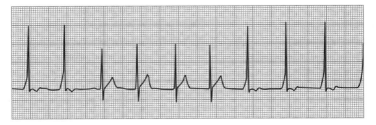

Figure 1.4 Wolff-Parkinson-White (WPW) Syndrome

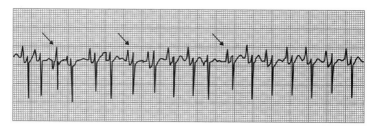

Figure 1.5 Multifocal Atrial Tachycardia

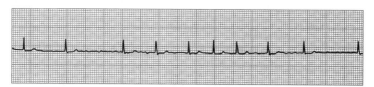

Figure 1.6 Atrial Fibrillation

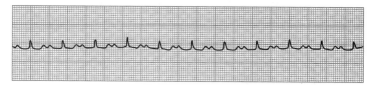

Figure 1.7 First-Degree Heart Block

ARRHYTHMIAS: IDENTIFICATION AND TREATMENT

Table 1.4 Arrhythmia Descriptions*

Atrial Ectopy	Early P wave with different morphology than others; ↑ risk SVT
Junctional Premature Beat	Early QRS with no P wave
Premature Ventricular Beat	Wide QRS, no preceding P wave
Junctional Ectopic Tachycardia	SVT with AV dissociation, ventricular rate > atrial rate
Heart Block	**First Degree:** every sinus beat conducted to ventricle, prolonged PR interval **Second Degree:** *Mobitz I:* gradual ↑ in PR leads to dropped beat; *Mobitz II:* abrupt nonconducted beat **Third Degree:** communication between atria and ventricles is completely disconnected

*See Figures also.

Table 1.5 Medications Used in the Treatment of Arrhythmias

Class 1A: Procainamide	Acts to ↑ QRS and ↑ QT interval; used in atrial fibrillation or flutter, monomorphic VT, and WPW Bolus: 5–15 mg/kg IV (max: 1000 mg) over 30 min; Infusion: 20–80 mcg/kg/min IV (draw levels 2 hours after change in rate, adjust so that levels are 4–10 mcg/mL)
Class 1B: Lidocaine, Mexiletine	Used in ventricular arrhythmias; **Lidocaine:** 1 mg/kg slowly infused IV, then 20–50 mcg/kg/min **Mexiletine:** 5–10 mg/kg/day PO, divided q 8 hours
Class 1C: Flecainide, Propafenone	↑ QRS duration; high proarrhythmic potential, use only in children with good ventricular function **Flecainide:** 2–6 mg/kg/day PO, divided q 8–12 hours **Propafenone:** 150–300 mg/m²/day PO, divided q 8 hours
Class II: Propranolol, Nadolol, Atenolol, Esmolol	**Propranolol** (nonselective): 0.5–4 mg/kg/day PO, divided tid or qid **Nadolol:** 0.5–1 mg/kg/dose PO q day **Atenolol** (cardioselective): 1–2 mg/kg dose PO q day (max, 2 mg/kg/day) **Esmolol:** 100 < 500 mcg/kg IV over 1 min, then 50–250 mcg/min
Class III: Amiodarone, Sotalol	↑ action potential duration and refractory period **Amiodarone:** Refractory pulseless VT/VF: 5 mg/kg rapid IV/IO push Stable tachycardias: 5 mg/kg IV over 20–60 min Oral dosing: 10–20 mg/kg/day PO q day or divided bid for 7–10 days then 5 mg/kg/day PO for 1–2 months, then wean as tolerated (min: 2.5 mg/kg/day); side effects include hypotension (IV form), corneal deposits, thyroid problems, pulmonary fibrosis, hepatitis, peripheral neuropathy, skin rash/discoloration. May use in children with poor ventricular function **Sotalol:** 80–200 mg/m²/day PO div q 8 hours; use only in children with good ventricular function
Class IV: Verapamil	Causes sinus slowing, ↑ PR interval **Dosing:** 0.1 mg/kg/dose IV over 2 min, may repeat 1× after 30 min; 3–4 mg/kg/day PO divided tid (max, 8 mg/kg or 480 mg/day). Beware hypotension, bradycardia in neonates; can ↑ conduction in WPW; don't use in children already on beta blocker
Adenosine	Used in narrow QRS tachycardias; also used to clarify diagnosis of atrial flutter. Give ***rapid IV push*** < 50 kg: 50–100 mcg/kg 1×, then q 1–2 min if needed > 50 kg: 6mg initially, then 12 mg q 1–2 min if needed
Digoxin	Slows AV conduction in atrial fibrillation or flutter; contraindicated in WPW syndrome **Dosing:** 8 mcg/kg/day PO divided bid

Reference: *Nadas' Pediatric Cardiology*, 2nd ed. Philadelphia: Elsevier/Saunders, 2006.

CONGENITAL HEART DISEASE

Table 1.6 Findings in Congenital Heart Disease (CHD)

Murmur	May or may not be heard depending on lesion type and size
Cyanosis	Central cyanosis (mucous membranes, lips, trunk) always pathologic. CHD-associated cyanosis usually does not improve with oxygen, gets worse with crying/agitation. Typically have ductal-dependent right-sided obstruction (inadequate blood to lungs)
Shock	More common presentation when **left-sided ductal-dependent lesion**, inadequate systemic perfusion when ductus closes (~ 2 weeks old)
CHF	Respiratory distress, crackles, ↑ respiratory rate, poor feeding, sweating, hepatomegaly, cardiomegaly. CHF found in large L → R shunts (critical AS, coarctation, VSD)
Blood Pressure Differential	Present in coarctation of the aorta or critical AS
Hyperoxia Test	Supply 100% FiO_2 for 10 minutes. Measure postductal ABG. If PaO_2 < 150 mmHg, congenital heart disease suspected. If PaO_2 > 150 mmHg, more likely pulmonary disease

ABG: Arterial blood gas; AS: Aortic stenosis; CHF: Congestive heart failure; PS: Pulmonic stenosis; VSD: Ventricular septal defect.

Table 1.7 Innocent Murmurs

	Description	Age at Auscultation
Branch Pulmonary Stenosis	Systolic, upper left sternal border, I-II/VI intensity, transmits to axillae and back. If persists, consider pulmonic stenosis.	Infants, up to 3–6 months
Still's Murmur (vibratory murmur)	Systolic, left lower-mid sternal border, I-III/VI, vibratory, low-frequency	3–6 yrs, occasionally in infants
Venous Hum: (turbulence in jugular vein)	Continuous, I-III/VI, right or left supra/infraclavicular areas. Changes with right and left rotation of head. Disappears when supine.	3–6 yrs
Carotid Bruit (can be significant stenosis)	Systolic, right supraclavicular and carotid, II-III/VI, occasional thrill	Any age
Pulmonary Ejection Murmur	Early-mid systolic ejection, I-III/VI, left upper sternal border, no radiation	8–14 yrs

Table 1.8 Pathologic Murmurs

	Description	Age at Auscultation
Patent Ductus Arteriosus	Continuous, II-V/VI, possible bounding pulses, louder with ↓ pulmonary resistance	Left infraclavicular
Ventricular Septal Defect	Holosystolic, "blowing," II-V/VI, louder with ↓ pulmonary resistance	Left lower sternal border
Atrial Septal Defect	Systolic, II-III/VI, widely split and fixed S2	Left upper sternal border
Pulmonic Stenosis	Systolic ejection, II-V/VI, S2 widely split, ejection click	Left upper sternal border and back
Aortic Stenosis	Systolic ejection, II-V/VI, ejection click, narrowly split S2, single S2 if severe AS	Right upper sternal border
Mitral Valve Prolapse	Late systolic murmur (II-III/VI), mid-systolic click	Mid-precordium→left axilla

Table 1.9 Left-Sided Ductal-Dependent Lesions*

Lesion	Comments	Stabilization
Coarctation of aorta	Usually narrowing at ligamentum arteriosum; +/− aneurysm proximal to coarct, +/− bicuspid aortic valve; pulse and BP differential between upper/lower extremities (nl BP 5–10 mmHg higher in lower extremity); CXR may show rib notching	• Consider intubation • PGE1 infusion at 0.05–0.1 mcg/kg/min. Titrate to palpable femoral pulses; up to 10% of infants will have apnea on infusion • Inotropic support if needed (dopamine/dobutamine) • Correction of acidosis and electrolyte abnormalities
Critical AS	Narrowing at aortic valve. ↑ with maternal phenytoin use	
Hypoplastic left heart syndrome	Underdeveloped LV, AV, MV, LA, aorta	
Interrupted aortic arch	1% of CHD	

*Presents with shock, diagnosis with echocardiogram.

AS: Aortic stenosis; ASD: Atrial septal defect; AV: Aortic valve; CHD: Congenital heart disease; Coarct: Coarctation of the aorta; HTN: Hypertension; LA: Left atrium; LV: Left ventricle; MV: Mitral valve; PS: Pulmonic stenosis; TA: Tricuspid atresia; TOF: Tetralogy of Fallot; TOGV: Transposition of the great vessels; VSD: Ventricular septal defect.

Table 1.10 Right-Sided Ductal-Dependent Lesions

Lesion	Comments	Stabilization
Tricuspid Atresia	1% of CHD	• Consider intubation • PGE1 infusion at 0.05–0.1 mcg/kg/min, titrate to oxygen sat 80–85%; up to 10% of infants will have apnea on infusion. • Inotropic support if needed (dopamine/dobutamine) • Correction of acidosis and electrolyte abnormalities
Pulmonic Stenosis	1% of CHD; ↑ with maternal phenytoin use	
Tetralogy of Fallot (see figure) ("blue tets": severe outflow tract obstruction, present early; "pink tets": ↑ cyanosis in first weeks)	• Large VSD • RV outflow tract obstruction overriding aorta • RVH **"Tet Spell":** ↑ R → L shunting; ↑ cyanosis, resp distress, grunting, and agitation. Treat with oxygen, knee–chest position, morphine, beta-blocker, and phenylephrine CXR: "Boot-shaped heart"	
TOGV	90% present in first day of life. Usually no murmur. May not be cyanotic if ASD, VSD, or PDA present. CXR: "egg on a string," left-sided aortic arch, prominent pulmonary vasculature (50%); ↑ in maternal diabetes	
Ebstein Anomaly	Tricuspid valve displaced into ventricle; associated with valve insufficiency and stenosis, *often associated with arrhythmia (do ECG)*. > 80% have ASD also. CXR: "globe-shaped," massively enlarged heart. ↑ in maternal lithium use	

ASD: Atrial septal defect; CHD: Congenital heart defect; CXR: Chest radiograph; ECG: Electrocardiogram; PDA: Patent ductus arteriosus; RVH: right ventricular hypertrophy; VSD: Ventricular septal defect.

Table 1.11 Congenital Heart Lesions That Present with CHF*

PDA	Machinery-like harsh murmur; dyspnea with feeding. Unlikely to close spontaneously after 1 year of age
TAPVR	Pulmonary veins attach to other venous structures and not the left atrium. Four forms: supracardiac, cardiac, infracardiac, mixed. + ASD. Mild–moderate cyanosis. PGE sometimes used to help initial stabilization, but BEWARE **PGE may worsen respiratory distress in infants with TAPVR**
Truncus Arteriosus	Large VSD + one large vessel that leaves the heart, one semilunar valve, pulmonary hypertension. Bounding pulses, +/− mild cyanosis, tachypnea, and diaphoresis
VSD	↑ in maternal diabetes, ETOH use Small: loud holosystolic murmur Large: poor weight gain, resp distress, diaphoresis

*Stabilize infants in CHF with digoxin, diuretics, and possibly ACE inhibitors/afterload reduction.

Table 1.12 Treatment of Congenital Heart Lesions

Small VSD	Manage conservatively if asymptomatic (no CHF or pulmonary HTN), adequate growth, and low PA pressure
Large VSD	Surgical closure recommended for most infants with large VSD Usually transatrial approach, subpulmonic defects approached through pulmonary valve Catheter-delivered devices more commonly used in kids > 1 year with muscular defects Right bundle branch block in almost all after transatrial repair
Pulmonic Stenosis	Balloon dilatation if peak gradient > 30 mmHg. No restrictions or endocarditis prophylaxis if lower gradients.
Tetralogy of Fallot	US usually adequate, catheterization rarely necessary for diagnostic details. Mild–moderate cyanosis often requires only supportive care until surgery. Rarely require PGE1 if RV outflow obstruction. Treat CHF if present. Avoid meds that cause systemic vasodilation. Treat "tet" spells (see above). Surgical repair typically at 3 months. Modified Blalock-Taussig shunt may be done urgently if refractory tet spells, or as a palliative measure if there's reason to defer definitive repair
Aortic Stenosis	Often progressive, may be associated with sudden death, repeated interventions are likely; all need endocarditis prophylaxis (high risk) **Categorized based on peak–peak gradients:** • < 25 mmHg: stable and nl ECG and nl stress test = no restriction • 25–49 mmHg: stable, nl ECG and nl stress test = no highly strenuous exercise • 50–79 mmHg: all warrant intervention. Balloon valvulotomy treatment of choice if no or mild AR
Aortic Regurgitation	Surgical intervention if syncope, CHF, angina, or arrhythmia
ASD	> 8 mm + significant left-to-right shunt → close when identified; ≤ 8 mm can be watched. If > 5 mm after several years → close to prevent pulmonary HTN and ↓ risk of atrial fibrillation and atrial flutter Correct surgically or with catheter device (clamshell, button, ASDOS, angel wings, and Amplatzer device)
PDA	Should be closed if failure to thrive or CHF (thoracotomy with ductal occlusion or VATS procedure). **Premature infants:** if ventilated and < 1000 g and in those > 1000 g if significant L → R shunt treat with indomethacin. May give 2 rounds; ~79% successful. Consider surgery if indomethacin unsuccessful
Coarctation of the Aorta	Uncomplicated coarctation with a consistent arm/leg systolic blood pressure gradient > 20 mmHg is indication for repair (most with surgery, some with balloon angioplasty +/− stent), ideally < 2 years old. Older at time of correction → ↑ risk HTN
Interrupted Aortic Arch	Surgical repair as soon as possible, after correction of acidosis. Correct additional abnormalities at the same time
TOGV (See figure)	PGE1 should be started (may hold if VSD allows mixing). Surgical repair early (first 2 weeks of life) with arterial switch procedure. Atrial septostomy may be unnecessary if surgery imminent or if there is a large VSD for mixing
Hypoplastic Left Heart Syndrome	**Norwood procedure:** Main pulmonary artery joined to upper portion of the aorta, allowing blood pumped from right ventricle to systemic circulation **Blalock-Taussig Shunt:** conduit used to connect subclavian artery to the pulmonary artery. **Sano shunt:** conduit made from single ventricle to pulmonary artery (more pulsatile flow than BT shunt) **Fontan Procedure** (also used in tricuspid atresia, pulmonary atresia with intact ventricular septum, double-inlet ventricle): blood diverted from vena cava to pulmonary artery without passing through ventricle

AR: Aortic regurgitation; AF: Atrial fibrillation; ASDOS: Atrial septal defect occlusion system; CHF: Congestive heart failure; ECG: Electrocardiogram; HTN: Hypertension; PGE1: Prostaglandin E1; RV: Right ventricular; VATS: Video-assisted thoroscopic surgery; VSD: Ventricular septal defect.

Table 1.13 Postoperative Complications After Congenital Heart Repair

Complication*	Workup/Notes
Thrombosis of shunt-conduit (↓ flow)	CXR to determine heart size and pulmonary vascularity are a good first step to determining problem
↑ shunt-conduit flow and CHF	
Dysrhythmias (atrial or ventricular)	ECG
Heart block	
Myocardial ischemia	ECG
Endocarditis	Echocardiogram, blood cultures
Postpericardiotomy syndrome	Fever, chest pain, and a pericardial effusion, +/− friction rub, ↑ heart size on CXR, confirm with echo. Usually resolves over weeks with NSAIDs and rest; pericardiocentesis if tamponade (rare)

*Complication less likely in transcatheter placement of occlusive devices for PDA, ASD, VSD.

Data from: Marx: Rosen's Emergency Medicine, 7th ed.; Chapter 169; Dolbec K - Emerg Med Clin North Am - 01-NOV-2011; 29(4): 811–27, vii.

CONGENITAL ARRHYTHMIAS

Table 1.14 Congenital Arrhythmias

Arrhythmia	Notes	Treatment
Supraventricular Tachycardia (SVT)	Presents with irritability, feeding intolerance, CHF if prolonged. Narrow complex tachycardia, no P waves, HR 220–300/min. Look for Wolff-Parkinson-White (WPW) with short PR interval and delta waves (slurred initial part of QRS)	• Vagal maneuvers • Adenosine 0.1 mg/kg, max 6 mg; repeat doses 0.2 mg/kg, max 12 mg. Successful in 90% of patients • Digoxin or procainamide alternatives • Do not use verapamil • Unstable: direct cardioversion 0.5–1 J/kg • Many outgrow by 1 year old • May need digoxin or propranolol treatment long term; ablation if persistent
Prolonged QTc	QTc > 500 milliseconds + symptoms are highly likely to have disease (immediate evaluation by cardiology); QTc > 440–500 milliseconds requires further evaluation urgently. At risk for developing torsades de pointes	• Avoid adrenergic stimulation (exercise, sudden waking, loud noise) • Treat with beta blockers • Consider placement of cardioverter-defibrillator • Screen all first-degree family members
Congenital Complete Heart Block	Usually diagnosed in utero; ↑ risk with maternal SLE	Permanent pacemaker required

Data from: Rosen's Emergency Medicine, 7th ed.; Chapter 169. Emerg Med Clin North Am 2011;29(4):811–827.

ANTIMICROBIAL PROPHYLAXIS FOR BACTERIAL ENDOCARDITIS

Table 1.15 Antibiotic Prophylaxis for Bacterial Endocarditis

Limited to dental, oral, respiratory tract, skin, or musculoskeletal procedures in patients at highest risk: Prosthetic heart valve, prior infective endocarditis, valvulopathy after cardiac transplantation or cardiac repair, unrepaired cyanotic congenital heart disease including shunts and conduits, repaired congenital heart disease with prosthetic material or device (within first 6 months post-repair)

Standard regimen	Amoxicillin 50 mg/kg (max 2 g) PO
Unable to take oral medications	Ampicillin 50 mg/kg (max 2 g) IV/IM; or Ceftriaxone 50 mg/kg (max 1 g) IM/IV
Allergic to penicillin (PCN)	Clindamycin 20 mg/kg (max 600 mg) PO; or Cephalexin† 50 mg/kg (max 2 g) PO; or Azithromycin or clarithromycin 15 mg/kg (max 500 mg) PO
Allergic to PCN and unable to take oral medications	Clindamycin 20 mg/kg (max 600 mg) IV/IM; or Cefazolin† or ceftriaxone† 50 mg/kg (max 1 g) IV/IM

Prophylaxis is no longer recommended for genitourinary or gastrointestinal tract procedures

Data from: American Heart Association Guidelines http://www.americanheart.org. *Circulation* 2007;116(15):1736.

† Avoid cephalosporins if prior penicillin-associated anaphylaxis, angioedema, or urticaria

HEART TRANSPLANTATION

Table 1.16 Postoperative Management of Heart Transplant Recipients

Indwelling catheters:	Monitor: • atrial filling pressures • pulmonary artery pressures • systemic arterial pressure
Monitor cardiac output:	• urine output • skin temperature • peripheral pulses strength

Data from: *Keane: Nadas' Pediatric Cardiology, 2nd ed.*; Chapter 60.

Table 1.17 Postoperative Immunosuppression of Heart Transplant Patients

Immunosuppressive Agents*
Cyclosporine (started at 0.1 mg/kg/h IV; target levels: < 6 mo after transplant: 250–300 ng/mL; 6–12 mo after transplant: 200–250 ng/mL; > 1 year after transplant: 125–150 ng/mL), or tacrolimus (target levels: < 6 months after transplant: 10–13 ng/mL; 6–12 months after transplant: 8–10 ng/mL; > 12 months after transplant: 5–8 ng/mL)
Mycophenolate mofetil (Start dosing at 300 mg/m²/day IV or 500 mg/m²/day PO divided bid, ↑ as tolerated to maintain level of 2.5–5 mcg/mL) or azathioprine
Corticosteroids
Plasmapheresis with nonspecific immunoglobulin G infusion has been used in few highly sensitized patients
Anti-infective Measures
Prophylactic antibiotics in immediate postoperative period
If evidence of prior CMV infection (donor or recipient): IV ganciclovir × 14 days then PO therapy × 3 mo
If CMV + donor and CMV − recipient: CMV IgG given early postop
EBV may → PTLD: treat PTLD with ↓ immunosuppression + ganciclovir; if unsuccessful consider rituximab (Rituxan)
Trimethoprim sulfamethoxazole: prophylaxis × 1 year for pneumocystis prophylaxis
Other Long-Term Medications
ACE inhibitors may be used prophylactically or to treat signs of nephrotoxicity/hypertension (due to calcineurin inhibitors)

*Target levels of immunosuppressive agents may need to be changed depending on rejection history and side effects. CMV: cytomegalovirus; EBV: Epstein-Barr Virus; PTLD: Post-transplant lymphoproliferative disease.

Data from: *Keane: Nadas' Pediatric Cardiology, 2nd ed.*; Chapter 60.

Table 1.18 Signs of Acute Rejection* in Heart Transplant Recipients

Fatigue	Fever
Nausea	Gallop
↓Appetite/poor feeding	Arrhythmia, ↑ HR
Abdominal pain	Hepatomegaly
Weight gain/edema	Signs of CHF
Treatment: Grade 1R: often observation and re-biopsy; Grade 2R: IV methylprednisolone at or PO prednisone; Grade 3R: bolus steroids and consider daclizumab, OKT3, antithymocyte globulin, methotrexate, or total lymphoid irradiation	

*Definitive diagnosis made by endomyocardial biopsy; most common in first 3–6 months post-transplant

Data from: *Keane: Nadas' Pediatric Cardiology, 2nd ed.*; Chapter 60.

Table 1.19 Presentation of Chronic Rejection (Coronary Arteriorpathy)* in Heart Transplant Recipients

Presyncope/syncope	Edema
Ectopy	Chest pain (rare)
Exercise intolerance	Asymptomatic

*Coronary angiogram recommended every 1–2 years post-transplant

Data from: *Keane: Nadas' Pediatric Cardiology, 2nd ed.*; Chapter 60.

SYNCOPE AND NEAR SYNCOPE

Table 1.20 Syncope and Near Syncope

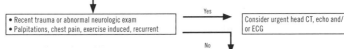

• *Syncope*: Transient loss of consciousness with resultant loss of muscle tone secondary to cerebral hypoperfusion, • *Near syncope*: Transient alteration in mental status without unconscious period

• Recent trauma or abnormal neurologic exam
• Palpitations, chest pain, exercise induced, recurrent   →(Yes)→   Consider urgent head CT, echo and/or ECG

No ↓

• **History and physical exam:** Assess hydration, blood pressure, medications, precipitating events, recent exercise
• **Past history:** Kawasaki disease, hypertension, congenital heart disease, palpitations
• **Family history:** Sudden cardiac death, early MI, Marfan's, long QT syndrome
• **Lab:** Blood glucose, pregnancy test, electrolytes, complete blood count
• **ECG:** Perform in all patients, unless clearly *not* cardiac. Consider Holter monitor

(Continued)

Table 1.20 Syncope and Near Syncope *(Continued)*

Differential Diagnosis	History and Exam	Lab/Radiology Findings	Treatment
Neurocardiogenic [Vasovagal (> 50%)]	• Prolonged standing • Prolonged fast • Emotional event • Rapid standing • Micturition • Defecation • Recent exercise	• Generally normal • Tilt-table test rarely used: (sensitivity 26–80%, specificity 90%) • Consider Holter	• None • Medications rarely necessary, but may be helpful
Supraventricular Tachycardia	• Palpitations • Normal exam	• ECG often normal • WPW: Delta wave • Holter monitor	• Cardiologist • Medication • Ablation
Long QT Syndrome	• Recurrent syncope (cold water to face) • Previous "seizures" • Family history of sudden death • Congenital deafness	• ECG: Long QTc • Screen family members	• β-blocker • Implantable defibrillator (ICD)
Aortic Stenosis	• Exercise syncope • Systolic murmur	• ECG: LVH	• Valvuloplasty • Avoid exercise
Seizure (5–10%)	• Tonic-clonic • Post-ictal state	• Abnormal EEG and/or electrolytes	• Anti-epileptics • Neurologist
Migraine (5%)	• Headache, aura • Family history positive	• Normal	• Identify triggers
Breath Holding Spell (2–5%)	• Toddler cries/holds breath until syncopal	• Normal	• Self-resolves by 5 years old
Hypertrophic Cardiomyopathy (incidence=1:500)	• Syncope or chest pain during exercise • Family history positive	• ECG: LVH • Echo diagnostic	• Exclusion from sports • ICD
Hyperventilation	• Anxiety, pain, etc	• ↓ $PaCO_2$	• Relaxation

ECG: electrocardiogram, Echo: echocardiogram, EEG: electroencephalogram, Holter: Holter monitor, ICD: Implantable defibrillator, LVH: left ventricular hypertrophy, MI: myocardial infarction, WPW: Wolff-Parkinson-White syndrome
Data from *Circulation.* 2006 Jan 17:113(2:316).

CHAPTER 2 ■ DERMATOLOGY

Indication: Imminent risk of complication from hemangiomas still in growth phase

HEMANGIOMA LOCATIONS HIGH-RISK FOR COMPLICATIONS

- Central nervous system with risk of spinal cord compression
- Periocular with associated risk of astigmatism or amblyopia
- Airway involvement
- Gastrointestinal, hepatic, or other diffuse hemangiomatosis with (or at risk for) congestive heart failure
- At risk of permanent disfigurement (facial, nose, ear, lip, genitals, ulcerating)

CONTRAINDICATIONS

- Medications: antiarrhythmics, calcium channel blockers, chlorpromazine, cimetidine, clonidine, digoxin, ergotamines, hydralazine
- Hypoglycemia: current or previous history
- Asthma or prior episode of reactive airway disease
- Decreased cardiac output (known, or with cardiac lesion predisposing to)
- PHACES association (**P**osterior fossa malformations, **H**emangioma, **A**rterial abnormalities, **C**ardiac anomalies/**C**oarctation of the aorta, **E**ar and Eye abnormalities, **S**ternal defects)

  Inpatient initiation indicated for: < 8 weeks old, comorbid condition of respiratory or cardiovascular system, inadequate social support

PRE-INITIATION EVALUATION SHOULD INCLUDE

- Baseline vital signs (HR, BP, temperature, respiratory rate)
- Electrocardiogram
- Echocardiogram
  - If concern for PHACES association, obtain cardiology and ophthalmology consultation, and ensure echocardiogram has adequately evaluated the aorta

INITIATION

- Monitor HR and BP prior to initiation, and 1 and 2 hours post each dose
- Blood glucose monitoring
  - BG q 8 hours (immediately prior to feeding)
  - Risk of hypoglycemia increased with prolonged fast or illness
  - Discontinue propranolol during illness

Table 2.1 Recommended Feeding Intervals While on Propranolol

Age	< 6 weeks old	6 weeks– 4 months	> 4 months old
Feeding Interval	Every 4 hours	Every 5 hours	Every 6–8 hours

DOSING (ADMINISTER WITH FEEDING)

- Propranolol (20 mg/5 mL solution): 1 mg/kg/day PO divided q 8 hours. If tolerated well, increase dose to 2 mg/kg/day PO divided by q 8 hours
  - Hold dose for hypoglycemia or bradycardia (HR < 100 for infant < 3 months old, HR < 90 for infant 3–6 months old, HR < 80 for infants 6–12 months old, HR < 70 for > 1 year olds)

DISCHARGES

- Inpatient monitoring of infants for 48–72 hours to allow propranolol to reach steady-state and look for potential complications
- Outpatient monitoring of vitals and blood glucose twice weekly initially

MANAGEMENT OF COMPLICATIONS

- Bradycardia
  - Asymptomatic: Continue to monitor BP every 5–15 minutes
  - Symptomatic
    - Atropine: 0.02 mg/kg IV (minimum dose 0.1 mg, max single dose 0.5 mg). Repeat in 5 minutes as needed
    - Epinephrine (1:10,000): 0.01 mg/kg IV (max single dose 1 mg)
- Hypotension
  - Normal saline 20 mL/kg IV, repeat as necessary
  - Epinephrine (1:10,000): 0.01 mg/kg IV (max single dose 1 mg)
- Hypoglycemia (BG < 70 mg/dL)
  - Asymptomatic: Recheck in opposite extremity
  - Symptomatic
    - Feed breast milk, formula, or oral sucrose
    - Neonate – 2 months old: D10% 2 mL/kg
    - Infant > 2 months old: D25% 4 mL/kg
- Bronchospasm
  - Albuterol 1.25–2.5 mg nebulized or 4–6 puffs of MDI (90 mcg/puff)
  - SQ epinephrine (1:1000): 0.01 mg/kg = 0.1 mL/kg/dose SQ

Reference: *Pediatrics*. 2013 vol. 131(1):128–140.

Abbreviations: BG: Blood glucose; BP: Blood pressure; HR: Heart rate; MDI: Metered dose inhaler; SQ: subcutaneously

BURNS

Table 2.2 Classification of Burn Thickness

	Superficial	Partial-Thickness	Full-Thickness
Color	Pink or red	Superficial = red, deep = yellow	White or brown
Blisters	None	Present	+/– eschar
Pain	Mild–moderate	Moderate–severe	Absent
Layers	Epidermis only	Epidermis plus dermis	Subdermis
Management	Moisturizers	Debride blisters	Refer
Burns progress over time, have multiple depths of injury within the same wound			

Table 2.3 Outpatient Management of Minor Burns

Clean with soap and warm water bid. Debride blisters			
	Bacitracin	**Silver Sulfadiazine**	**Mafenide Acetate**
Indication	Small area; superficial second degree; facial burns	Partial (second degree) or full-thickness	Eschar and burns near cartilage
Action	Bacteriostatic	Bactericidal	Anti-pseudomonal
Contraindication	Allergy to bacitracin	Sulfa allergy; G6PD; infants→kernicterus	Allergy to mafenide acetate
Side Effect	Local irritation	Can delay healing and permanently stain	Severe pain; metabolic acidosis

Table 2.4 Estimation of Body Surface Area (BSA)

Age (in years)	< 1	1	5	10	15
Head	19%	17%	13%	11%	9%
One Thigh	5%	6.5%	8.5%	9%	9.5%
One Leg (below knee)	5%	5%	5.5%	6%	6.5%

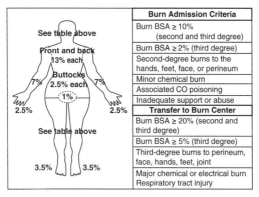

Burn Admission Criteria
Burn BSA ≥ 10% (second and third degree)
Burn BSA ≥ 2% (third degree)
Second-degree burns to the hands, feet, face, or perineum
Minor chemical burn
Associated CO poisoning
Inadequate support or abuse
Transfer to Burn Center
Burn BSA ≥ 20% (second and third degree)
Burn BSA ≥ 5% (third degree)
Third-degree burns to perineum, face, hands, feet, joint
Major chemical or electrical burn Respiratory tract injury

Figure 2.1 Burn Quantification and Admission Criteria

Reprinted with permission, *Tarascon Pediatric Emergency Pocketbook*, 6th edition, Jones and Bartlett Learning, Sudbury, MA.

Table 2.5 Evaluation and Treatment of Moderate to Severe Burns

Airway	Evaluate risk of inhalation injury. Clues include facial burns, singed eyebrows/facial hair, hoarseness, stridor, black-tinged sputum or matter in nostrils, respiratory distress. Early intubation recommended. **EARLY RISKS:** acute CO poisoning, airway obstruction, pulmonary edema. **24–48 hours after injury:** ARDS; **DAYS-WEEKS LATER:** pneumonia, pulmonary embolism
Carbon Monoxide Poisoning	Treat with 100% oxygen (severe burns require hyperbaric oxygen). **MILD:** (< 20% HbCO): short of breath, headache, nausea, and ↓vision acuity, subtle mental status changes; **MODERATE** (20–40% HbCO): agitation, nausea, ↓vision, cognitive function; **SEVERE:** (40–60% HbCO): hallucinations, ataxia, coma
Access/Fluid Support	Peripheral IV can be placed through burned skin if necessary. Multiple lines or central access recommended. Central line if > 30% TBSA burned. Monitor adequacy of resuscitation via *vitals, urine output, blood gas, hematocrit, and serum protein* **Day 1: Parkland formula (fluid required for resuscitation): (4 mL lactated Ringer solution) × (weight in kg) × (% BSA burned) PLUS maintenance fluids.** Example: 20 kg child with 15% TBSA burns: $4 \times 20 \times 15 = 1200$ mL LR over 24 hours. *Give half of calculated total over the first 8 hr (calculate from time of injury); other half of calculated total over the next 16 hours.* **Day 2: Add 5% dextrose to LR, infuse half total infused in day 1 over 24 hours**
Albumin (Goal albumin level 2 g/dL)	**30–50% TBSA:** (0.3 mL of 5% albumin) × (weight in kg) × (% BSA burn) infused over 24 hr; **50–70% TBSA:** (0.4 mL of 5% albumin) × (weight in kg) × (% BSA burn) infused over 24 hr; **70–100% of TBSA:** (0.5 mL of 5% albumin) × (weight in kg) × (% BSA burn) infused over 24 hr.
Packed Red Blood Cells	Consider infusion of PRBCs if Hgb < 8 mg/dL or hematocrit < 24% (< 30% if ongoing infection, blood loss, or anticipated surgical procedures)
Fresh Frozen Plasma (FFP)	If evidence of elevated PT, PTT, or INR and continued bleeding or in anticipation of significant invasive procedure; may also use for volume resuscitation in young children (< 2 yrs), < 72 hours from burn + > 20% TBSA + inhalation injury
Initial Visualization	Remove clothes; cool water may be applied to small areas, but not large burn areas (risk hypothermia); room should be kept warm (28–33°C), make sure patient is adequately covered during transport
Pain Control	Morphine sulfate: 0.05–0.1 mg/kg IV (max of 2–5 mg) q 2 hr *or* morphine sulfate: 0.3–0.6 mg/kg PO/PR q 4 hr; Prior to dressing changes: 0.3–0.6 mg/kg PO 2 hr before change PLUS morphine IV 0.05–0.1 mg/kg IV just prior to procedure
Anxiety	Lorazepam 0.05–0.1 mg/kg/dose IV every 6–8 hr; Prior to dressing change: Lorazepam 0.04 mg/kg IV/ PO or midazolam 0.01–0.02 mg/kg IV (0.05–0.1 mg/kg if intubated). When possible taper anxiolytics 25%/dose over 1–3 days
Nutrition	PO feeds may start as early as 2 days after injury. Start NG feeds with appropriate formula or supplement. IV + PO to equal total fluid goal. ↑↑ Metabolic demands with burn and other complications. Provide calories at 1.5 × basal metabolic rate; Protein: 3–4 g/kg/day. Supplement with multivitamin, B vitamins, vitamin C, vitamin A, zinc. Some centers use B blockers to ↓ metabolic stress or oxandrolone: 0.1 to 0.2 mg/kg/day to ↑ protein synthesis (controversial)
Topical Treatment	Silver sulfadiazine (deep penetration), Silvadene® cream (deep penetration, wash residue off each bid dressing change), mafenide acetate (wash residue off each bid dressing change), 0.5% silver nitrate solution (superficial penetration, change q day, beware hyponatremia), AQUACEL Ag (2nd degree burns, stays on × 10 days), Accuzyme ointment (enzyme that debrides burn)
Systemic Antibiotics	Controversial; some centers use prophylactic penicillin or erythromycin, others do not
Tetanus prophylaxis	Ensure tetanus vaccine is up to date

Excision and Grafting	Promptly required in large 3rd-degree and deep/large 2nd-degree burns. Autografts, allografts, xenografts, and synthetic skin coverings may be used
Wound Membranes	Porcine xenograft, Biobrane®, Acticoat®, AQUACEL-Ag®, semipermeable membranes, impregnated gauzes, and hydrocolloid dressings. Check wound 2×/week. Often used for 2nd-degree burns; remain on for 7–10 days
Long-Term Considerations	Scars, contractures, itching, alopecia, sin cancer, neuropathic pain, PTSD, anoxic brain injury, long-term airway or pulmonary disease, and many more possible complications

Data from:
Nelson Textbook of Pediatrics, 19th ed., Philadelphia: Elsevier/Saunders, 2011: Chapter 68: Burn Injuries.
Am J Clin Dermatol. 2002;3(8):529.
Ann Plast Surg. 2005;55(5):485.

ECZEMA HERPETICUM

- Superinfection with herpes simplex virus HSV in child with eczema
- Appears as vesicles or punched-out lesions on a red base + fever and toxicity
- Initiate treatment, then confirm diagnosis with PCR, Tczank smear, and/or culture
- Consult ophthalmology urgently if periocular or ocular involvement suspected
- **Treatment:**
  - Cool, wet compresses to lesions
  - Ensure hydration, as skin may slough
  - Acyclovir 1500 mg/m^2/day (or 10 mg/kg/dose) IV q 8 hours
    - Adult dose: 250 mg IV TID
  - Consider anti-staphylococcal antibiotics as well

References: *Prim Care* 2008;35(1):105–117; Habif, *Clinical Dermatology, 5th ed.*, Chapter 12. St. Louis: Mosby, 2009.

STEVENS-JOHNSON SYNDROME (SJS) AND TOXIC EPIDERMAL NECROLYSIS (TEN)

- Fever, stinging eyes, dysphagia
- Lesions start a few days later at trunk, face, palms, soles (red macules that quickly coalesce, painful skin) → erythema/erosions or oral, genital, ocular, GI, and respiratory mucosa → epidermal detachment (+ Nikolsky sign)
- In SJS < 10% of body surface area is detached; in TEN > 30% is detached. Overlap of the two syndromes between 10–30%
- Long term sequelae include hyper- or hypopigmentation, nail problems, conjunctival keratinization, keratoconjunctivitis sicca
- Most commonly caused by drugs: TMP-SMX, carbamazepine, phenytoin, phenobarbital, cephalosporins, penicillins, allopurinol, quinolone, NSAIDs
- **TREATMENT:**
  - Stop offending drug ASAP
  - Admit to PICU or burn unit
  - Nonadherent dressing *without* topical sulfa-based creams
  - Supportive care with fluids and pain control
  - Consider early administration of high-dose immunoglobulin (IVIG) in severe cases (controversial; some studies suggest possible benefit, 2–3 g/kg)
  - Consult ophthalmology; may require topical steroid or lubricants
  - Nutritional support
  - Systemic steroids controversial
    - Use caution, as may increase risk for sepsis

Reference: *Med Clin North Am*. 2010;94(4):727–742.

ADRENAL INSUFFICIENCY

DEFINITION/PRESENTATION OF CONGENITAL ADRENAL HYPERPLASIA (CAH)

- Group of autosomal recessive disorders (Incidence: 1:10,000–1:20,000)
- Classic CAH is 21-hydroxylase deficiency (95% of cases)
  - Inability to convert 17-hydroxyprogesterone (17-OHP) to 11 deoxycortisol
  - Accumulation of 17-OHP; tested for on newborn screen in most states
  - Cortisol precursors diverted to androgen synthesis
    - Virilization of females
    - Precocious puberty
  - 75% of cases have salt wasting due to aldosterone deficiency
    - Neonatal salt loss → failure to thrive → hypovolemia → shock
    - Elevated plasma renin activity (PRA) and a reduced ratio of aldosterone to PRA indicate impaired aldosterone synthesis

Table 3.1 Post-Infancy 17-OHP Values in Diagnosis of CAH

Test	17-OHP Results		
	Classic CAH	Non-Classic CAH	Likely Unaffected
Early morning "baseline"	> 300 nmol/L	6–300 nmol/L	< 6 nmol/L (possible NCCAH)
Post-ACTH stimulation test*	> 300 nmol/L	31–300 nmol/L	< 50 nmol/L (possible heterozygote)

*ACTH stimulation test using 0.125–0.25 mg cosyntropin

MEDICAL TREATMENT OF CAH IN GROWING PATIENTS

- Hydrocortisone (use tablets, avoid suspension) 10–15 mg/m^2/day PO divided tid
- In infants with salt wasting, add:
  - Fludrocortisone acetate 0.05–0.2 mg/day daily or divided bid, *and*
  - Sodium chloride 1–2 g/day (17–34 mEq/day) PO divided tid–qid
    - Due to insufficient quantities in breast milk and infant formula

MEDICAL TREATMENT OF CAH IN ADULT PATIENTS

- Hydrocortisone 15–25 mg/day PO divided bid–tid, *or*
- Prednisone 5–7.5 mg/day PO divided bid, *or*
- Prednisolone 4–6 mg/day PO divided bid, *or*
- Dexamethasone 0.25–0.5 mg PO daily, *or*
- Consider fludrocortisone 0.05–0.2 mg PO daily for elevated PRA or reduced aldosterone to PRA ratio

Reference: *J Clin Endocrinol Metab.* 2010;95(9):4133–4160.

Abbreviations: 17-OHP: 17-hydroxyprogesterone; CAH: congenital adrenal hyperplasia; NCCAH: non-classical congenital adrenal hyperplasia; PRA: plasma renin activity

CUSHING SYNDROME

Table 3.2 Causes of Cushing Syndrome

Endogenous	**ACTH dependent**: Cushing's disease (ACTH overproduction in pituitary, usually caused by ACTH-secreting pituitary microadenoma, most common cause of syndrome in children > 7 yrs); ectopic ACTH production is rare (small cell cancer of lung, carcinoid tumors in bronchus, pancreas, or thymus; medullary carcinomas of the thyroid, pheochromocytoma; other neuroendocrine tumors). CRH overproduction very rare **ACTH independent**: adrenal adenoma, carcinoma or hyperplasia; most common cause of Cushing's in prepubertal child is adrenal lesion
Exogenous	Exogenous administration of glucocorticoids (pulmonary, autoimmune, dermatologic, hematologic diseases) or ACTH (seizure disorder)
Associated with other disorders	**Primary pigmented adrenocortical nodular disease (PPNAD):** genetic disorder (AD, Carney Complex), associated with multiple endocrine problems, lentigines, and myxomas **Massive macronodular adrenal hyperplasia (MMAD):** massive adrenals with cortisol-producing adenomas **McCune–Albright syndrome (MAS):** usually presents < 6 months old, continuous non-ACTH dependent stimulation of adrenal cortex

Table 3.3 Diagnosis of Cushing Syndrome

Document hypercortisolism	**24-hour urinary free cortisol (UFC)* excretion** *and/or* **Low-dose dexamethasone suppression test** (1 mg of dexamethasone at 11 PM, measure serum cortisol the following morning at 8 AM.) If > 1.8 mcg/dL, further workup necessary. (If both tests negative, likely rule out Cushing syndrome UNLESS periodic hypersecretion)
Distinguish between pseudo-Cushing and Cushing syndrome (normal height gain consistent with pseudo-Cushing)	*Dexamethasone-CRH test:* Treat with dexamethasone (0.5 mg adjusted for weight for children < 70 kg) q 6 hours × 8 doses then oCRH. Measure ACTH, cortisol, and dexamethasone levels at baseline (−15, −5, and 0 min) and 15 minutes after the administration of oCRH. The patient with pseudo-Cushing syndrome will exhibit low or undetectable basal plasma cortisol and ACTH and have a diminished or no response to oCRH stimulation. Cortisol > 1.4 mcg/dL (38 nmol/L) 15 minutes after oCRH suggests Cushing syndrome
Distinguish ACTH-dependent disease from the ACTH-independent syndrome	*Modified Liddle's/high-dose dexamethasone suppression test:* (120 mcg/kg, maximum dose 8 mg) at 11 PM, measure plasma cortisol level the next AM. 20% suppression of cortisol from baseline highly predictive of Cushing's Disease versus adrenal tumor. If non-suppression of serum cortisol and/or negative imaging studies, and/or suspected adrenal disease do: *Classic Liddle's* (dexamethasone 30 mcg/kg/dose; maximum 0.5 mg/dose q 6 hours × 8 doses, then dexamethasone 120 mcg/kg/dose; maximum 2 mg/dose q 6 hours × 8 doses). ↓ cortisol, UFC, and 17OHS in 85% with Cushing's Disease *oCRH stimulation test:* ↑ plasma ACTH and cortisol after oCRH in 85% of patients with Cushing disease. Most with ectopic ACTH do not respond to oCRH.
Imaging	• If suspect Cushing's disease: do pituitary MRI with contrast • If suspect adrenal lesion, do CT of adrenals • If suspect ectopic ACTH, do CT or MRI neck, chest, abdomen, and pelvis or nuclear medicine study

*Falsely elevated 24-hour UFC (pseudo-Cushing state) can be caused by emotional stress, severe obesity, pregnancy, excessive exercise, depression/anxiety, poorly controlled diabetes, alcoholism, anorexia/malnutrition, narcotic withdrawal, and high water intake.

Data from: *NEJM*. 1986;314(21): 1329.

Table 3.4 Treatment of Cushing Syndrome

ACTH-secreting pituitary adenoma (Cushing's disease)	Trans-sphenoidal surgery (TSS) > 90% success rate; < 1 % mortality. Postop complications: transient DI, SIADH, hypothyroidism, GH deficiency, hypogonadism, bleeding, meningitis. Radiation if surgery fails
Benign adrenal tumors	Transperitoneal, retroperitoneal removal, or laparoscopic adrenalectomy
Adrenal carcinoma	Surgical removal, mitotane (adrenocytolytic, adjuvant); chemotherapy; radiation Glucocorticoid antagonists or steroid synthesis inhibitors may be needed for hypercortisolism
Bilateral nodular adrenal disease (PPNAD and MMAD)	Bilateral total adrenalectomy (can result in Nelson syndrome ↑ pigmentation, ↑ ACTH levels, and a growing ACTH-producing pituitary tumor)
To control hypercortisolism (if other treatments fail or source not identified)	Mitotane, aminoglutethimide, metyrapone, trilostane, and ketoconazole may also be used alone or in combinations to control hypercortisolism

Table 3.5 Postoperative Glucocorticoid Replacement Therapy

Operation	Recommended Glucocorticoid Regimen
TSS in Cushing disease, excision of autonomously functioning adrenal adenoma, unilateral adrenalectomy for a single adrenocortical tumor	Stress dose steroids postoperatively, then physiologic replacement dose: Hydrocortisone 12–15 mg/m^2/day PO divided into 2–3 daily doses)
Bilateral total adrenalectomy	Stress dose steroids postoperatively, then Physiologic replacement dose: Hydrocortisone 12–15 mg/m^2/day PO in 2–3 divided doses, AND Fludrocortisone 0.1–0.3 mg PO daily

TSS: Trans-sphenoidal surgery.

Table: 3.6 Stress Dose Hydrocortisone Dosing

Indications	Fever (> 38.5°C), gastroenteritis with dehydration, surgery with general anesthesia, major trauma
Infants and children	1–2 mg/kg/dose bolus IV/IM, then 25–150 mg/day (3–4 × daily dose) in divided doses q 6–8 hours
Older children	1–2 mg/kg/dose bolus IM/IV, then 150–250 mg/day (3–4 × daily dose) in divided doses q 6–8 hours
Adult	IV, IM: 100 mg IV bolus, then 300 mg/day in divided doses q 8 hours or as continuous infusion for 48 hours PO (once stable): 50 mg q 8 hours for 6 doses, then taper to 30–50 mg/day in divided doses

Data from: Stratakis CA. *Endocrinol Metab Clin North Am.* 2012;41(4):793-803; Speiser PW. *J Clin Endocrinol Metab.* 2010;95(9):4133-4160.

Symptoms: Obesity with short stature, facial plethora, headaches, hypertension, hirsutism, amenorrhea, delayed puberty, virilization (pubertal), acne, violaceous striae, bruising, and acanthosis nigricans

DIABETIC KETOACIDOSIS

CRITERIA FOR DIAGNOSIS OF DIABETIC KETOACIDOSIS (DKA)
- BG > 200 mg/dL
- pH < 7.3 and/or serum bicarbonate < 15 mEq/L

INITIAL MANAGEMENT OF DKA
- Initiate insulin drip (IV regular insulin) at 0.05–0.1 units/kg/hour
  - *Do not* give initial bolus of IV regular insulin

- Volume replete with NS or LR bolus 10 mL/kg over 1 hour
  ○ Gradual volume repletion may decrease risk of cerebral edema
  ○ Repeat 10 mL/kg NS or LR bolus × 1 ONLY if poor circulation
  ○ After initial isotonic fluid bolus, initiate IVF of 0.9% NS or LR at 1.5–2 times maintenance (NOT to exceed 3000 mL/m^2/day)
    – Do not replace urinary losses
- Avoid bicarbonate therapy except in patients with pH < 6.9 with poor perfusion or at risk for cardiac arrest

Table 3.7 Subsequent Management of DKA: Intravenous Regular Insulin

Blood Glucose	Insulin drip* (initial 0.05–0.1 units/kg/hour)
≥ 500 mg/dL	Increase rate by 10–20%
301–500 mg/dL	Do not adjust rate of insulin drip Goal BG decrease: 50–75 mg/dL/hour If BG decrease by > 90 mg/dL/hour, add 5% dextrose to IVF
151–300 mg/dL	Add 5–10% dextrose to IVF If rapid decline, decrease insulin drip rate by 10–20%
100–150 mg/dL	Decrease insulin drip rate by 20–50% Add 10% dextrose to IVF
76–99 mg/dL	Hold insulin drip for at least 1 hour Monitor for symptoms of hypoglycemia
≤ 75 mg/dL	Stop insulin drip Give glucose bolus: 2.5–5 mL/kg of D10%W or 1–2 mL/kg of D25% (dilute D50%W 1:1 with sterile water to make D25%W) If concerned for prolonged hypoglycemia (subq insulin given), add 10% dextrose to IVF to run at 1.2–3 ml/kg/hr = 2–5 mg/kg/min

*Assumes ongoing acidosis. Once acidosis resolves, switch to subcutaneous insulin.

Table 3.8 Subsequent Management of DKA: Potassium

Potassium Level	Potassium in IV Fluid Replacement
< 3.3 mEq/dL	Separate KCl infusion of 1–2 mEq/kg to run over 4 hours
3.4–4.5 mEq/dL	40 mEq/L added to IVF
> 4.5 mEq/dL	Serum K will drop rapidly with insulin infusion. Follow levels hourly and add KCl to IVF once < 4.5 mEq/dL

Table 3.9 Subsequent Management of DKA: Phosphorus

Phosphorus Level	Management
≥ 1 mg/dL	No replacement recommended. Watch for weakness as approaching 1 mg/dL
< 1 mg/dL	Add 20–30 mEq/L potassium phosphate to IVF*

*Phosphorus replacement may lead to decreased serum calcium. Monitor closely.

Table 3.10 Monitoring Therapy While on Insulin Drip

Blood glucose	Hourly × 4–6 hours. Subsequent frequency based on reassessment of patient condition, insulin needs, degree of acidosis
Electrolytes	Hourly × 3–4 hours, then every 2 hours × several. Subsequently every 4–6 hours once clinically stable
Venous pH	Hourly × 3–4 hours, then every 2–4 hours until pH > 7.3

Table 3.11 Insulin Types

Insulin Type (by speed of onset)	Name	Onset (hours)	Peak (hours)	Duration (hours)	Peak Low BG risk
Rapid-acting	Lispro or aspart	5–10 min	0.5–2	2–3	2–3 hours
Fast-acting	Regular	0.5–1	2–5	6–8	3–7 hours
Intermediate-acting	NPH or lente	1–3	5–8	8–18	4–16 hours
Long-acting	Ultralente	3–4	8–15	22–26	8–18 hours
Very Long-acting	Glargine (*Lantus*®) or detemir (*Levemir*®)	1.5–4	None	20–24	5–10 hours

Mixed insulin solutions (70/30) should *not be used* for management of children unless significant barriers to diabetic control exist. These preparations *do not* take into account variable glucose levels, meal volumes, and exercise.

CRITERIA TO TRANSITION TO SUBCUTANEOUS INSULIN

- Venous pH > 7.30 *or* serum HCO_3 > 15 mEqL
- BG < 200 mg/dL
- Anion gap normalized (10–14 mEq/L)
- Tolerating oral intake (no nausea or vomiting)

Give basal insulin (glargine or detemir) SQ, then discontinue IV insulin in 2 hours

References: *Pediatrics.* 2004;113:e133; *Diabetes Care.* 2006;29:1150; *Am J Med.* 1999;106:399.

Abbreviations: BG: blood glucose; IV: intravenous; IVF: intravenous fluids; NS: normal saline; LR: lactated Ringer's solution; SQ: subcutaneous

TYPE 1 DIABETES MELLITUS IN CHILDREN (T1DM)

EPIDEMIOLOGY:

Affects 170/100,000 kids age < 19 yo, mean onset age 8–12 yo, 1:1 ♂:♀.

DIAGNOSIS:

(1) Random/casual blood glucose (BG) > 200 mg/dL (11.1 mmol/L) + symptoms, *or*

(2) Fasting blood glucose > 126 mg/dL (7 mmol/L) + symptoms, *or*

(3) 2-hr blood glucose ≥ 200 mg/dL after 75 gram (g) oral glucose tolerance test + symptoms, *or*

(4) Two abnormal blood glucoses or HbA1c on two separate days without symptoms, *or*

(5) HbA1c ≥ 6.5 *and* symptoms

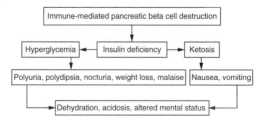

Figure 3.1 Pathophysiology of T1DM

NEW ONSET T1DM:

If no evidence of acidosis at diagnosis, inpatient or outpatient intensive education at specialty center equally effective, without ↑ risk to patient.

Cochrane Reviews 2007(2). No:CD004099.

- **TOTAL DAILY INSULIN DOSE (TDD)**
  - 40–50% long-acting insulin, 50–60% short-acting insulin
  - Preadolescents: 0.5–0.75 units/kg/day
  - Adolescents: 0.75–1 unit/kg/day (may require as much as 1.25 unit/kg/day at peak growth)
  - *"Honeymoon" period*: Residual endogenous insulin decreases exogenous needs
  - **Basal-bolus technique**: Patient must be taught to count carbohydrates (carb)
    - ○ Long-acting insulin for basal needs given once or twice daily
    - ○ Rapid-acting insulin 5 may require as much as 1.25 unit/kg 15 mins before meals (consider giving "picky eaters" insulin *after* eating to limit hypoglycemic risk)
    - ○ Meal insulin: Carb ratio may vary by age from 1:30 in children to 1:5 in adolescents (adolescents have ↑ insulin resistance, particularly in AM from ↑ growth hormone)

Table 3.12 T1DM Therapy Goals

Age	Hemoglobin A1C	Bedtime Glucose	Pre-meal Glucose
< 6 years old	7.5–8.5%	110–200 mg/dL	100–180 mg/dL
6–12 years old	≤ 8%	100–180 mg/dL	90–180 mg/dL
13–19 years old	≤ 7.5%	90–150 mg/dL	90–130 mg/dL

- **CORRECTION DOSE**
  - Additional rapid-acting insulin to correct hyperglycemia (see Table 3.11)
  - **Insulin sensitivity** (1800 rule): 1800/TDD = expected drop in BG (mg/dL) from 1 unit rapid-acting insulin
  - Do not give correction dose more than q 2 hr (or duration of given insulin used)
  - Consider half of correction dose at bedtime
  - Unless ill or ketotic, no correction overnight given risk of hypoglycemia

- **BLOOD GLUCOSE (BG) MONITORING**
  - Before meals and bedtime. 2 AM check for 1 wk after changing basal insulin and no hypoglycemia
  - 2-hour postprandial BG results used to adjust rapid-acting insulin:carb ratio
  - Overnight BG and multiday trends useful in adjusting basal insulin
  - *Sick-day*: Increase BG and ketone monitoring as hypo- and hyperglycemia common insulin needs generally ↑, but may ↓ while ill. Poor PO intake = ↑ risk hypoglycemia
  - *Ketones*: Check urine or serum ketones if BG > 250 mg/dL × 2, or if ill/emesis
    - ○ If ketones present, consider correction dose and monitor for signs of DKA
  - *Diet*: Goal ~50–55% carbs, 15–20% protein, 30% fat. OK to eat > 3 meals/day

Table 3.13 T1DM Long-Term Considerations/Screening

Depression	25–33% prevalence; factor in poor compliance/recurrent DKA
Retinopathy	Age ≥ 10 and T1DM > 3–5 years: Annual ophthalmologic exam
Nephropathy	Age ≥ 10 and T1DM ≥ 5 years: Annual urine microalbumin: creatinine. If abnormal, consult nephrology and consider ACE inhibitor. Blood pressure and lipid control crucial. Avoid smoking.
Thyroid disease	Thyroid stimulating hormone (TSH) at diagnosis and q 1–2 years
Celiac disease	Screen at diagnosis, and for weight loss, failure to gain weight, or gastrointestinal symptoms.
Eating disorders	Consider in underweight patients or those with recurrent DKA.

Data from:
Diabetes. 2005;54(4):1100–1107.
J Clin Endo Metab. 2007;92(3):815–816.
Diabetes Care. 2010;33:511–561.

Hypoglycemia:

- Signs/symptoms: Irritability, headache, lethargy, hunger, tremor, sweating, palpitations, difficult to arouse, seizures. Infants have subtle symptoms.
- BG < 70 mg/dL or symptomatic:
  - ○ "15/15 rule" = eat 15 g rapidly absorbed carb (4 oz. juice), recheck BG in 15 mins.
  - ○ If next meal > 30 mins away, add protein (peanut butter).
- **Glucagon**: For severe hypoglycemia with loss of consciousness or seizure.
  - ○ < 20 kg = 0.5 mg, > 20 kg = 1 mg IM.

Exercise: ↑ hypoglycemic risk during and after exercise (including overnight).

- Check BG q 30 min during, q 15 min after prolonged exercise *and* at 2 AM.
- If on long-acting insulin, snack (15 g carb) prior to and q 30 min during prolonged exercise.
- Patients on insulin pump: ↓ basal by 30–70% prior to exercise.

References: *Diabetes* 2005;54(4):1100–1107; *J Clin Endo Metab* 2007;92(3):815–816; *Diabetes Care* 2005;28:186–212; *Diabetes Care.* 1999;22(1):133–136.

GROWTH HORMONE STIMULATION TESTING

- Random GH measurement cannot diagnose deficiency because is pulsatile
- Prior to GH stimulation testing, review growth history and labs. Should have bone age, TSH, FT4, and karyotype (female), IGF-1, IGFBP-3
- Pretreating with sex steroids can help improve specificity of test. Treat females with conjugated estrogens 5 mg PO the night prior AND morning of the test, OR 50 to 100 µg/day ethinyl estradiol × 3 days prior to testing. For boys, use 100 mg of depot testosterone 3 days before testing
- TWO different provocative tests required to be positive in order to make diagnosis
- Obese patients have lower GH levels

Table 3.14 Growth Hormone Stimulation Testing Options

Test	How to Administer	Notes
Arginine	0.5 g/kg 10% arginine HCl in 0.9% NaCl (max 30 g) IV over 30 minutes; measure serum GH at 0, 15, 30, 45, 60 minutes	Most commonly used
Levodopa	< 15 kg: 125 mg 10–30 kg: 250 mg > 30 kg: 500 mg; measure GH at 0, 60, 90 min	Nausea
Insulin	0.05 to 0.1 unit/kg IV; measure GH at 0, 15, 30, 60, 75, 90, 120 minutes	*Beware hypoglycemia, monitor closely
Glucagon	0.03 mg/kg (max 1 mg); measure GH at 0, 30, 60, 90, 120, 150, 180 minutes	Nausea
Clonidine	0.15 mg/m^2; measure GH at 0, 30, 60, 90 minutes	Hypotension, somnolence
GHRH	1 mcg/kg IV	Flushing

*Growth hormone < 10 mcg/L generally considered to be cutoff for positive test.
Data from: *Williams textbook of endocrinology*, p985–996 and *Pituitary*, 2008;11(2):115, *J Clin Endocrinol Metab*. 2000 Nov; 85(11):3990–3.

THYROID ABNORMALITIES

HYPOTHYROIDISM

Testing indicated for: Child with enlarged thyroid; new-onset growth failure, cold intolerance, fatigue, constipation, dry skin; or follow-up newborn screen

Table 3.15 Causes of Hypothyroidism

Type	History/Exam	Notes
Primary congenital	Usually detected on newborn screen; caused by thyroid dysgenesis/agenesis or dysmorphogenesis	↑ TSH ↓ T4 ↑ chance false positive if checked before 3 days old
Transient congenital	Often asymptomatic and identified on newborn screen; may present with Goiter in neonate; transient hypothyroxinemia* (↓ T4, normal TSH) common in premature infants	Caused by iodine deficiency or excess, maternal thyroid-stimulating hormone receptor (TSHR) antibodies, maternal use of antithyroid drugs, DUOX 2 (dual oxidase 2) mutations, prematurity, maternal hyperthyroidism, drugs
Inborn error in thyroid hormone synthesis	Autosomal recessive, most commonly thyroperoxidase enzyme deficiency	Pendred syndrome: *SLC26A4 mutation*, goiter + bilateral progressive hearing loss
Hashimoto's thyroiditis	Autoimmune, chronic lymphocytic thyroiditis, usually euthyroid initially and present with thyromegaly; may be hypothyroid or transient toxic thyroiditis	+ antithyroglobulin and/or antithyroperoxidase antibodies. Most common cause of hypothyroidism in childhood
Less common causes	Iodine deficiency (developing countries), post-radiation, postoperative, TSH deficiency	

Table 3.16 Workup of Hypothyroidism

TSH	Most useful single test; ↑ in primary congenital hypothyroidism, pituitary hormone resistance, TSH-secreting tumors; ↓ in Graves', thyrotoxicosis. Normal range 0.5–5.0 IU/mL
Thyroglobulin	Protein made only by thyroid gland, precursor to T3 and T4. Undetectable levels suggest absent thyroid tissue (congenital or postoperative).
Antithyroglobulin antibodies (ATA) or antithyroperoxidase antibodies (more specific)	Present in Hashimoto's, Graves', euthyroid, Hashimoto's encephalopathy, type I diabetes, Addison's disease. Do not treat based on + antibodies alone
T3	Converted from T4 primarily by the liver; mainly used in diagnosis of hyperthyroidism
Free T4	Free T4 is more reliable than total T4. Normal range 0.9–1.6 ng/dL

Data from: *Indian J Endocrinol Metab.* 2011 Jul;15(Suppl 2):S117-20.

Treatment:
Congenital hypothyroidism: Levothyroxine (75–100 mcg/m²/day) initiated as soon as possible
Hashimoto disease (autoimmune thyroiditis): Levothyroxine 50–100 mcg/m²/day (if ↓ T4, ↑ TSH); propranolol if toxic thyroiditis. Follow labs regularly (may not treat) if euthyroid

References: *Indian J Endocrinol Metab.* 2011;15(Suppl 2):S117-S120; *J Clin Endo Metab.* 2011;96(10):2959–2967.

HYPERTHYROIDISM

Testing indicated for: more than one of the following: hyperactivity, declining school performance, heat intolerance, tachycardia, unintentional weight loss

Table 3.17 Causes of Hyperthyroidism in Children

Graves' disease	Most common cause of hyperthyroidism in children; autoantibodies stimulate thyroid gland; + thyroid stimulating antibodies (>95% sensitivity and specificity), usually ↑ T4 and T3, ↓ TSH. Usually treated with methimazole or PTU; if fails, consider ablative therapy or surgery
Neonatal Graves' disease	1% of babies born to mothers with Graves' disease may have hyperthyroidism (often fetal thyroid US and maternal antibody titers followed). Usually symptoms manifest within 10 days of birth including excessive irritability, restlessness, ↑ appetite, ↑ stooling, tachycardia, heart failure, hematologic abnormalities, craniosynostosis. May monitor mild cases. Moderate–severe cases treated with antithyroid drugs, beta-blockers, iodine, iodinated contract materials; rarely, digoxin or glucocorticoids may be used
Hashimoto's thyrotoxicosis	↑ antithyroglobulin and antithyroid peroxidase antibodies, but thyroid-stimulating antibodies negative. Thyroid ¹²³I uptake scan: uptake usually low/patchy distribution (in Graves' disease, uptake is elevated/diffuse)
Exogenous thyroxine ingestion	Acute symptoms of accidental ingestions similar to hyperthyroidism, outcomes are usually good. Chronic ingestion can lead to thyrotoxicosis

Reference: *Thyroid.* 1999;9(7):727–733.

Table 3.18 Medications Used in Hyperthyroidism

Methimazole	0.4–0.7 mg/kg/day once daily dosing	May take 6–12 weeks for preformed T4 to drop, symptoms may persist this long. Dose to keep T4 in normal range; as TSH ↑, wean dose to stop. Side effects: rash, bitter taste, nausea, headache; less common: arthritis, agranulocytosis, hepatitis
PTU*	PTU 5–7 mg/kg/day divided tid	
Propranolol	Propranolol, 80 mg/m²/day	Used in moderate to severe cases, cardiac involvement
Iodine	Transiently decrease T4 synthesis. Lasts approximately 2 weeks	Lugol iodine solution (6.3 mg elemental iodine/drop). Saturated solution of potassium iodide (SSKI) (38 mg KI/drop)
Iodinated contrast solutions	Release iodine and inhibit conversion of T4 to T3	Sodium iopanoic acid (333 mg iodine/capsule); sodium ipodate (308 mg iodine/capsule)
Sodium iodide I-131 (Hicon, Iodotope)	1–2 doses for radioablation	
Hydrocortisone (Solu-Cortef, Cortef)	Stress dose steroids (see section on adrenal insufficiency)	Used for thyroid storm, protects from adrenal insufficiency, ↓ autoantibodies, and ↓ T4 to T3 conversion

*Black box warning for severe liver injury and acute liver failure; only use for patients who cannot tolerate other treatment options. May consider in women in first trimester pregnancy and breastfeeding mothers.

Data from: http://www.thyca.org/pediatric/treatment-pap.htm#overview, http://emedicine.medscape.com/article/920283-workup.

THYROID MASS

- Overall, thyroid nodule in child has a 30% chance of malignancy. Increased risk if child has received radiation therapy for other cancer
- Thyroid scan: "Cold" nodules more likely to be malignant; "hot" nodules almost always benign
- Papillary cancers most common; follicular less common (consider MEN syndrome)
- Neck ultrasound prior to surgery to evaluate nodes
- Treatment usually surgical (including removal of groups of nodes where metastatic nodes found) + radioactive iodine (several weeks after surgery)
- Surgery complications: laryngeal nerve damage, hypocalcemia from damaged parathyroids, bleeding, infection

References: Thyroid Cancer Survivor's Association: http://www.thyca.org/pediatric/treatment-pap.htm#overview

Medscape Reference: Pediatric Graves' disease workup. http://emedicine.medscape.com/article/920283-workup

CHAPTER 4 ■ FLUIDS AND ELECTROLYTES

ACID–BASE DISTURBANCES

Table 4.1 Normal Arterial Blood Gas Values

pH	7.35–7.45
HCO_3^-	20–28 mEq/L
PCO_2	35–45 mmHg

Table 4.2 Anion Gap (AG)

$AG = [Na^+] - [Cl^-] - [HCO_3^-]$ Normal = 4–11

Table 4.3 Expected Compensation in Acid–Base Disorders

Metabolic acidosis	$PCO_2 = 1.5 \times [HCO_3^-] + 8$
Metabolic alkalosis	With each 10 mEq/L ↑ in $[HCO_3^-]$ → PCO_2 ↑ by 7
Acute respiratory acidosis	With each 10 mmHg ↑ in PCO_2 → $[HCO_3^-]$ ↑ by 1
Chronic respiratory acidosis	With each 10 mmHg ↑ in PCO_2 → $[HCO_3^-]$ ↑ by 3.5
Acute respiratory alkalosis	With each 10 mmHg ↓ in PCO_2 → $[HCO_3^-]$ ↓ by 2
Chronic respiratory alkalosis	With each 10 mmHg ↓ in PCO_2 → $[HCO_3^-]$ ↓ by 4

ACID–BASE ANALYSIS
- First determine if patient has acidemia (pH < 7.35) or alkalemia (pH > 7.45). (*patient with mixed disturbance or chronic respiratory alkalosis with complete metabolic compensation may have normal pH)
- Determine if HCO_3^- and CO_2 are ↑ or ↓

Table 4.4 Types of Metabolic Acidosis

pH < 7.35 and ↓ HCO_3^- → metabolic acidosis
If CO_2 normal → Simple metabolic acidosis
If ↓ CO_2 → metabolic acidosis + respiratory alkalosis
If ↑ CO_2 → metabolic acidosis + respiratory acidosis

Table 4.5 Types of Respiratory Acidosis

pH < 7.35 and ↑ PCO_2 → respiratory acidosis
If HCO_3^- normal → simple respiratory acidosis
If ↑ HCO_3^- → respiratory acidosis + metabolic alkalosis
If ↓ HCO_3^- → respiratory acidosis + metabolic acidosis

Table 4.6 Types of Metabolic Alkalosis

pH > 7.45 and ↑ HCO$_3^-$ → metabolic alkalosis
If PCO$_2$ normal → simple metabolic alkalosis
If ↑ PCO$_2$ → metabolic alkalosis + respiratory acidosis
If ↓ PCO$_2$ → metabolic alkalosis + respiratory alkalosis

Table 4.7 Types of Respiratory Alkalosis

pH > 7.45 and ↓ PCO$_2$ → respiratory alkalosis
If HCO$_3^-$ normal → simple respiratory alkalosis
If ↓ HCO$_3^-$ → respiratory alkalosis + metabolic acidosis
If ↑ HCO$_3^-$ → respiratory alkalosis + metabolic alkalosis

- Then determine if compensation is adequate based on expected compensations chart above. If the compensation is not adequate, then a mixed respiratory and metabolic disorder is present. If it is adequate, then it is a simple disturbance.
- If both metabolic acidosis + respiratory acidosis are present OR metabolic alkalosis + respiratory alkalosis are present, it is a mixed disorder.

METABOLIC ACIDOSIS

Table 4.8 Etiologies of Metabolic Acidosis

Normal Anion Gap
Diarrhea Renal tubular acidosis (RTA)
Elevated Anion Gap
Lactic acidosis (shock, inborn errors of metabolism, medication, liver failure) Ketoacidosis (diabetes, kidney failure, starvation) Poisonings (salicylate, ethylene glycol, methanol, toluene) Inborn errors of metabolism

TREATMENT OF METABOLIC ACIDOSIS:

- Treat underlying disorder
- If chronic, untreatable metabolic acidosis, treat with oral base therapy (oral NaHCO$_3$ tablets for older children, sodium citrate or potassium citrate if solution needed for younger children)
- Acute, uncorrectable metabolic acidosis may be treated with sodium bicarbonate therapy 1 mEq/kg bolus or added to IVFs (NaHCO$_3$ or sodium citrate, ↓ NaCl)
- Tris-hydroxymethyl aminomethane (THAM) may be considered in patients with a metabolic acidosis and a respiratory acidosis
- Consider hemodialysis in patients with metabolic acidosis + renal failure (especially if ↑ K), methanol or ethylene glycol intoxication (in addition to fomepizole, which inhibits alcohol dehydrogenase)

METABOLIC ALKALOSIS

Table 4.9 Etiologies of Metabolic Alkalosis

Chloride-responsive*
Vomiting or NG suction Diuretics Diarrhea Chloride-deficient formula Cystic fibrosis
Chloride-nonresponsive*
Adrenal hyperplasia ↑ Renin Cushing syndrome Licorice ingestion

*Chloride-responsive alkalosis typically has a urine Cl^- < 15 mEq/L; chloride-nonresponsive has urine Cl^- > 20 mEq/L

RESPIRATORY ACIDOSIS

Table 4.10 Etiologies of Respiratory Acidosis

CNS or PNS Abnormalities	↓ Chest Wall Movement
↑ ICP (brain tumor, head trauma, infection, stroke) Congenital central hypoventilation syndrome (Ondine's curse) Guillain-Barré syndrome Tick paralysis Myasthenia gravis Multiple sclerosis Spinal cord injury Botulism Spinal muscular atrophies Poliomyelitis	Flail chest Ascites, abdominal tumors, scoliosis
	Medications
	Narcotics Barbiturates Benzodiazepines Propofol Paralyzing agents (vecuronium, succinylcholine) Aminoglycosides Organophosphates (pesticides)
Pulmonary Causes	**Upper Airway Obstruction**
Asthma Bronchiolitis Pneumothorax Bronchopulmonary dysplasia (BPD) ARDS Cystic fibrosis Pulmonary embolus	OSAS Laryngospasm Aspiration Angioedema Vocal cord paralysis Tumor (intrinsic or extrinsic) Tonsillar hypertrophy Infection: peritonsillar abscess, croup, bacterial tracheitis

TREATMENT OF RESPIRATORY ACIDOSIS

- Treat underlying cause
- Naloxone (*Narcan*) if indicated (opioid overdose: 0.01 mg/kg IV; repeat with 0.1 mg/kg IV if necessary)
- Supplemental oxygen
- Mechanical ventilation if indicated (try to avoid if chronic respiratory acidosis; if intubate child with chronic respiratory acidosis aim for their baseline CO_2, slowly)

RESPIRATORY ALKALOSIS

Table 4.11 Etiologies of Respiratory Alkalosis

Pulmonary Causes	CNS Causes
Pneumonia Pulmonary edema Pulmonary embolism Hemothorax Pneumothorax ARDS	Subarachnoid hemorrhage Encephalitis or meningitis Trauma Brain tumor Stroke
Asthma	**Systemic Causes**
Severe anemia High altitude Laryngospasm Aspiration Carbon monoxide poisoning Pulmonary embolism Interstitial lung Mechanical ventilation/ECMO	Fever Pain Psychogenic Liver failure Sepsis Pregnancy Hyperammonemia
Cardiac Causes	**Medications**
Cyanotic heart disease Congestive heart failure	Salicylate intoxication Theophylline Progesterone Exogenous catecholamines Caffeine

Data from: *Nelson's Textbook of Pediatrics*. Philadelphia: Elsevier, 2011, pp. 229–242.

TREATMENT OF RESPIRATORY ALKALOSIS

- Treat underlying cause

HYPOCALCEMIA

Table 4.12 Symptoms of Hypocalcemia

Carpopedal spasms	Lethargy	Poor feeding
Muscle cramps	Seizures	Abdominal distension
Paresthesias	Hypotension	Chvostek's/Trousseau's sign
Tremulousness	Asymptomatic	Tetany (iCa < 1.1 mmol/ L)

Table 4.13 Causes of Hypocalcemia

Hypoparathyroidism ($\downarrow$ PTH, $\downarrow$ or nl phosphate; $\uparrow$ ca with PTH challenge); postop, autoimmune or congenital **Pseudohypoparathyroidism** ($\uparrow$ PTH, no response to PTH challenge) or pseudo-pseudohypoparathyroidism **Vitamin D metabolism** disorders ($\uparrow$ PTH, no response to PTH challenge) **Familial hypercalciuric hypocalcemia** (CaSR gene) **Hyperphosphatemia** (renal failure, tumor lysis, rhabdomyolysis, exogenous phosphate) **Sepsis**	Malabsorption **Renal tubular defects, renal failure** (urine Ca/creatinine > 0.3 with hypocalcemia is abnormal) **DiGeorge syndrome** **Hypomagnesemia, severe hypermagnesemia** (neonate after Mg containing tocolytics used) **Chemotherapy complications** (cisplatin, 5-fluorouracil) Complication of **EDTA** chelation, excessive **fluoride** administration, **furosemide** **Osteoblastic metastases** **Pancreatitis**

WORKUP OF HYPOCALCEMIA

- **Corrected [Ca] = Total [Ca] + (0.8 × [4.5 − albumin level])**
- Serum electrolytes including plasma calcium, phosphate, glucose, magnesium
- Ionized calcium level
- Alkaline phosphatase
- 25-hydroxyvitamin D and 1,25-dihydroxyvitamin D
- Parathyroid hormone levels
- Urine calcium, magnesium, phosphorus, creatinine, pH, glucose, protein levels
- Lymphocyte and T cell subset analysis (DiGeorge)
- CXR (evaluate for thymic shadow, absent in DiGeorge)
- Ankle/ wrist x-ray (evaluate for rickets)
- ECG (prolonged QTc or ST, T wave abnormalities)
- Genetic testing (CaSR, GNAS, AIRE, VDR, mitochondrial DNA, 22q11 deletion)[1]

SPECIAL CONSIDERATIONS IN CALCIUM DISTURBANCES

- Low serum albumin or pH alteration can cause ↓ total Ca, but ionized Ca should be normal (acidosis: ↓ Ca bound to albumin)
- Hypocalcemia may lead to ↓ Mg, and correcting both is important.
- Hypomagnesemia may lead to hypocalcemia by affecting PTH release.
- Phosphate: usually high in renal failure, hypoparathyroidism, and phosphate loading. Usually low in rickets and vit D deficiency.
- If concurrent acidemia, treat hypocalcemia first

TREATMENT OF HYPOCALCEMIA

- If serum Ca < 7.0 mg/dL or iCa < 0.8 *and symptomatic*: 10% calcium gluconate 1 mL/kg IV over 15 minutes then 0.5 to 1.5 mg/kg/hr until initiate oral calcium supplementation. Goal serum level is 8.0 mg/dL.
- Ca gluconate causes less tissue necrosis than Ca chloride
- Too rapid administration can cause cardiac arrest
- Do not administer in same line as bicarbonate or phosphate
- Treat other electrolyte abnormalities
- Hypoparathyroidism or pseudohypoparathyroidism: calcitriol (20–60 ng/kg/day) and supplemental oral calcium (30–75 mg elemental Ca/kg/day)
- Oral calcium options: Calcium glubionate (liquid form): contains 115 mg of elemental calcium/5 mL; calcium carbonate (liquid or tab, 40% elemental calcium (1 g of calcium carbonate = 400 mg of elemental calcium)

HYPERCALCEMIA

Table 4.14 Symptoms of Hypercalcemia

Irritability	Polyuria/polydipsia/nocturia	Dehydration
Mood changes	Short QTc	Weakness
Headache	Decreased appetite	Nephrocalcinosis on renal US
Constipation, abdominal pain	Hypertension	Anxiety

Table 4.15 Causes of Hypercalcemia

Primary hyperparathyroidism (consider multiple endocrinopathy like MEN I or II, or familial HPT) **Secondary hyperparathyroidism** (associated with chronic renal failure, lithium, thiazides) **Acute renal failure** **Familial hypocalciuric hypercalcemia (FHH)** (can confirm findings in parent) **Hyperthyroidism**	**Vitamin D excess** (nutritional or associated with granulomatous disease: sarcoidosis, TB, Crohn's) **Exogenous calcium administration** **Immobilization** **Medication side effects** (theophylline, vitamin A, thiazide diuretics) **Hyperphosphatemia** **Associated with malignancy** **Milk alkali syndrome** (excessive milk or antacid intake)

WORKUP OF HYPERCALCEMIA

- **Corrected [Ca] = Total [Ca] + (0.8 × [4.5 − albumin level])**
- Serum electrolytes including plasma calcium, phosphate, glucose, magnesium
- Ionized calcium level
- Alkaline phosphatase
- 25-hydroxyvitamin D (elevated in excessive exogenous intake of vitamin D) and 1,25-dihydroxyvitamin D (elevated if kids with granulomatous, chronic inflammatory, or lymphatic disease)
- Parathyroid hormone levels (increased in primary or secondary hyperparathyroidism)
- Urine calcium, magnesium, phosphorus, creatinine, pH, glucose, protein levels
- PTHrP (PTH-related peptide); elevated in hypercalcemia associated with malignancy

Table 4.16 Acute Treatment of Hypercalcemia

Total Serum Calcium (mg/dL)	Treatment
< 12 mg/dL *and* asymptomatic	May be deferred until cause evaluated
> 12 mg/dL *and/or* symptomatic	IV fluids (NS 2× maintenance) Diuretics (furosemide) Bisphosphonates or calcitonin Dialysis in resistant cases

Table 4.17 Long-Term Treatment of Hypercalcemia by Etiology

Etiology	Treatment
Primary hyperparathyroidism	Surgery
Secondary hyperparathyroidism	Calcitriol, lower serum phosphate, maintain calcium in normal range
Immobilization	Low calcium and vitamin D intake, aggressive hydration, mobilization ASAP
Granulomatous disease, inflammatory disease, vitamin D ingestion	Glucocorticoids (inhibit 25-hydroxyvitamin D-1 alpha hydroxylase activity)

Data from: http://www.hawaii.edu/medicine/pediatrics/pedtext/s15c06.html accessed 9/26/12

Reference: *Ann Endocrinol (Paris)*. 2005 Jun;66(3):207–215.

DEHYDRATION

PRINCIPLES OF ORAL REHYDRATION THERAPY

Successful in most children with mild–moderate dehydration
- **Allow continued breastfeeding**
- Do not change from or dilute standard infant formula

- Use commercially available ORS or prepare per instructions at rehydrate.org
  ○ 1 level tsp salt + 8 level tsp sugar + 1000 mL clean water
  ○ 50–100 mL/kg PO/NG over 3–4 hours in frequent, small aliquots
  ○ For each episode emesis or diarrhea, child needs additional fluid as follows
    – Child < 10 kg: 60–120 mL
    – Child > 10 kg: 120–240 mL

Table 4.18 Assessment of Percentage Dehydration

Sign/Symptom	< 5% (mild)	5–9% (moderate)	> 10% (severe)
Fluid deficit	< 50 mL/kg	~100 mL/kg	> 100 mL/kg
Activity	Normal	Irritable or lethargic	Lethargic or listless
Pulse	Normal	Tachycardic, +/– weak	Thready
Blood pressure	Normal	Normal	Decreased
Capillary refill	Normal	Prolonged	Very prolonged
Mucous membranes	Moist/tears	Dry/decreased tears	Dry/no tears
Skin	Normal	Dry, no tenting	Tenting, cold, mottled
Urine	Normal	Decreased UOP, dark	Minimal UOP
Eyes/fontanelle	Normal	Slightly sunken	Markedly sunken

Table 4.19 Oral Rehydration Solutions (ORS)

Solution	CHO (g/dL)	Na (mEq/L)	K (mEq/L)	Base (mEq/L)	Osmolality
WHO/UNICEF	2	90	20	30	310
Pedialyte	3	50	25	30	200
Infalyte	2.5	75	20	30	310
Rehydralyte	2.5	75	20	30	310

Table 4.20 Inappropriate "Clear Liquids" for Rehydration

	CHO (g/dL)	Na (mEq/L)	K (mEq/L)	Base (mEq/L)	Osmolality
Gatorade*	5.8	45.8	12.5		280–340
Apple juice	12	0.4	26	0	700
Chicken broth	0	2	3	3	330
Milk	4.9	22	36	30	260

*Inappropriate CHO:Na ratio impairs water absorption, may ↑ osmotic diarrhea
Data from: Pediatrics 1996; 97:424; MMWR.2003; 52 (RR-16):1–16

- Resume normal diet as soon as possible. Do not restrict diet (avoid BRAT diet)
- PO zinc sulfate (age < 6 months: 10 mg, age > 6 months: 20 mg × 10–14 days) may ↓ diarrhea
- Avoid: Unnecessary lab work, antidiarrheal agents, antibiotics, and phenothiazines
- Consider intravenous 20 mL/kg bolus of normal saline for severe dehydration
- IV ondansetron may ↓ emesis.
- Avoid promethazine in children age < 2 and use with extreme caution in older children. Risk of respiratory depression.
- For patients with dehydration and electrolyte abnormalities, see specific electrolyte abnormality for evaluation and management
- For patients requiring IV fluid resuscitation and rehydration, see Section on IV Fluid basics

References: *Pediatrics.* 1996;97:424; *MMWR.* 2003;52(RR-16):1–16; *Pediatrics.* 2002;109: e62; WHO/UNICEF. Management of acute diarrhea. 2004. http://www.unicef.org/publications/index_21433.html

Abbreviations: BRAT: bananas, rice, applesauce, toast; CHO: carbohydrate; IV: intravenous; K: potassium; Na: sodium; NG: nasogastric tube; PO: orally; sg: specific gravity; UNICEF: United Nations Children's Fund; UOP: urine output; WHO: World Health Organization

HYPERKALEMIA

DEFINITION: serum potassium > 6.0 mEq/L; severe hyperkalemia: > 7.0 mEq/L

Table 4.21 Causes of Hyperkalemia

Hemolysis	Blood transfusion	**Medications:**
Tissue ischemia or necrosis	Exogenous administration	Succinylcholine
↑ WBC	Acidosis	Digitalis
Hypoaldosteronism	Malignant hyperthermia	Excessive fluoride
GI bleeding	Heel-stick blood draw	Beta-blockers
Tumor lysis syndrome	Rhabdomyolysis	ACE inhibitors
Hyperkalemic periodic paralysis	Exercise	Angiotensin II blockers
Renal failure	Adrenal insufficiency	K+-sparing diuretics
Renal tubular acidosis	Kidney transplant	Calcineurin inhibitors
↑ Platelets	Lupus nephritis	NSAIDs
Congenital adrenal hyperplasia	Sickle cell disease	Trimethoprim
		Heparin
		Yasmin (oral contraceptive pill)

Data from: *Cochrane Database Syst Rev* 2005: CD003235; Arch Dis Child. 2012;97(4):376–380.

SIGNS/SYMPTOMS OF HYPERKALEMIA:

- **ECG:** Peaked T waves initially; ST-segment depression, ↑ PR interval, flattened P wave, wide QRS complex. Can lead to VF, asystole
- Paresthesias, fasciculations, weakness usually *after* ECG changes

EVALUATION OF HYPERKALEMIA:

- Comprehensive metabolic panel, venous K measurement, CBC, acid–base evaluation, CPK, urinalysis, urine K+
- Transtubular K gradient (TTKG): [K] urine/ [K] plasma × (plasma osmolarity/urine osmolarity). Urine osm must be > serum osm. TTKG < 8 suggests defect in renal K excretion(↓ aldosterone or no response to aldosterone)
- Check ECG if K > 6.0 mEq/L

Table 4.22 Treatment of Hyperkalemia

Aggressiveness of treatment depends on K+ level, specific ECG changes, and underlying etiology	
Treatment	Dose
Calcium gluconate 10%	1 mL/kg/dose IV (100 mg/kg/dose) over 5 min
NaHCO₃	1–2 mEq/kg IV over 10 min
Insulin + glucose	Regular insulin 0.1 units/kg IV *PLUS* 25% glucose 2 mL/kg over 30 min Alternative: continuous infusion D25W 1–2 mL/kg/hr with regular insulin 0.1 units/kg/hr Check glucose hourly while on continuous insulin infusion
Nebulized albuterol	10–20 mg via MDI or nebulized solution
Loop diuretic	Furosemide 0.5–2 mg/kg/dose IV, IM, PO q 6–12 hr
Sodium polystyrene sulfonate (*Kayexalate*)	1 g/kg PO q 6 hr (unapproved: 1 g/kg PR q 2–6 hr). Avoid in patients with abnormal bowel function/constipation. Suspension: 15 g/60 mL
Dialysis (peritoneal or hemodialysis)	For severe or refractory cases with renal failure

Data from: *Cochrane Database Syst Rev* 2005: CD003235; *Arch Dis Child*. 2012;97(4):376-3800.

References: *Arch Dis Child*. 2012;97(4):376–380.

HYPERNATREMIA

Definition: Serum Na > 145–150 mEq/ L

Table 4.23 Causes of Hypernatremia

Sodium excess	IV administration of NaHCO₃ or hypertonic saline, baking soda or seawater ingestion, Munchausen-by-proxy syndrome, improper mixing of infant formula, hyperaldosteronism
Free water deficit	Diabetes insipidus (central or nephrogenic), inadequate water intake (difficulty with breastfeeding, neglect, gingivostomatitis or other illness causing decreased PO intake), ↑ insensible losses (prematurity, phototherapy, fever)
↓ Water and + sodium	GI losses (vomiting/diarrhea/NG suction); skin losses (burns); renal losses (kidney disease, diuretics, ATN, diabetes mellitus)

ATN: Acute tubular necrosis

Data from: *Nelson's Textbook of Pediatrics*, Philadelphia: Elsevier, 2011 pp. 212-215.

Table 4.24 Findings in Hypernatremia

Signs/Symptoms	Possible Complications
• Typically have signs of dehydration (initial losses from intracellular space, so early in course signs are less severe) • CNS: Irritability, restlessness, lethargy • ↑ glucose, ↓ calcium	• Subarachnoid, subdural, and parenchymal hemorrhages (water moves out of neurons, veins tear) • Central pontine and extrapontine myelinolysis • Thrombosis (dural, peripheral, and renal veins)

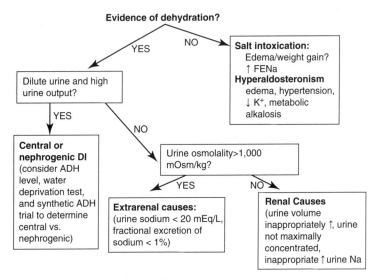

Figure 4.1 Algorithm for Evaluation of Hyponatremia

TREATMENT:

- **WARNING:** Correcting chronic/subchronic hypernatremia too quickly can result in cerebral edema, seizures, coma (idiogenic osmoles created to ↑ intracellular osm). Monitor serum sodium frequently during correction
- **GOAL:** Decrease the serum sodium by < 12 mEq/L every 24 hr (0.5 mEq/L/hr) AFTER intravascular volume has been restored with NS boluses (not LR because has lower Na content). NS boluses aimed at normalizing hypotension, tachycardia, signs of poor perfusion
- **Calculate free water deficit:** body weight (kg) × 0.6 L/kg [1 − (145/current Na)]
- **Estimate free water deficit** by: 3–4 mL/kg of free water required to decrease serum Na by 1 mEq/L
- Typical fluids for correction are D5¼ or D5½ NS at 20% greater than maintenance rate. May also need to replace ongoing losses
- **Acute** iatrogenic hypernatremia/sodium intoxication may be corrected more rapidly; can use D5W, add furosemide if volume overload. Dialysis if severe

Reference: *Nelson's Textbook of Pediatrics.* Philadelphia: Elsevier, 2011, pp. 212–215.

HYPOKALEMIA

Table 4.25 Causes of Hypokalemia

Alkalosis Diarrhea Cystic fibrosis (CF) Refeeding syndrome Anorexia Laxative abuse Periodic paralysis Renal tube acidocis Diabetic ketoacidosis Interstitial nephritis Hypomagnesemia	Syndromes: EAST, Liddle, Gitelman, Bartter Renovascular disease Renin-secreting tumor Adrenal hyperplasia Cushing's syndrome Licorice ingestion Emesis NG suction	**Medications:** Albuterol Alpha agonists Aminoglycosides Amphotericin Barium Cesium chloride Cisplatin Furosemide Hydroxychloroquine Insulin Kayexalate Penicillin Theophylline Toluene

Reference: *Nelson's Textbook of Pediatrics*. Philadelphia: Elsevier, 2011, pp. 222–224.

SIGNS/SYMPTOMS:

- **ECG:** flattened T wave, a depressed ST segment, U wave, (between T and P waves). Children with congenital heart disease at ↑ risk VF and torsades; ↑ risk for children on digitalis (SVT, VT, heart block)
- Weakness and muscle cramps
- K < 2.5 mEq/L may lead to paralysis, constipation, and/or urinary retention
- Polyuria/polydipsia
- Poor growth if chronic hypokalemia

EVALUATION:

- Comprehensive metabolic panel, acid–base evaluation, Ca^+, Mg^+, phosphorus
- Urinary K^+ (24-hr urine collection, a spot potassium:creatinine ratio, a fractional excretion of potassium, or calculation of the TTKG [See hyperkalemia]). (Urine K^+ > 15 mg/L; TTKG > 4 suggest renal losses)
- If plasma renin activity < 0.5 ng/mL/hr and direct renin assay < 15 mU/LPRA, check aldosterone levels and 11-deoxycorticosterone (DOC)
- If plasma renin activity high, suggests renal parenchymal disease, pheochromocytoma, or glucocorticoid excess
- ↑ aldosterone likely primary hyperaldosteronism
- If ↑ DOC, check cortisol, ACTH, 17-OHP, evaluate for adrenal etiologies

TREATMENT:

- If hypokalemia is caused by intracellular shifts (not total-body depletion), correcting underlying problem often corrects K^+
- Use caution with K^+ administration (especially if renal impairment). If total-body depletion, consider oral K^+ 2–4 mEq/kg/day (max 120–240 mEq/day in divided doses)
- IV K^+ (usually KCl): 0.5–1 mEq/kg over 2–4 hr (max 30 mEq/infusion)
  - ○ Maximum IV rate 0.5 mEq/kg/hr unless in ICU setting or critically ill
    - – Rapid administration can lead to ventricular arrhythmias
  - ○ Consider KAcetate or KPhosphate if other abnormalities present as well
- Correct ↓ Mg concurrently

HYPOMAGNESEMIA

Normal magnesium is 1.5–2.3 mg/dL

Table 4.26 Causes of Low Serum Magnesium

Diarrhea (infection, IBD, celiac disease, cystic fibrosis, small bowel resection, pancreatitis)	**Medications:** Aminoglycosides
Primary aldosteronism	Amphotericin
IV fluids	Cisplatin
Diabetes	Cyclosporine
Genetic syndromes (Bartter and Gitelman cause renal losses)	Loop diuretics Mannitol
Hypomagnesemia with secondary hypocalcemia	Pentamidine
Chronic kidney disease	Thiazide diuretics
Poor oral intake/chronic malnutrition	Hypercalcemia
Infants of diabetic mothers	Exchange transfusion

Data from: *Nelson's Textbook of Pediatrics*. Philadelphia: Elsevier, 2011 p. 225e.1–225e.3.

SIGNS/SYMPTOMS OF HYPOMAGNESEMIA:

- ↓ Mg^+ causes ↓ Ca^{++}
- Flattened T wave and ↑ ST segment length. Arrhythmias possible especially if preexisting cardiac disease

DIAGNOSIS OF HYPOMAGNESEMIA:

- If diagnosis is not clear from history, fractional excretion of Mg^+ can help determine whether renal or non-renal causes
- $FE[Mg] = (U_{Mg} \times P_{Cr})/ ([0.7 \times P_{Mg})] \times U_{Cr}) \times 100$; if FE_{Mg} is > 4% in presence of ↓ serum Mg, likely due to renal Mg wasting

TREATMENT OF HYPOMAGNESEMIA:

- Magnesium sulfate 25–50 mg/kg (0.05–0.1 mL/kg of a 50% solution; 2.5–5.0 mg/kg of elemental magnesium) IV over 4 hours
- Side effects of infusion may include flushing, diaphoresis
- Oral long-term therapy: Slow-Mag (60 mg elemental magnesium/tablet) and Mag-Tab SR (84 mg elemental magnesium/tablet)

HYPERMAGNESEMIA

CAUSES OF HYPERMAGNESEMIA:

- Usually due to excessive intake (laxative, enemas, cathartics used in drug overdoses, antacids, TPN) or infant born to mothers treated with Mg SO_4
- Less common causes include renal failure, familial hypocalciuric hypercalcemia, DKA, lithium ingestion, milk-alkali syndrome, tumor lysis syndrome

SYMPTOMS OF HYPERMAGNESEMIA:

- Hypotonia, weakness, decreased reflexes, poor suck, somnolence, flushing, hypotension, nausea, vomiting, and hypocalcemia
- ECG may show prolonged PR, QRS, and QT intervals
- Mg > 15 mg/dL can cause 3rd-degree heart block and cardiac arrest

TREATMENT OF HYPERMAGNESEMIA:

- Usually clears spontaneously if normal renal function
- Loop diuretics

- Dialysis for ↑↑ Mg with renal failure
- Cardiac emergency: 100 mg/kg of intravenous calcium gluconate via push or over 3–5 minutes (comes as 100 mg/mL solution, therefore dose is 1 mL/kg)

Reference: *Nelson's Textbook of Pediatrics*. Philadelphia: Elsevier, 2011, pp. 225e.1–225e.3.

HYPONATREMIA

Definition: Serum sodium < 135 mEq/L (135 mmol/L)

Table 4.27 Causes of Hyponatremia

Low Serum Osmolarity	
SIADH	Sodium < 120 mEq/L; euvolemic; urine Na ± usually > 40 mEq/L; low/normal serum, urea, uric acid, K^+. Treated with fluid restriction; IV fluids should be NS or 3% NaCl; add loop diuretic to hypertonic saline if necessary.
Diuretic use	Loop or thiazide diuretics
Excessive free water intake	Dilute formula, fresh water swimming, psychogenic polydipsia, iatrogenic, tap water enema
Renal disease	ATN, post-obstructive diuresis, PKD, Type II RTA
CNS disease	Cerebral salt wasting
↓ Aldosterone	21-hydroxylase deficiency, pseudo-hypoaldosteronism I, UTI/ obstruction
Endocrine causes	Adrenal insufficiency, hypothyroidism
Hypervolemic causes	Capillary leak (sepsis) Cirrhosis Congestive heart failure Nephrotic syndrome Renal failure
Hypovolemic causes	Diarrhea, vomiting, excessive sweating, burns
Normal Serum Osmolarity (pseudohyponatremia)	*Does not happen on machines used for ABG determination*
Hyperlipidemia	Hypertriglyceridemia, hypercholesterolemia
Hyperproteinemia	Multiple myeloma, intravenous immunoglobulin
High Serum Osmolarity	
Hyperglycemia	1.6–mEq/L (1.6–mmol/L) ↓ in serum; sodium for every 100 mg/dL (5.6 mmol/L) ↑ in glucose above normal; usually do not have symptoms of hyponatremia **Corrected Na = Measured Na + 1.6 ([glucose] − 100 mg/dL) / 100**
Mannitol, sucrose	

Workup of hyponatremia:
- Serum electrolytes and comprehensive metabolic panel
- Urine electrolytes and urine osmolarity
- Assess volume status (volume depleted or volume overloaded)?
- Medications?
- Other medical conditions or symptoms?

Table 4.28 Presentation of Hyponatremia

Early	Mild headache, nausea
Later	Vomiting, weakness, behavioral changes, impaired responsiveness
Late	Signs of cerebral herniation including seizures, decorticate posturing, respiratory arrest*, dilated pupils

*Higher brain-to-skull size in children lowers their threshold for symptoms and increases risk of complications. Children with hyponatremia are at much higher risk of long-term brain damage or death if they also experience a hypoxic event during hyponatremia.

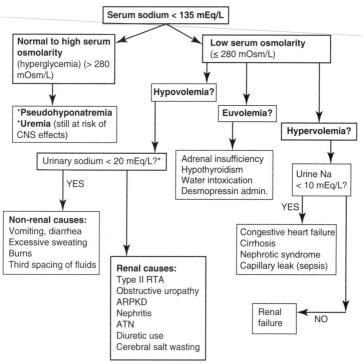

* Timing of urinary sodium measurement in relation to fluid administration, diuretic dosing, should be taken into consideration

Figure 4.2 Algorithmic Evaluation of Hyponatremia

Table 4.29 Diagnostic Criteria for SIADH

Urine osmolality > 100 mOsm/kg (urine osmolarity usually > plasma)
Serum osmolality < 280 mOsm/kg
Serum sodium < 135 mEq/L
Urine sodium > 30 mEq/L
Rule out other causes of hyponatremia
Water restriction leads to correction of hyponatremia

Table 4.30 Treatment of Hyponatremia

Monitor pulse oximetry, treat hypoxia (can worsen cerebral edema)
If severe symptoms (i.e., seizures, coma), bolus with hypertonic saline: 1 mL/kg of 3% NaCl will ↑ serum Na ~ 1 mEq/L. Often improve after 4–6 mL/kg 3% NaCl, may require 10–12 mL/kg. Give bolus over 60 minutes
WARNING: If corrected too rapidly, can lead to central pontine myelinolysis (disorientation, agitation, paralysis, death) Unless critically ill, correct serum sodium by < 12 mEq/L/24 hr or < 18 mEq/L/48 hr
For patients with hyponatremic dehydration, see section on dehydration. Treat hypovolemia (tachycardia, hypotension, poor perfusion) with NS bolus
Hypervolemic hyponatremia: water and sodium restriction, may use diuretics. Tolvaptan (ADH antagonist) can be helpful in heart failure and cirrhosis
Treat underlying cause when possible
Treatment of SIADH: fluid restriction; furosemide + Na± supplementation; tolvaptan; PO urea

Data from: *Nelson's Textbook of Pediatrics*, Philadelphia: Elsevier, 2011, pp. 215–219.

INTRAVENOUS FLUID HYDRATION

Table 4.31 Maintenance Fluid Requirements per 24 Hours

Child's Weight	Maintenance Fluid Requirement in 24 Hours
< 10 kg	100 mL/kg
10–20 kg	1000 mL + 50 mL/kg over 10 kg
> 20 kg	1500 mL + 20 mL/kg over 20 kg

Table 4.32 Maintenance Fluid Requirements per Hour

Child's Weight	Maintenance Fluid Requirement in per Hour
< 10 kg	4 mL/kg/hr
10–20 kg	40 mL/hr + 2 mL/kg/hr for each kg > 10
> 20 kg	60 mL/hr + 1 mL/kg/hr for each kg > 20

Table 4.33 Increased Fluid Requirements Guidelines

Indication	Fluid Adjustment
Fever	Controversial, as intact ADH secretion may make increased fluids unnecessary: Consider ↑ total fluids by 10–15% for each 1°C over 38°C or 1 mL/kg/hr for each 1°C > 38°C
Burns	See section on burns

Table 4.34 Contents of Typical IV Fluid Preparations

Fluid	Na	Glucose	pH	K+	Ca++	Osmolarity
0.45% NS	77 mEq/L		5.3			144 mOsm/L
0.9% NS	154 mEq/L		5.3			310 mOsm/L
0.2% NS	34 mEq/L		5.3			
D5W		5 g/dL	4.7			250 mOsm/L
D10W		10 g/dL	4.6			505 mOsm/L
LR	130 mEq/L		6.3	4 mEq/L	3 mEq/L	275 mOsm/L

NS: normal saline; D: dextrose; W: water; LR: lactated Ringer's solution

Table 4.35 IV Solution Choice by Age and Clinical Situation

Clinical Picture	Solution
< 1 month old patient	D5 ¼ NS + 20 mEq KCl/L
> 1 month old patient, Na+ ≥ 138 mEq/L	D5 ½ NS + 20 mEq KCl/L
> 1 month old and Na+ < 138 mEq/L, or post-operative	D5 NS + 20 mEq KCl/L
Hypokalemia or ↑ K requirements	May add up to 40 mEq KCl/L
Acidosis	May add K acetate to IVF instead of KCl

*Leave out KCl if not urinating

Table 4.36 IVF Management in Dehydration

20 mL/kg NS or LR bolus over 10–15 minutes
Repeat bolus if necessary to replete deficit, up to 60–80 mL/kg total
If electrolyte abnormalities present, see section on specific electrolyte abnormality
Dehydration: (see also table on clinical determination of dehydration) *Calculate total fluid deficit* - Mild dehydration: 4% deficit (40 mL/kg deficit) - Moderate dehydration: 8% deficit (80 mL/kg deficit) - Severe dehydration: 12% deficit (120 mL/kg deficit) *Then subtract total fluids given during boluses above. You are left with estimate of patient's current deficit, and this will guide your maintenance fluid administration. If hyper- or hyponatremia present, see related section.*

Table 4.36 IVF Management in Dehydration (*Continued*)

Over the next 24 hours: - First 8 hours: 50% deficit + maintenance - Next 16 hours: 50% deficit + maintenance
Ongoing losses: - Replace stool output if stool > 30 mL/kg/day - Replace 1:1 stool losses with ½ NS + 20 mEq KCl/L in addition to maintenance IVF

Table 4.37 Intravenous Management of Acute Hypoglycemia

	Neonate	Child
Threshold glucose (mg/dL)	< 40 mg/dL or symptomatic	< 70 mg/dL or symptomatic
Emergency treatment	$D_{10}W$ (0.10 g/mL) 2 mL/kg IV/IO	$D_{25}W$ (0.25 g/mL) 2 mL/kg IV/IO

Data from: http://www.cc.nih.gov/ccc/pedweb/pedsstaff/ivf.html; Family Practice Notebook. Pediatric dehydration management. Retrieved from http://www.fpnotebook.com/peds/FEN/PdtrcDhydrtnMngmnt.htm, accessed 5/7/14.

PHOSPHATE ABNORMALITIES

Table 4.38 Normal Serum Phosphorus

Newborn	4.8–8.2 mg/dL
1–3 yrs	4.0–6.5 mg/dL
4–11 yrs	3.7–5.6 mg/dL
12–15 yrs	2.9–5.4 mg/dL
16–19 yrs	2.3–4.7 mg/dL

Table 4.39 Note About Phosphorus

Phosphorus is mostly intracellular. ↓ Phos can indicate intracellular shifts or total body depletion. May have significant Phos depletion despite normal serum levels.

Table 4.40 Causes of Hypophosphatemia

Prematurity Refeeding syndrome Hypophosphatemic rickets Metabolic acidosis Vitamin D deficiency	Total parenteral nutrition Hungry bone syndrome Antacids Diuretics Respiratory alkalosis Sepsis	Glycosuria Hyperparathyroidism Bone marrow or kidney transplantation Glucocorticoids Dialysis

SIGNS/ SYMPTOMS:
- Phosphorus is required for ATP synthesis and glycolysis
- Acutely, phosphorus < 1.5 can cause hemolysis, ↓ oxygen delivery, rhabdomyolysis, altered mental status, cardiac arrhythmias, seizures

TREATMENT:
- No treatment necessary in mild cases
- Oral phosphorus can cause diarrhea (2–3 mmoL/kg/day in divided doses)
- IV Na phosphorus or K phosphorus (0.08–0.16 mmoL/kg over 4–6 hr)

HYPERPHOSPHATEMIA

Table 4.41 Causes of Hyperphosphatemia

Renal failure	Rhabdomyolysis	Acute hemolysis
Diabetic ketoacidosis	Lactic acidosis	Iatrogenic
Enema use	Vitamin D intoxication	Infants ingesting cow's milk
Hyperthyroidism	Hypoparathyroidism	Tumor lysis syndrome

Data from: *Nelson's Textbook of Pediatrics*. Philadelphia: Elsevier, 2011, pp. 228–229. *Pediatric Hospital Medicine*. Philadelphia: Lippincott Williams and Wilkins, 2008, p. 770.

SIGNS/SYMPTOMS:

- Hypocalcemia (see section on hypocalcemia)
- Systemic calcification (when serum phosphorus [mg/dL] × Ca [mg/dL] > 70); conjunctival, pulmonary calcifications, and nephrocalcinosis

DIAGNOSIS:

- Comprehensive metabolic panel, calcium, phosphorus, CBC
- Consider uric acid, lactate dehydrogenase, bilirubin, TSH, FT4, and CPK

TREATMENT:

- If normal renal function and mild, phosphorus intake reduction (↓ dairy, ↓ soda) may be adequate. Increase fluids/forced diuresis
- If ongoing phosphorus exposure (tumor lysis, rhabdo), add oral phosphorus binder (aluminum hydroxide 50 mg/kg q 8 hr, calcium carbonate 45–65 mg/kg/day divided q 6 hr PO [dose as elemental calcium]), calcium acetate with food + maintain high urine flow with ↑ fluids, consider furosemide
- If chronic use of phosphorus binders is necessary, use calcium carbonate or calcium acetate or sevelamer hydrochloride (avoid aluminum toxicity)
- Risk of hypercalcemia with calcium-based phosphorus binders
- Dialysis may be necessary if poor renal function

CHAPTER 5 ■ GASTROENTEROLOGY

ABDOMINAL PAIN

Key elements to history and physical exam:

- **Trauma**: Consider emergent evaluation for hematoma, hemorrhage, perforation, contusion
- **Emesis**: Partial list of differential diagnoses
  - Bilious: Small or large bowel obstruction, mid gut volvulus
  - Bloody (large or small volume): Esophagitis, gastritis, Mallory-Weiss tear (esophageal or gastric tear after vomiting), gastric or duodenal ulcer, esophageal varices, foreign body, iron toxicity
  - "Coffee grounds": Resolved bleeding from gastric ulcer, esophagitis, gastritis, Mallory Weiss tear, or iron toxicity
  - Food or gastric acid: Gastroenteritis, early in obstructive processes
- **Peritoneal irritation**: Suggested by guarding, rebound, or percussion tenderness. Warrants urgent evaluation
  - Acute appendicitis: Commonly presents with severe abdominal pain (periumbilical → right lower quadrant), anorexia, vomiting, fever, involuntary guarding, leukocytosis
  - Bowel perforation
- **Quality of stool**: Partial list of differential diagnoses
  - Watery: Infectious gastroenteritis, fever, intra-abdominal abscess
  - Decreased stool frequency: Obstruction or constipation
  - Hard stool: Constipation
  - Greasy (steatorrhea): Pancreatic insufficiency, pancreatitis
  - "Currant jelly": Intussusception
  - Acholic (pale, lacking pigmentation): Biliary atresia or other bile obstruction, liver disease
  - Bloody: Anal fissure, hemorrhoid(s), colitis (infectious, IBD), polyp, HSP, Meckel's diverticulum
  - Melanotic: Upper gastrointestinal bleed such as from gastric or duodenal ulcer

Table 5.1 Differential Diagnosis of Acute Abdominal Pain by Location of Pain

Nonspecific/Diffuse Abdominal Pain: AGE, constipation, perforation, intussusception, IBD, DKA, functional abdominal pain, lead poisoning, porphyria, Henoch-Schönlein purpura		
Right Upper Quadrant Hepatitis, cholecystitis, AGE, cholelithiasis, cholangitis, pyelonephritis, gastritis, pneumonia, nephrolithiasis, pleural effusion, pericarditis, pancreatitis, constipation	*Epigastric* Gastritis, AGE, gastroesophageal reflux, peptic ulcer disease, pancreatitis, pneumonia, pericarditis, constipation	*Left Upper Quadrant* Constipation, pancreatitis, pyelonephritis, pneumonia, pericarditis, nephrolithiasis, pleural effusion, AGE, splenomegaly, hydronephrosis
	Peri-umbilical AGE, constipation, early appendicitis, UTI, obstruction, fever, functional abdominal pain, pancreatitis, lead/iron toxicity, IBD, mesenteric adenitis, small bowel volvulus	

(Continued)

Table 5.1 Differential Diagnosis of Acute Abdominal Pain by Location of Pain *(Continued)*

Right Lower Quadrant	*Suprapubic*	*Left Lower Quadrant*
Appendicitis, AGE, IBD, constipation, ovarian pain, ectopic pregnancy, testicular torsion, hernia, intussusception	Cystitis, constipation, PID, UTI, AGE/ colitis, uterine issues (imperforate hymen, etc.)	Constipation, AGE, colitis, IBD, ovarian pain, ectopic pregnancy, hernia, testicular torsion, sigmoid volvulus

AGE: Acute gastroenteritis; DKA: Diabetic ketoacidosis; HSP: Henoch-Schönlein purpura; IBD: inflammatory bowel disease; PID: pelvic inflammatory disease; UTI: urinary tract infection

Table 5.2 Physical Exam Maneuvers in Acute Abdominal Pain

McBurney Point Tenderness	Percussion/palpation of RLQ elicits tenderness two thirds of distance from umbilicus to anterior superior iliac spine (ASIS)
Psoas Sign	Pain with either maneuver below: 1. Place patient on left side. Stabilize hip and extend right thigh 2. While supine, have patient raise right leg against resistance
Obturator Sign	Flex hip and knee to 90° each. ↑ pain with internal rotation of thigh
Rebound Tenderness	Release of deep palpation causes sudden ↑ pain

RLQ: right lower quadrant

Table 5.3 If Diagnosis Unclear by Exam and Labs, Consider Imaging in Evaluation of Acute Appendicitis:

Ultrasound	PPV = 91%	NPV = 88%	If negative, consider computed tomography
CT with Contrast	PPV = 92%	NPV = 98%	IV, PO, and/or rectal contrast[i]

CT: computed tomography; NPV: negative predictive value; PPV: positive predictive value

CHOLESTASIS

- Direct bilirubin > 1 mg/dL (if tbili < 5 mg/dL), or direct bilirubin > 20% TSB
- All infants 2 weeks of age with noted jaundice (unless exclusively breastfed without dark urine or light [acholic] stools, and follow-up scheduled within a week) should have total and direct bilirubin checked
- Differential diagnosis includes: Biliary atresia, neonatal hepatitis, sepsis (particularly urinary tract infection), choledochal cyst, Alagille syndrome, inspissated bile, alpha-1 antitrypsin deficiency, hypothyroidism, cystic fibrosis, total parenteral nutrition, tyrosinemia, galactosemia
- If signs of sepsis or specific metabolic/genetic disease, treat appropriately (antibiotics, alpha-1 antitrypsin assay, urine succinylacetone [tyrosinemia], and liver function testing)
- If otherwise well, obtain abdominal ultrasound to evaluate for extrahepatic bile ducts (absence implies biliary atresia) and choledochal cyst
- If abdominal ultrasound normal, refer to gastroenterologist or pediatric surgeon for liver biopsy
- Scintigraphy controversial due to known incidence of both false-positive and false-negative results
- For biliary atresia, better outcomes with earlier portoenterostomy (Kasai procedure), where a Roux-en-Y limb of the jejunum is anastomosed to the porta hepatis

References: *J Ped Gastro Nutr.* 2004;39:115–128; *Pediatrics.* 2008;121:e1438–e1440.

FECAL IMPACTION

WORKUP

- Abdominal X-rays if unable to do rectal exam or history consistent with constipation but exam normal
- Barium or air contrast enema, rectal manometry, and/or rectal biopsy if suspect Hirschsprung's disease
- Consider thyroid-stimulating hormone (TSH), thyroxine (T4), calcium, celiac antibodies, lead level, colonic transport study, sweat chloride, and/or psychological/behavioral evaluation if clinically indicated. In refractory cases, consider MRI of lumbosacral spine (tethered cord, sacral agenesis, tumor)

Table 5.4 Historical Clues to Ask About

Weight loss/anorexia	Vomiting		Encopresis	Delayed meconium
Onset in infancy	Rectal pain/bleeding			Withholding behavior
Family history of hypothyroidism, Hirschsprung's, cystic fibrosis, celiac disease				

Table 5.5 Differential Diagnosis of Constipation

*Nonorganic**	Low-fiber diet, dehydration, psychosocial, withholding
Anatomic Causes	Imperforate anus, anal stenosis, displaced anus, mass
Metabolic Causes	Hypothyroidism, hypercalcemia, hypokalemia, diabetes
Spinal Cord Anomalies	Tethered cord, spinal trauma or mass
Food Intolerance	Gluten enteropathy, cow's milk protein intolerance
Other Disorders	Cystic fibrosis, Hirschsprung's, NF, CP, prune belly, gastroschisis, Down syndrome, connective tissue disease
Drugs	Opiates, phenobarbital, antacids, antidepressants, iron
Infection/Toxic	Botulism, lead/heavy metal ingestion, vitamin D

*Most common cause, even in infants; CP: Cerebral palsy; NF: Neurofibromatosis

Table 5.6 Physical Exam Red Flags in Constipation

Abdomen distended	Patulous anus	Displaced anus	Failure to thrive
Absent anal wink	Explosive stool	Occult blood	Anal skin tags
Back: Midline hair tuft or deep sacral dimple, pigment changes, no lumbar-sacral curve		Neuro: Muscle atrophy/flat buttocks, ↓ strength/tone lower extremities, altered deep tendon reflexes	

Data from: *J Pediatr Gastroenterol Nutr.* 2006;43(3):e1–13 and Heyman, M. *Arch Pediatr Adolesc Med.* 1988;142(3):340–342.

Table 5.7 Disimpaction

Age Group	Suggestions
Infants	• Enemas not recommended • Glycerin suppositories may be used occasionally
Older Kids/Adolescents	*ORAL:* Polyethylene glycol 3350 (*MiraLax*), mineral oil[†] (> 5 years) *RECTAL:* No consensus about digital disimpaction; mineral oil, saline, phosphate soda enemas; bisacodylsuppository (avoid tap water, soap suds, magnesium enemas)

Data from: *J Pediatr Gastroenterol Nutr.* 2006;43(3):e1–13 and Heyman, M. *Arch Pediatr Adolesc Med.* 1988;142(3):340–342.

INPATIENT MANAGEMENT OF FECAL IMPACTION

- Place nasogastric tube with confirmatory radiograph
- Clear liquid diet
- Consider intravenous hydration to run at maintenance to prevent dehydration, especially if patient refusing to take clear liquid diet
- Initiate polyethylene glycol 25 mL/kg/hr (max 1000 mL/hr) by nasogastric tube until rectal effluent clear
- If infusion needed ≥ 48 hours, check electrolytes, though rarely abnormal
- Confirm efficacy of clean out with physical exam and abdominal radiograph

Table 5.8 Medications Commonly Used in the Treatment of Constipation

Medication	Dose	Notes
Phosphate Enemas (*Fleet*)	*2–11 years*: 2.25 oz pediatric enema PR *> 12 years*: 4.5 oz enema PR	Avoid in children < 2 years old, history of kidney or cardiac disease
Mineral Oil Enema	*2–11 years old*: 30–60 mL *> 12 years*: 60–150 mL PR	Avoid if ostomy or appendicitis
Polyethylene Glycol Solution (*GoLYTELY*)	25 mL/kg/hr (max 1000 mL/hr) by nasogastric until clear	Usually inpatient (for disimpaction)
Mineral Oil[†]	1–3 mL/kg/d divided qd–tid	Children > 4 years old only
Lactulose (10 g/15 mL syrup)	*Infants*: 2.5–10 mL PO daily *Older children*: 1–3 mL/kg/day divided bid (max 60 mL/day)	Avoid in galactosemia and diabetes mellitus
Magnesium Citrate (1.745 g/30 mL)	*> 2 years*: 2–4 mL/kg/day PO div qd–bid; max 150 mL/day	Avoid in renal dysfunction, acute abdomen
Malt Soup Extract (*Barley Malt Extract*)	*Infants*: 1–2 teaspoons in 2–4 oz formula or water qd–bid	
Polyethylene Glycol 3350 (*MiraLax*)	8.5–17 gm in 8 oz water daily	As with all medications, avoid prolonged use.

†Risk of lipoid pneumonia if aspirated. Use only in neurologically normal children > 4 years old.
Data from: *J Pediatr Gastroenterol Nutr*. 2006;43(3):e1-13.

Table 5.9 Maintenance

Infants	*Dietary Changes*: 2–4 oz/day of apple, prune, pear juice	*Medications*: Lactulose, corn syrup, sorbitol, barley malt extract (AVOID mineral oil or stimulant laxatives)	
Older Children/ Adolescents	*Dietary Changes*: High-fiber diet (age in years) + 5 = goal grams of fiber/day; stay hydrated; add high sorbitol juices	*Behavioral Changes*: Unhurried time on toilet after meals Do not withhold Do not scold	*Medications*: Mineral oil, Mg hydroxide, lactulose, sorbitol, polyethylene glycol 3350 (*MiraLax*)

Data from: *J Pediatr Gastroenterol Nutr*. 2006;43(3):e1–13 and Heyman, M. *Arch Pediatr Adolesc Med*. 1988;142(3):340–342.

References: *J Pediatr Gastroenterol Nutr*. 2006;43(3):e1–13; *Arch Pediatr Adolesc Med*. 1988;142(3):340–342.

GASTROINTESTINAL (GI) BLEEDING

DEFINITIONS AND PRESENTATION:

- Upper GI (UGI) Bleed: Bleeding from GI tract proximal to ligament of Treitz
  - Generally presents with melena (dark, black, foul-smelling, tarry stool), hematemesis, or "coffee-ground" emesis
  - Can present with hematochezia (bright red blood per rectum [BRBPR]) if very brisk upper GI bleed
- Lower GI (LGI) Bleed: Bleeding from GI tract distal to ligament of Treitz
  - Generally presents with hematochezia

Table 5.10 Differential Diagnosis of Gastrointestinal (GI) Bleeding

Age	Upper GI (UGI) Bleed	Lower GI (LGI) Bleed
< 1 month old	• Ingested maternal blood, esophagitis, bleeding disorder, gastritis, gastric ulcer	• Cow's milk/soy protein intolerance, anal fissure, ingested maternal blood, infection, bowel ischemia (necrotizing enterocolitis, volvulus), upper GI bleed (very rapid transit)
1 month–2 years old	• Gastritis, esophagitis, ulcer	• Anal fissure, cow's milk/soy protein intolerance, infection, ischemia, intussusception, polyps, Meckel's diverticulum
2–5 years old	• Gastritis, esophagitis, ulcer, varices, bleeding diathesis, Mallory-Weiss tear, nasopharyngeal bleed	• Fissure, infection, foreign body, polyp, Meckel's, intussusception, bowel ischemia, IBD • Mimics: Red food ingestion (jello, rehydration solutions), medication (cefdinir)
> 5 years old	• Peptic ulcer, gastritis, esophagitis, Mallory-Weiss tear, nasopharyngeal bleed	• Infection (bacterial, viral, parasitic), IBD, Meckel's, red food/medication ingestion, polyp, hemorrhoid, fissure

GI: Gastrointestinal; IBD: Inflammatory bowel disease; NEC: Necrotizing enterocolitis

DIAGNOSTIC APPROACH TO GI BLEEDING

- Good history and physical examination helps narrow above differential diagnoses and guides further investigation
- Lab evaluation: Complete blood count with differential. Stool culture if indicated. Complete metabolic panel. Consider coagulation studies
- In neonates with hematochezia, Apt test differentiates maternal from fetal blood (mix fresh stool with water [1:5], centrifuge and add NaOH. After 2 minutes, adult Hb turns brown, fetal Hb remains pink)
- UGI Bleed: Consider endoscopy or upper gastrointestinal series (fluoroscopy after ingesting water soluble contrast)
- LGI Bleed: Consider air or water-soluble contrast enema if considering intussusception; consider Meckel's scan for painless BRBPR

Table 5.11 Bacterial Causes of Acute Diarrhea

Pathogen	Transmission	Presentation	Treatment	Other
Campylobacter	• Poultry, dogs, cats, contaminated water, fecal material; person to person less common	• Variable; +/– fever, cramps in 66%, bloody stool in > 50% • 80% of cases last < 1 week • Incubation 1–7 days	Most do not require abx Erythro- or azithromycin × 5–7 days ↓ duration sx	• Eradication after 2–3 days of antibiotics • ↑ risk GBS and intussusception
Escherichia Coli	• Person–person, contaminated water and food, unpasteurized milk • *0157:H7:* Ground beef, petting zoos, apple cider, raw fruits and vegetables (alfalfa) • Incubation: 1–8 days • Excreted up to 2 weeks	• *Enterohemorrhagic E Coli:* Fever (33%), severe abdominal pain, bloody stools • 0157:H7: 8% of patients develop hemolytic uremic syndrome (HUS) • Other types: "Traveler's diarrhea" days → weeks of watery diarrhea and cramps, self-limited	• Treat severe disease with TMP- SMX, azithromycin or ciprofloxacin for 3 days • Antibiotics for 0157:H7: No proven benefit. Meta-analysis did not confirm ↑ risk of HUS if used	• *HUS:* Onset < 2 weeks after illness: Renal failure, hemolytic anemia, ↓ platelet. • If labs normal 3 days after resolution, low risk of HUS • ↑ risk diabetes mellitus after HUS
Shigella	• Person–person, contaminated water	• Tenesmus, high-fever (40°C), watery, mucoid, or bloody diarrhea • ↑ serum and stool WBC, bandemia	• Know local susceptibilities as national ↑ resistance ampicillin (60%), TMP/SMX (41%) • Ceftriaxone, cipro remain options	• Consider treating mild disease to prevent spread • ↑ risk seizures, HUS • Vit A if malnourished • Avoid antidiarrheals
Salmonella	• Poultry and eggs cause ~50% disease. Excreted in stool × 5 weeks • Reptiles (turtles < 4 cm)	• Incubation 6 hours to 3 days, moderate to severe watery diarrhea, fever ~38.5–39°C	• Treat infants < 3 months and asplenic patients with ampicillin or TMP/SMX • Avoid antidiarrheals	• Rare: Meningitis osteomyelitis, sepsis • ↑ shedding if treated with antibiotic
Yersinia Enterocolitica	• Pork, milk, contaminated water	• Acute-onset abdominal pain, fever, diarrhea (watery-mucousy)	• ↓ excretion with antibiotics (Bactrim, tetracycline)	• Mesenteric adenitis mimics appendicitis
C Difficile	• Recent antibiotic use	• Mild–severe diarrhea (+/–blood)	• Metronidazole PO	• Vancomycin PO

Abx: Antibiotics; GBS: Guillain-Barré syndrome; HUS: Hemolytic uremic syndrome; PO: Orally; pt: Patient; Rx: Treatment; sx: Symptoms; TMP/SMX: Trimethoprim-sulfamethoxazole

Data from *J Pediatr* 2010;156:761–765; *JAMA* 2002;288(8):996–1001; and CDC. NARMS for Enteric Bacteria, 2008.

INTUSSUSCEPTION

Table 5.12 Intussusception

Pathology	• Telescoping of bowel (proximal → distal segment) • Engorged veins, edema leads to ischemia (and pain)
Epidemiology	• 95% ileocolic (at ileocolic junction) • 5% ileoileal: Associated with Meckel diverticulum and HSP • 80% patients < 2 years old, male:female = 2:1

Clinical Signs
(< 10%
  patients have
  ≥ 3 of these)
	• Paroxysms of severe, crampy abdominal pain (symptom-free periods in between pain paroxysms)
	• Vomiting (occasionally bilious)
	• Bloody stool: ~70% patients + for occult or gross blood. "Currant jelly stool" is a late sign
	• Right upper quadrant mass

Diagnosis	• Air or contrast enema: diagnostic +/− therapeutic • Ultrasound sensitive (especially for ileoileal), x-rays low yield
Treatment Options	• **Air or hydrostatic enema:** 70–90% success if ill < 48 hours, < 50% success if ill > 48 hours. Consider prophylactic antibiotics (cefoxitin 30–40 mg/kg × 1 for pts > 3 months) prior to enema
	• **Surgical reduction:** First line for patients with perforation, shock, peritonitis, or ileoileal intussusception

HSP: Henoch-Schönlein purpura

PANCREATITIS

PRESENTATION

- Severe abdominal pain (epigastric > back), vomiting, anorexia, pleural effusion
- Elevated pancreatic enzymes (amylase, lipase) 3× greater than normal
- Hemorrhagic: Cullen's sign (periumbilical ecchymosis) and Grey-Turner sign (flank ecchymosis)
- Imaging: Not necessary for diagnosis
  ○ Abdominal ultrasound shows pancreatic changes ~33–50% of patients
    – Useful to evaluate for gallstones
  ○ Computed tomography or ultrasound useful several days into illness if concern for pancreatic necrosis or pseudocyst
  ○ Magnetic resonance imaging of pancreatic duct (MRCP) may help define pancreatic divisum or ductal stricture in recurrent pancreatitis

ETIOLOGIES

- Biliary/Obstructive (10–30%): Choledocholithiasis, sludging in gallbladder, pancreatic divisum, sphincter of Oddi dysfunction, ERCP-related
- Medication (~25%): Valproic acid, L-aspariginase, prednisone, 6-mercaptopurine, tetracycline, estrogens, furosmide
- Traumatic (10–40%): Motor vehicle accident, falls, sports injuries, child abuse
- Systemic illness (30+%): Sepsis, viral syndrome, bacterial infections, collagen vascular disease, cystic fibrosis, ulcerative colitis, hemolytic uremic syndrome
- Metabolic (2–7%): Diabetic ketoacidosis, hypertriglyceridemia, hypercalcemia
- Hereditary (5–8%): PRSS1 or SPINK1 gene mutation, cystic fibrosis
- Idiopathic (13–4%)

GENERAL TREATMENT GUIDELINES

- Fluid resuscitation: 0.9% saline 20 mL/kg
- Ondansetron (*Zofran*): 0.1–0.15 mg/kg/dose (max 8 mg/dose) IV or PO q 8 hours
- Pain control
  - Morphine: 0.05–0.1 mg/kg/dose IV q 2 hours as needed
  - Ketorolac (*Toradol*): 0.5 mg/kg/dose (max 30 mg/dose) IV q 6 hours
    - Monitor renal function and do not exceed 5 days of therapy
- Feeding: Historically, patients were kept NPO until symptoms and laboratory markers resolved. Adult data suggest that early enteral feeds (either jejunal or continuous nasogastric) with elemental or semi-elemental formula improve outcomes (decreased infections, necrotizing pancreatitis, surgical interventions) over total parenteral nutrition (TPN)
- Antibiotics: Only if severe or necrotizing pancreatitis

ETIOLOGY-SPECIFIC TREATMENT OF PANCREATITIS

- Choledocholithiasis: Endoscopic removal of stone (ERCP) for obstruction lasting 2–3 days, cholangitis, or worsening disease
- Sludge: Unclear if treatment with ursodeoxycholic acid beneficial
- Medication: Removal or avoidance of offending medication
- Hypercalcemia: Evaluate for hyperparathyroidism (serum calcium and intact PTH)
- Systemic: Treat underlying cause

COMPLICATIONS OF PANCREATITIS

- Early complications: Systemic disease (only ~5% children with pancreatitis)
  - Shock, sepsis, ARDS, pleural effusions, renal insufficiency/failure, pneumonia, gastrointestinal bleeding
- Late complications: Pancreatic pseudocyst (10–20% patients) or necrosis
  - Treatment: Drain for infection or persistent symptoms
- Mortality rare, more common in patients with underlying systemic illness
- Ranson criteria are not useful in pediatrics. Other scoring systems proposed, but not yet in widespread use
- Recurrent pancreatitis occurs in 15–35% of patients

ARDS: acute respiratory distress syndrome; ERCP: endoscopic retrograde cholangiopancreatography; Hb, hemoglobin; MRCP: magnetic resonance cholangiopancreatography; NPO: nothing per orem; PTH: parathyroid hormone; TPN: total parenteral nutrition

References: *JPGN*. 2011;Mar 52(3):262–270; *Pancreas*. 2010;39(2):248–251; *Dig Surg*. 2006;23:336; DeBanto JR. *Am J Gastro*. 2002;97:1726–1731.

OSTOMY CARE

- Average ileostomy output 0–15 mL/kg/day, 90% is water
- Difficult to define "diarrhea" with ileostomy, but consider treatment if losses > 1000 mL/day (or 30 mL/kg/day), higher than normal output, or more watery consistency than baseline
- Small intestine cannot conserve NaCl; losses average of 30–40 mEq/day
- At risk for hypomagnesemia, $\downarrow$ B_{12}, and folic acid deficiencies
- Postoperatively often treated with proton pump inhibitor (PPI)
- In the setting of $\uparrow$ ostomy output, replace effluent 1:1 with normal saline
- Loperamide has been used to $\downarrow$ intestinal transit and $\downarrow$ output (2–4 mg PO max 8–16 mg/day)
- If high output despite loperamide, consider codeine or diphenoxylate and atropine (Lomotil: beware of overdose potential and atropine side effects)

VOMITING

Table 5.13 Differential Diagnosis of Vomiting in Children

Vomiting usually associated with diarrhea*	Vomiting +/– associated diarrhea	Vomiting alone
Viral gastroenteritis (rotavirus, adenovirus, calicivirus, norovirus) Bacterial enteritis (*Campylobacter, Shigella, Salmonella*) Protozoal infection (*Giardia, Cryptosporidia*) Food poisoning *(Staphylococcus* toxin) Cow's milk protein allergy Celiac disease Inflammatory bowel disease	Urinary tract infection Eating disorders Medication side effect Cholecystitis Hepatitis Pneumonia Acute otitis media/upper respiratory infection Toxic ingestion Psychogenic Irritable bowel syndrome	Pyloric stenosis (in infants) Appendicitis Increased intracranial pressure (head injury, pseudotumor cerebri, hemorrhage, tumor, hydrocephalus) Meningitis, encephalitis Migraine; cyclic vomiting syndromes GI obstruction (intussusception, atresia, malrotation, volvulus, Hirschsprung's disease, mass, strangulated hernia, etc.) Metabolic disease Gastroesophageal reflux (GER) Pancreatitis Pregnancy Diabetic ketoacidosis (DKA) Uremia Foreign body ingestion Peptic ulcer disease

*May present with vomiting alone.

Table 5.14 Red Flags in a Vomiting Child

Associated with acute abdominal pain	Nuchal rigidity / photophobia / neurologic signs
Projectile vomiting	Absence of associated diarrhea
High fever	Blood or bile in emesis
Persistent tachycardia or hypotension	Altered mental status

EVALUATION OF VOMITING

Workup will depend on clinical history and examination. If a specific diagnosis is being considered, see section on that diagnosis (e.g., meningitis, acute abdominal pain, intussusception)

TREATMENT

- Treatment will depend on cause of vomiting
- Rehydration and fluid maintenance are of prime importance
- Once cause of vomiting identified, consider trial of ondansetron, though not routinely recommended in treatment of gastroenteritis as not FDA-approved in pediatrics except for in prevention and treatment chemotherapy-associated and postoperative nausea/vomiting

Table 5.15 Non-FDA-Approved Dosing of Ondansetron for Vomiting Associated with Acute Gastroenteritis in Children > 6 Months of Age

IV dosing	0.1–0.15 mg/kg IV q 8 hours as needed (maximum: 8 mg/dose)
PO dosing	Weight 8–15 kg: 2 mg PO as a single dose Weight > 15–30 kg: 4 mg PO as a single dose (max 12 mg/day) Weight > 30 kg: 6–8 mg PO as a single dose (max 16 mg/day)

Data from: http://www.aafp.org/afp/2007/0701/p76.html#afp20070701p76-t4; accessed 1/20/13; http://www.mdconsult.com/das/pharm/body/397019133-3/0/full/453?infotype=1 accessed 1/20/13.

References: *Am Fam Physician.* 2007;76(1):76–84.

DYSFUNCTIONAL UTERINE BLEEDING

- Normal menstruation: 2–7 days bleeding (20–80 mL blood loss)/21- to 45-day cycle
- Follicular phase: Follicle-stimulating hormone (FSH) leads to maturation of follicle and ↑ estrogen, which thickens endometrium. Estrogen and luteinizing hormone (LH) surges lead to ovulation
- Luteal phase: Corpus luteum (residual follicle) makes progesterone (stabilizes endometrium) and estrogen. If no conception, corpus luteum involutes, hormone levels drop, and endometrial lining sloughs, resulting in typical menstrual bleeding
- Adolescent DUB: Abnormal endometrial sloughing without structural pathology (differs from post-adolescent DUB). Often result of anovulation in first 2–3 years after menarche
- Menorrhagia: Prolonged or heavy bleeding at regular intervals
- Metrorrhagia: Uterine bleeding at irregular intervals
- Menometrorrhagia: Prolonged or heavy bleeding occurring at irregular intervals

Table 6.1 Differential Diagnosis of Adolescent Dysfunctional Uterine Bleeding

Anovulatory Cycles	Endometrial sloughing after prolonged unopposed estrogen. Diagnosis of exclusion; can be stress or exercise induced
Disorders of Coagulation	Von Willebrand's disease (vWD), thrombocytopenia, Factor XI deficiency, platelet function defect, renal/liver failure, lupus
Endocrine Abnormalities	Hypo- or hyperthyroidism Androgen disorders: Polycystic ovarian syndrome (PCOS), non-classic 21-hydroxylase deficiency
Pregnancy-Related Causes	Pregnancy (including ectopic); spontaneous, threatened, or incomplete abortion; hydatidiform mole
Anatomic Abnormality	Retained tampon or intrauterine device, laceration (trauma, rape, abuse), bicornate uterus, transverse septum, polyp
Infections	Sexually transmitted infection (STI)
Breakthrough Bleeding	Progestin-only or low-dose estrogen combined oral contraceptives, implanted and injectable contraception; recently started new hormonal contraception

Table 6.2 Evaluation of Adolescent Dysfunctional Uterine Bleeding

First assess hemodynamics and determine site of bleeding: Gastrointestinal, urinary tract, uterine, vaginal, cervical (external exam only in virginal girls)	
History	Menstrual, sexual history, medication, systemic symptoms, prior bleeding (epistaxis, dental work, etc.)
Exam	Pelvic exam, sexual maturity rating, dermatologic manifestations of other illness (thin hair, hirsutism, acanthosis nigricans, petechiae, acne), thyroid exam, breasts (for galactorrhea)
Family History	Polycystic ovarian syndrome or bleeding diathesis

(Continued)

Table 6.2 Evaluation of Adolescent Dysfunctional Uterine Bleeding *(Continued)*

Laboratory (before therapy)	Pregnancy test, complete blood count (CBC), erythrocyte sedimentation rate, sexually transmitted infection screening For chronic anovulation or irregular menstrual cycles: Thyroid, liver, and renal function tests, LH, FSH For recurrent/severe bleeding or onset with menarche: Coagulation studies, von Willebrand (vWD) panel (FVIII, vWD antigen and activity, vWD multimers: test prior to exogenous estrogen. Also test blood type as type O may have low vWD antigen) For signs of hyperandrogenism: Testosterone (total and free) and dehydroepiandrosterone sulfate 17-hydroxyprogesterone (17-OHP) to rule out congenital adrenal hyperplasia Iron studies if indicated
Radiology	Pelvic ultrasonography for uterine structural abnormalities or if pregnant

Table 6.3 Light Bleeding and Normal Hemoglobin (> 11–12 gm/dL)

- 60 mg elemental iron daily, menstrual calendar, reevaluation
- Initiate combined oral contraceptive (COC), if desired

Data from: *ACOG.* 2000 Mar; *Obstet Gynecol Clin.* 2008; 35(2); *Obstet Gynecol Clin.* 2009; 36(1).

Table 6.4 Moderate Bleeding or Hemoglobin (9–11 gm/dL)

- COC (35 mcg estrogen) tid × 3 days, bid × 4 days then qd for remainder of pack skipping placebo week into second pack
- Allow withdrawal bleeding monthly once hemoglobin stable
- Continue COCs 3–6 months
- Consider naproxen 250–500 mg PO bid to reduce flow
- Begin iron therapy as above

- *If estrogen contraindicated (hypercoagulable state)* use progestin-only therapy
  Micronized oral progesterone: 100–200 mg daily for first 12 days of month
  Does not reliably prevent ovulation, therefore not effective birth control

Data from: *ACOG.* 2000 Mar; *Obstet Gynecol Clin.* 2008; 35(2); *Obstet Gynecol Clin.* 2009; 36(1).

Table 6.5 Severe Bleeding or Hemoglobin (< 9 gm/dL)

- *If hemodynamically stable and able to tolerate COC:* Treat as "moderate bleeding"
- *Severe anemia or hemodynamically unstable:* Admit, intravenous fluids +/– blood transfusion, rule out coagulopathy
- Initiate COC therapy and perform taper as noted for "moderate bleeding." Can ↑ estrogen to 50 mcg/pill. May need antiemetic
- Severe nausea, vomiting, or uncontrolled bleeding: Begin IV equine estrogen (*Premarin* = 25 mg every 4–6 hours for up to 6 doses) and antiemetics
- If bleeding does not stop with IV estrogen, consider hysteroscopy and/or dilation and curettage
- Once bleeding controlled: Begin new packet combination COC. Use continuously, *without* placebo (first 21 days of packet), for 3 months. Can use cyclic progestin therapy instead of COC: Medroxyprogesterone 10 mg orally daily × 12 days/month, or norethindrone acetate 5–10 mg orally daily × 12 days/month
- Allow withdrawal bleeding q 3 months to prevent excessive endometrial buildup

Data from: *ACOG.* 2000 Mar; *Obstet Gynecol Clin.* 2008; 35(2); *Obstet Gynecol Clin.* 2009; 36(1).

Table 6.6 Management of Bleeding Secondary to Hormonal Contraception

- Increase estrogen content of combined COCs (from 20 mcg to 30–35 mcg daily)
- Bleeding secondary to progestin-only contraception will respond to addition of conjugated estrogen for 5–7 days + nonsteroidal anti-inflammatory drug. Initially controls active bleeding, but ongoing risk of future spotting

Data from: *ACOG.* 2000 Mar; *Obstet Gynecol Clin.* 2008; 35(2); *Obstet Gynecol Clin.* 2009; 36(1).

Table 6.7 Management of Bleeding Secondary to Coagulopathy

- Continuous use of COC *without* placebo (first 21 days of packet) × 3–6 months. Allow withdrawal bleeding (use of placebo pills) 1 week q 3–6 months, *or*
- Depot medroxyprogesterone acetate (DMPA): 150 mg intramuscular or 104 mg subcutaneously q 12 weeks
- DDAVP (1-desamino-8-D-arginine vasopressin) and antifibrinolytic agents (aminocaproic acid [*Amicar*®]) likely have a role in patients with vWD, platelet function disorders, and other bleeding diatheses

Data from: *ACOG.* 2000 Mar; *Obstet Gynecol Clin.* 2008; 35(2); *Obstet Gynecol Clin.* 2009; 36(1).

OVARIAN TORSION

Table 6.8 Ovarian Torsion

Pathophysiology	Ovary +/− fallopian tube twist → disruption of circulation → ovarian edema and necrosis Up to 30% of premenarchal girls with torsion have no cyst or mass, presumed to have an elongated utero-ovarian ligament Risk factors: Ovarian cyst, malignancy, benign tumor
Symptoms	Constant or intermittent lower abdominal/pelvic pain; leukocytosis (59–82%), fever (19–29%), nausea and vomiting (50–73%)
Radiologic findings	Ultrasound with Doppler most commonly used, but not sensitive or specific enough to be definitive Consider abdominal CT if peritonitis present, or concern for appendicitis Consider laparoscopy if suspicious despite normal radiologic studies
Treatment	Detorsion 80–95% salvage rate, even if ovary/tube appear necrotic Consider cystectomy or aspiration if cyst present Oophorectomy should only be considered if ovary/tube highly friable or necrotic, or if mass highly suspicious for malignancy found
Outcome	Complications include ↓ fertility, peritonitis, pulmonary embolism, death

Data from: *Ultrasound Clin.* 2007;2(1):155-166, *J Pediatr Surg.* 2009;44(6):1212-16; *Eur J Pediatr Surg.* 2010;20(5):298-301; *J Pediatr Surg.* 204;39(5):750.

PELVIC INFLAMMATORY DISEASE

Table 6.9 Pelvic Inflammatory Disease

Symptoms	Lower abdominal pain, pelvic pain, cramps, dyspareunia, dysuria, bleeding, vaginal discharge, and fever. Asymptomatic infection or Fitz-Hugh-Curtis syndrome (perihepatitis and RUQ pain) may also occur
Risk factors	History of PID or GC/chlamydia, current douching, recent IUD, bacterial vaginosis, low SES
Symptoms	Lower abdominal pain and cervical motion or uterine tenderness (may not be present if normal appearing cervix and no WBC on saline prep smear) Temperature > 38.3°C and + cervical or vaginal discharge may be present
Workup	ESR/CRP (↑) Gonorrhea and Chlamydia NAAT (nucleic acid amplification test) of urine or cervical swab CBC with differential (↑ WBC) Ultrasound or other imaging if indicated based on exam Offer testing for HIV, hepatitis B and C, and bacterial vaginosis

(*Continued*)

Table 6.9 Pelvic Inflammatory Disease (*Continued*)

Indications for admission	• Teenager • If consideration being given to surgical emergency such as appendicitis • If patient is pregnant (↑ risk of maternal morbidity and preterm delivery) • Inadequate response to PO antibiotics • Patient cannot tolerate oral therapy • Severe pain, vomiting, or high fever • Tubo-ovarian abscess
Inpatient treatment	Cefotetan 2 g IV q 12 hours or cefoxitin 2 g IV q 6 hours PLUS Doxycycline 100 mg PO or IV q 12 hours OR Clindamycin 900 mg IV q 8 hours PLUS Gentamicin 2 mg/kg IV/IM, then 1.5 mg/kg IV/IM q 8 hours Once there has been clinical improvement × 24 hours, may switch to doxycycline 100 mg PO bid (complete total of 14 days of treatment) and consider discharge
Outpatient treatment	Once there has been clinical improvement × 24 hours, may switch to doxycycline 100 mg PO bid (complete total of 14 days of treatment) and consider discharge

Data from: *MMWR*. 2010;59(RR–12):63–65; *Med Clin North Am.* 2008;92(5):1083–1113.

HYPERCOAGULABLE STATE

Table 7.1 Categorization of Hypercoagulable States

Inherited	Activated protein C resistance (Factor V Leiden mutation) Protein C or S deficiency Prothrombin gene mutation G20210A Antithrombin III deficiency
Acquired	Immobilization (postoperative, long travel) Estrogen containing contraceptives Pregnancy Obesity Trauma
Other	Hyperhomocysteinemia (MTHFR C677T variant) Systemic lupus erythematosus Indwelling central venous catheter Antiphospholipid syndrome Sickle cell disease

MTHFR: Methylenetetrahydrofolate reductase

RISK FACTORS:

Combination of more than one thrombophilia risk factors significantly increases risk. Anticardiolipin antibodies and Factor V Leiden increased risk by 5-fold

LABS (CONSULT HEMATOLOGIST):

Consider complete blood count, d-dimer, fibrinogen, PT, PTT (prolonged with lupus anticoagulant), protein C, S, antithrombin III and homocysteine assays, prothrombin (Factor II), Factor V Leiden and MTHFR gene mutation analysis, anticardiolipin, IgG and IgM, lupus anticoagulant, and antinuclear antibodies

Table 7.2 Treatment of Venous Thromboembolism (in consultation with hematologist)

Pediatric	Acute: • LMWH*[ε]: enoxaparin 1 mg/kg SQ q 12 hours Chronic: • LMWH*[ξ]: enoxaparin 0.5 mg/kg SQ q 12 hours, or • VKA (warfarin): start 0.1–0.2 mg/kg PO daily × 2 days. Usual dose • 0.05–0.34 mg/kg PO daily (max 10 mg/dose). Goal INR (2.0–3.0). Monitor weekly. Reverse with vitamin K
Neonatal	Acute: • Remove CVL/UVC • UH**: Start 75–100 units/kg IV; usual dose ~28 units/kg/hr IV × 3–5 days • LMWH*[ε]: enoxaparin 1.5 mg/kg SQ q 12 hours Chronic: • LMWH*[ξ]: enoxaparin 0.75 mg/kg SQ q 12 hours

≠Avoid thrombolytics unless limb-/organ-threatening thrombosis

*Discontinue if platelets < 100,000; reversal of enoxaparin overdose with 1 mg protamine sulfate/mg of enoxapain injected in last 8 hours

¥Goal aPTT to correspond with anti-FXa level 0.35–0.7 U/mL

[ε]Goal anti-FXa level for *acute* therapy: 0.5–1 U/mL 4 hours after injection

[ξ]Goal anti-FXa level for *chronic* therapy: 0.1–0.3 U/mL checked every 3–4 weeks on stable dose

aPTT: activated partial thromboplastin time; anti-FXa: anti Factor Xa assay; CVL: central venous line; INR: international normalized ratio; IV: intravenous; LMWH: low molecular weight heparin; UH: unfractionated heparin; UVC: umbilical venous catheter; VKA: vitamin K antagonist (warfarin, *Coumadin*)

Data from: Muwakkit SA et al. *Pediatr Neurol.* 2011 Sep;45(3):155–8; Kenet G et al. *Stroke* 2000 Jun;31(6):1283–8.

ALTEPLASE (TPA) FOR OCCLUDED CATHETER

(1) Determine type, brand, and size of catheter
   a. For catheter lumen volume, refer to the Catheter Priming Volume table
(2) Determine the patient's weight is < 30 kg: alteplase (1 mg/mL) dose volume = 110% of catheter lumen volume plus 0.25 mL for priming the stopcock. (Maximum dose = 2 mL)
   a. < 30 kg: TPA (1 mg/mL) dose volume = 110% of catheter lumen volume plus 0.25 mL for priming the stopcock. (Maximum dose = 2 mL)
   b. > 30 kg: TPA (1 mg/mL) dose volume = 2 mL
(3) Wait 30 minutes
(4) Attach 10-mL syringe and attempt to aspirate 5 mL
   a. If able to aspirate at least 3 mL, flush with 10 mL normal saline and go to Step 7
   b. If unable to aspirate at least 3 mL, wait an additional 90 minutes and repeat Step 4 and 5
(5) If no results after 90 minutes, give a second dose of alteplase (repeat Steps 2–4)
(6) If no results after the second dose of alteplase, consider third dose vs. removing line
(7) If venous catheter is cleared, resume catheter use or "heparin lock" with appropriate heparin dose for line (see next section)

HEPARIN FOR MAINTAINING VENOUS LINE PATENCY*

No routine heparin flush to a lumen is needed while intravenous fluid is continuously being infused through that lumen

Only use 5 mL syringe or larger on central venous line (CVL) in neonates

Only use 10 L syringe or larger on CVL in infants and children

Additional flushes can be given if residual blood noted in catheter, after blood draw from catheter, or after drug / PRBC administration*

*Beware when approaching systemic heparinization doses (50 units/kg q4 hours)

1. Peripheral intravenous catheter (PIV): Use preservative free 10 unit/mL heparin
   a. Neonates: 5 units (0.5 mL) IV q6 hours
   b. Infants and children: 30 units (3 mL) IV q8 hours
2. Central venous line (Broviac®) not running continuous IV fluid
   a. Patient weight ≤ 10 kg use 10 units/mL heparin: 30 units (3 mL) IV daily
   b. Patient weight > 10 kg use 100 units/mL heparin: 300 units (3 mL) IV daily
3. Implanted subcutaneous port device (Port-a-Cath®, Medi-Port®)
   a. Monthly flush to maintain patency, or with de-accessing port device (removal of needle after use):
      i. Patient weight ≤ 10 kg use 10 units/mL heparin: 50 units (5 mL) IV
      ii. Patient weight > 10 kg use 100 units/mL heparin: 500 units (5 mL) IV

BLEEDING DISORDERS

Table 7.3 Differential Diagnosis of Bleeding

Type of Bleeding	Commonly Associated Disorder
Mucosal	Platelet disorder, von Willebrand disease (vWD)
Intramuscular, Intraarticular	Hemophilia A (Factor VIII deficiency), Hemophilia B (Factor IX deficiency)
Menorrhagia	vWD (30%), dysfunctional uterine bleeding
Epistaxis	Trauma, foreign body, rhinitis, vWD

Table 7.4 Most Likely Hematologic Causes of Purpura*

Neonatal	Maternal ITP, drug use, intrauterine infection, alloimmune thrombocytopenia, thrombocytopenia-absent radii (TAR) syndrome
1–4 years	Idiopathic thrombocytopenic purpura (ITP)
4–7 years	ITP, Henoch-Schönlein purpura

*Always assess for trauma, abuse, liver disease, sepsis, vasculitis, renal failure

Data from: *Am Fam Phys* 2001;64:419–28.

Table 7.5 Lab Analysis

Check PT, PTT, mixing studies‡, fibrinogen, platelets. Consult hematologist. Also consider vWD panel*, PFA-100, thrombin time, factor levels		
PT	**PTT**	**Differential Diagnosis**
Nl	↑	Factor VIII or IX deficiency; lupus anticoagulant† (Factor XII causes ↑ PTT, but rare bleeding)
Nl	Nl or ↑	vWD, uremia, medication effect, platelet defect
↑	Nl	Factor VII or vitamin K deficiency; liver disease
↑	↑	Vitamin K deficiency; liver disease; Deficiency in Factor II, V, X; disseminated intravascular coagulation (inpatient)
Coagulation studies are specimen sensitive. Always consider lab error.		

Nl: normal, PT: prothrombin time, PTT: partial thromboplastin time, PFA-100: platelet function analysis.

*VWD Panel: includes vW antigen, ristocetin cofactor (function), Factor VIII, and multimeric analysis.

‡Mixing study: Patients blood mixed 1:1 with normal serum. In factor deficiency, PT or PTT will correct to normal. If PT or PTT remains prolonged, patient has †Lupus anticoagulant (circulating antibody that prolongs PTT, but patient is actually hypercoaguable)

Data from: Berman et al, *Pediatric Decision Making*, Mosby 2003.

ANEMIA

Initial evaluation of diet and blood loss history. If mild anemia, give trial of iron. If moderate or persistent, check CBC, reticulocyte count, blood type, and antibody screen.

Table 7.6 Normal RBC Indices per Age (mean and +/– 2 SD)

Age	Hb (g/dL)	Hct (%)	MCV (fL)	Blood Loss
Newborn	16.5 +/– 3	51 +/– 9	108 +/– 10	Related to trauma, GI bleed, hemorrhage, menorrhagia Neonates have additional sites: placental abruption, feto-maternal transfusion (Kleihauer-Betke test), twin-twin transfusion, cephalohematoma
2 weeks	16.5 +/– 4	51 +/– 12	105 +/– 19	
2 months	11.5 +/– 2.5	35 +/– 7	96 +/– 19	
3–6 months	11.5 +/– 2	35 +/– 6	91 +/– 17	
0.5–2 years	12 +/– 1	36 +/– 3	78 +/– 8	
2–6 years	12.5 +/– 1	37 +/– 3	81 +/– 6	
6–12 years	13.5 +/– 2	40 +/– 5	86 +/– 9	
♀ > 12 years	14 +/– 2	41 +/– 5	90 +/– 12	
♂ > 12 years	14.5 +/– 1.5	43 +/– 6	88 +/– 10	

Table 7.7 Altered Production—Low Retic Count

Microcytic	• **Fe deficiency**: Most common. ↑ RDW, ↓ RBC#. Premature infants have low stores. Lab: Fe, TIBC, ferritin, free erythrocyte protoporphyrin • Chronic inflammation → ESR; lead intoxication → lead level
Normocytic	• Transient erythroblastopenia of childhood, aplastic crisis, chronic renal disease, leukemia, Diamond-Blackfan (isolated RBC aplasia) lab: Creatinine and bone marrow biopsy
Macrocytic	• Folate/vitamin B_{12} deficiency, hepatic disease, Fanconi's anemia

Table 7.8 Increased Destruction—High Retic Count

Intrinsic	• Membrane: Hereditary spherocytosis, elliptocytosis (↑ MCHC) **Lab:** osmotic fragility • Enzyme: G6PD (X-linked), pyruvate kinase deficiency • Hemoglobinopathy (qualitative): Sickle cell, SS, SC, S-β thal, Heinz body anemia **Lab:** Hb electrophoresis • Hemoglobinopathy (quantitative): Thalassemia: normal = 4 alpha chains. # alpha chain deletions: 1 = silent, 2 = microcytic anemia, 3 = Hb H, 4 = hydrops fetalis; β thal major: Transfusion dependent; β thal minor: → HbA2; β thal intermedia: two abnormal β globin genes, → HbA2, but variable transfusion needs **Lab:** Hb electrophoresis, globin gene map
Immune	• Alloimmune (ABO/Rh incompatibility in infants), transfusion reaction, autoimmune, drug related • **Lab:** direct and indirect Coombs, cold agglutinins
Extrinsic	• Hemolytic uremic syndrome, disseminated intravascular coagulation, burns, mechanical heart valve, ECMO, vasculitis

Table 7.9 Iron Studies in Microcytic Anemias*

Iron Studies (normals)	Iron Deficiency	Chronic Disease	Lead Toxicity
Serum Fe (22–184 mcg/dL)	Low	Low	Normal–high
TIBC (100–400 mcg/dL)	High	Low–normal	Normal
Ferritin (varies by age)	Low	High	Normal–high

*Best test of iron deficiency is response to iron administration regardless of MCV

Table 7.10 Quick Reference for Treatment of Iron Deficiency Anemia

- Elemental Fe 6 mg/kg/day leads to ↑ retic in 3–5 days and ↑ Hb within 1 week. If Hb not ↑ in 1 month, consider other etiologies.
- Limit milk to ≤ 500 mL/day, as calcium inhibits Fe absorption.
- Encourage additional vitamin C, which facilitates Fe absorption.

Weight	Volume Fe Drops (15 mg Elemental Fe/0.6 mL)	Weight	Volume Ferrous Sulfate Elixir (44 mg elemental Fe/5 mL)
5–7 kg	0.6 mL (1 dropper) daily	11–13 kg	4 mL daily
7–10 kg	0.9 mL (1.5 dropper) daily	13–17 kg	5 mL daily
10–13 kg	1.2 mL (2 droppers) daily	17–24 kg	3 mL bid
• Divided dosing is encouraged		24–31 kg	4 mL bid

Abbreviations for Tables 7.5 through 7.8: CBC: complete blood count, Fe: iron, G6PD: glucose-6-phosphate dehydrogenase, Hb: hemoglobin, Hct: hematocrit, MCHC: mean corpuscular hemoglobin concentration, MCV: mean corpuscular volume, retic: reticulocyte count, TIBC: total iron binding capacity

BLOOD TRANSFUSIONS

Table 7.11 Approximate Risk of Being Infected with Selected Agents After Blood Transfusion

Infection	Chances of Acquiring
Syphilis	< 1:100,000
Hepatitis A	1:1,000,000
Hepatitis B	1:30,000–1:250,000
Hepatitis C	1:100,000
HIV-1 and -2	1:500,000–1:2,000,000
HTLV I and II	1:600,000
Bacterial contamination	1:2000 to 3000 units (platelets) 1:30,000 units (RBCs)
Tick-borne bacteria, parasites, prions	Not known

Table 7.12 Blood Products and Administration Guidelines

Product/Characteristic	Usual Dose	Indications
Packed Red Blood Cells (PRBCs)	10 mL/kg over 1–2 hours will ↑ Hb 2.5 g/dL. 1 unit ~250–350 mL	Standard RBC transfusion
Washed Red Blood Cells	Same as PRBCs	Poor renal function, hyperkalemia, history of anaphylaxis with transfusion, paroxysmal nocturnal hemoglobinuria, fetal transfusion
Frozen Deglycerolized Red Blood Cells	Same as PRBCs	IgA-deficient, + anti-IgA antibodies, and no IgA-deficient product; intrauterine transfusions; paroxysmal nocturnal hemoglobinuria
Apheresis Platelets (single donor) (may consider when ↓ platelets or platelet dysfunction)	10 mL/kg IV over 30–60 min ↑ platelets by 50,000. 1 unit ~200 mL	IgA-deficient patients with anti-IgA antibodies require IgA-deficient donor
Fresh Frozen Plasma (FFP) (use when ↑ PTT/ INR)	10–15mL/kg IV over 15–30 min ↑ factors levels by 10–20%	IgA-deficient patients with anti-IgA antibodies require IgA-deficient FFP
Cryoprecipitate (use for ↓ factor VIII, vWF fibrinogen)	1 unit ~7 mL; 1 unit per 5 kg ↑ fibrinogen by ~50	Can put in FFP or NS
CMV-Negative Components		Intrauterine transfusions, infants < 6 months old, bone marrow or solid organ transplant candidate, or recipients of a CMV-negative graft, congenital or acquired immunodeficiencies
Leukoreduced Components	< 5 × 10⁶ residual WBCs per unit	Prevents CMV transmission, nonhemolytic febrile transfusion reactions, WBC alloimmunization and platelet refractoriness in some patients

(Continued)

Table 7.12 Blood Products and Administration Guidelines *(Continued)*

Product/Characteristic	Usual Dose	Indications
Irradiated Components		< 6 months old, pediatric malignancies, intrauterine or neonatal exchange transfusions, recipients of components from designated donors, cross-matched or HLA-matched platelets, chemotherapy or irradiation, candidate for BMT or current BMT patient, congenital immunodeficiency
Partially Phenotypically Matched RBCs		Ongoing transfusion needs, RBC sensitization → + antibody formation

Table 7.13 Indications for Transfusion of Blood Products

Red Blood Cells (infant)	Premature + stable: Hgb < 7 mg/dL Premature + ill: • No oxygen requirement: Hgb < 10 g/dL • + oxygen requirement: Hgb < 12 g/dL • Heart disease, ↓ BP, apnea: Hgb < 12 g/dL Term baby < 4 months old: • Cyanotic heart disease: Hgb < 13 g/dL • Pre- or postop; shock; ↓ BP: Hgb < 10 g/dL • Apnea, ↑ HR, poor weight gain: < 7 g/dL
Red Blood Cells (older child/teen)	• Acute blood loss > 15% not responding to other fluids/interventions • Postoperative + symptoms of anemia: Hgb < 10g/dL • Severe heart or pulmonary disease: Hgb < 12 g/dL • Receiving chemotherapy or irradiation: Hgb < 7–8 g/dL • Chronic anemia, not symptomatic: Hgb < 6–7 g/dL • Sickle cell disease complication: See section on sickle cell disease
Platelets (infant)	Premature infant + stable: < 30,000/mcL Premature infant + sick: < 50,000/mcL Term infant < 4 months old: < 20,000/mcL
Platelets (older child/ teen)	NOT BLEEDING *but:* Platelet count < 10,000/mcL *and* planned LP Platelet count < 50,000/mcL *and* planned invasive procedure BLEEDING *and:* -Platelet count < 50,000/mcL -Qualitative platelet defect
FFP	INR > 1.5–2× normal, planned invasive procedure • Diffuse microvascular bleeding + PT or PTT > 1.5× normal • Warfarin overdose + bleeding *or* planned procedure • Patient with TTP + transfusion • Patient with single-factor deficiency is bleeding and individual factor replacement not available. • Vitamin K deficiency + bleeding
Cryoprecipitate	• Fibrinogen < 100 mg/dL + invasive procedure • Qualitative fibrinogen disorder + bleeding or procedure C • Von Willebrand disease or hemophilia A (Factor VIII deficiency) + active bleeding or invasive procedure + no response to DDAVP/factor

Data from: PEDIATRIC TRANSFUSION GUIDELINES accessed online 1/19/13 http://www.ucdmc.ucdavis.edu/pathology/services/clinical/clinical_pathology/
transfusion/xiii-12(6).pdf; OHSU PIC handbook accessed online 1/19/13 http://www.ohsu.edu/xd/health/services/doernbecher/research-education/
education/med-education/upload/PICU-Handbook.pdf.

TRANSFUSION REACTIONS

If transfusion reaction is suspected, stop transfusion immediately.

Table 7.14 Transfusion Reactions

Type of Reaction	Signs/Symptoms	Intervention*
Acute Hemolytic Reaction (rapid destruction of RBC within 24 hours of transfusion when recipient is given incompatible blood; e.g., type O patient receives type A, B or AB blood)	Sense of impending doom; fever, chills, back and chest pain, ↑ HR, ↓ BP; hemoglobinuria, shock, oliguria, nausea, flushing, dyspnea	Isotonic fluid bolus 20 mL/kg Furosemide 1–2 mg/kg IV if oliguria present Monitor urine until clear of hemoglobin Treat hypotension and shock if present
Delayed Hemolytic Reaction (usually in patient who have developed antibodies from previous transfusions or pregnancy)	Falling hematocrit and positive direct antiglobulin (Coombs) test (DAT). +/– fever, +/– hemoglobinuria; 24 hours–1 month after transfusion	Specific treatment not usually required Future transfusions may require antibody product
Allergic Transfusion Reaction	Urticaria, mucous membrane involvement, anaphylaxis Antigens in transfusate react with pre formed antibodies in recipient	Diphenhydramine 1–2 mg/kg IM or IV Aminophylline 3 mg/kg/dose IV over of 20 minutes if needed Epinephrine IM, IV, SC if needed
Febrile Non-Hemolytic Transfusion Reaction (1 in 8 transfusions)	Temperature increase ≥ 1°C or 2°F and chills Occurs during or within 4 hours of transfusion	Treat/pretreat with antipyretics Severe shaking chills can be treated with diphenhydramine or meperidine (Demerol)
Transfusion-Related Acute Lung Injury (TRALI) (acute onset of noncardiogenic pulmonary edema)	Acute respiratory distress, no volume overload or signs of heart failure Hypoxemia, bilateral infiltrates on CXR	Usually resolves in 72 hours, but can be fatal Mechanism unknown (? Due to antibodies in transfused blood)
Volume Overload	Dyspnea, orthopnea, severe headache ↑ HR, ↑ BP, CHF, pulmonary edema	Slow infusion rate May require diuretics: (furosemide 1 mg/kg IV)
Bacterial Contamination	Hypotension, shock, fever > 39°C or rise of 2°C over pre transfusion values, chills, nausea and vomiting, and respiratory distress	Respiratory and circulatory support Broad-spectrum antibiotics Culture donor and recipient blood
Hypotensive Reaction	Systolic or diastolic BP drops by at least 10 mmHg; NO other signs/ symptoms of transfusion reaction	Stop transfusion Supportive care
Graft Versus Host Disease (T-lymphocytes in transfused blood attack recipient)	Rash, fever, diarrhea, ↓ WBC, ↓ platelets; ↑ LFTs Generally occurs 3–4 weeks after transfusion	Immunosuppressive agents (corticosteroids, cytotoxic agents, intravenous immune globulin); treatment not often successful
Non-Immune Hemolysis (Hemolysis due to improper handling or storage of product)	May see symptoms similar to immune-mediated hemolysis Hemoglobinemia ↑ serum K+, arrhythmias	Supportive
Post-Transfusion Purpura (Recipient develops antibodies against transfused platelets → severe thrombocytopenia)	↓↓ Platelets 5–48 days after transfusion More common in females than males	Intravenous immune globulin If IVIG doesn't help, consider plasmapheresis with FFP replacement Consider glucocorticoids Platelet transfusion ineffective

(Continued)

Table 7.14 Transfusion Reactions (*Continued*)

Type of Reaction	Signs/Symptoms	Intervention*
Air Embolism	Cough, dyspnea, chest pain; shock	Supportive care
Metabolic Derangements	Citrate toxicity, ↑ K+, ↓ Ca++, ↓ core body temperature, respiratory alkalosis	Supportive care
Iron Overload	Chronic transfusion recipients	Cardiac and hepatic toxicity

*Whenever a transfusion reaction is suspected, STOP transfusion, disconnect IV line, check infusing bag of product for patient name and information. Once patient is stable, contact your blood bank and determine if post-transfusion sample should be taken from patient. Follow instructions from blood bank for management of current bag of product (may require investigation)

Data from: http://www.pathology.med.umich.edu/bloodbank/manual/bbch_7/index.html accessed 1/19/13; http://www.wadsworth.org/labcert/ blood_tissue/forms/factsheetsfinalweb0908.pdf accessed 1/19/13.

SICKLE CELL DISEASE

Mutations of β globin: HbSS (65%), HbSC, HbS-β-thalassemia

At diagnosis: Begin antipneumococcal prophylaxis and folic acid (tables) and refer to pediatric hematologist.

Table 7.15 Penicillin Prophylaxis in Sickle Cell Disease

Penicillin V* (PCN)	• *Newborn–3 years*: 125 mg PO bid • *3 years to at least 5 years old*: 250 mg PO bid • *Children > 5 yrs old*: PCN prophylaxis can be discontinued if no previous invasive *S. pneumo*. If febrile ≥ 39°C, should take 250 mg PCN and seek medical care.

*Use erythromycin for penicillin-allergic patients.

Table 7.16 Folic Acid Supplementation in Sickle Cell Disease

Folic Acid†	< 6 months	6 months–1 year	1–2 years	> 2 years
	0.1 mg/day	0.25 mg/day	0.5 mg/day	1 mg/day

†Some centers use 1 mg/day for all ages, others supplement after aplasia only.

Table 7.17 Sickle Cell Disease Treatments Determined by Hematologist

Hydroxyurea (no peds FDA indication)	15 mg/kg/d. Titrate by 5 mg/kg/d q 12 weeks to max 35 mg/kg/d.
	• ↓ pain crises, acute chest syndrome and hospitalization. • Increases life-span[1] • Hematologist to manage, frequent CBC to monitor bone marrow suppression
Blood Transfusion (use sickle-negative blood)	• For acute anemia related to splenic sequestration, aplasia of parvovirus or folate deficiency, or hyperhemolysis • Exchange transfusion for acute chest syndrome or stroke • Chronic transfusion for stroke prevention, abnormal transcranial Doppler ultrasound, or organ damage • Often indicated prior to anesthesia

Reference: *Pediatrics*. 2002;109(3):526–535.

FEVER

• Rates of bacteremia, sepsis, and meningitis have fallen with widespread pneumococcal vaccination but are still significant; therefore, patients with temperature > 38.3–38.5°C should receive **immediate** evaluation (clinic or ED), including history, physical exam, CBCd, blood culture, CXR, and other tests driven by presenting symptoms and signs.

- Ceftriaxone 50 mg/kg IV/IM (max 2 g) should be given as soon as possible
  - If allergic to ceftriaxone, give clindamycin 10–15 mg/kg IV (max 1.6 g) and admit for subsequent dosing
  - If clinically unstable, or suspect meningitis, give vancomycin 15 mg/kg IV (max 1 g)
- Admit all patients who are unwell appearing, have temperature > 40°C, low (< 5000/mm^3) or elevated (> 30,000/mm^3) WBC count, very young (more difficult to determine clinical deterioration at home), or those with unreliable families/transportation

References: *Pediatrics.* 2013 Jun;131(6):1035-41; *J Pediatr Hematol Oncol.* 2002;24(4):279.

ACUTE CHEST SYNDROME (ACS)

- Definition: Varying definitions exist, but generally, a new pulmonary infiltrate combined with fever, chest pain, hypoxia, dyspnea or tachypnea
- Pathogenesis: Multifactorial, and includes anything that leads to local hypoxemia, including ventilation-perfusion mismatch, infection (Chlamydia, Mycoplasma, viruses), bronchospasm, pain crisis in ribs, fat embolism, pulmonary infarct, and postoperative pain. Lower steady-state Hb and higher steady-state fetal Hb are thought to be somewhat protective against ACS, presumably due to lower blood viscosity
- Treatment:
  - Supplemental oxygen to keep SpO$_2$ 92–99%
  - Consider incentive spirometry hourly while awake to recruit alveoli
  - Maintain euvolemia: Dehydration leads to sickling. Overhydration leads to pulmonary edema, both of which can make ACS worse
  - Empiric antibiotics
    - Ceftriaxone 50–75 mg/kg/day div daily to bid (max 2 g/dose)
      - Clindamycin or vancomycin as above if ceftriaxone allergic
    - Azithromycin 10 mg/kg PO/IV day 1, then 5 mg/kg/day × 4 days
  - Transfusion improves oxygenation, consider early in course of ACS
    - Simple transfusion if Hb > 10% below baseline and increasing oxygen requirement: 4 mL/kg raises Hb 1 gm/dL. Goal ~11 g/dL
    - Exchange transfusion if elevated Hb, severe ACS (progressive or severe hypoxemia, multi-lobar disease), or previous severe ACS
      - Goal HbS < 30% total Hb, keeping total Hb < 10 g/dL
  - Bronchodilators if history of asthma or exam suggests bronchospasm
  - Noninvasive positive pressure ventilation with CPAP or BiPAP if indicated
  - Pain control (see section on acute pain crisis)

References: *Pediatrics.* 2011;128(3):484; *Pediatr Blood Cancer.* 2012 Aug;59(2):358–364

ACUTE PAIN CRISIS/VASO-OCCLUSIVE CRISIS (VOC)

- Ketorolac 0.5 mg/kg (max 30 mg) IV × 1, then 0.5 mg/kg (max 15 mg/dose) IV q 6 h × max of 3–5 days. Avoid concomitant NSAIDs or renal-toxic meds
- Opioids (monitor for excessive sedation or hypoventilation, doses vary significantly depending on previous exposure, start with lower doses for opiate-naïve patients)
  - Morphine 0.05–0.2 mg/kg/dose IV q 1–4 hours (max 15 mg/dose)
  - Hydromorphone 0.015 mg/kg/dose IV q 2–6 hours (max 0.5–1 mg/dose)
  - For patients old enough to manage independently, consider patient-controlled analgesia (see table below)
- Achieve euvolemia: Replete deficit with isotonic fluids (10–20 mL/kg NS or LR). Subsequently monitor IV + PO with goal of achieving 1× maintenance fluid needs
- Psychosocial support
- Transfusions provide little benefit

Table 7.18 Patient-Controlled Analgesia for Sickle Cell Pain in Pediatric Patients

Drug	Initial Patient-Administered Dose	Initial Opiate-Naïve Basal Rate	Lockout Interval
Morphine	0.01–0.02 mg/kg	0.005 mg/kg/hour	10 minutes
Hydromorphone	2–4 mcg/kg	1 mcg/kg/hour	8 minutes
Fentanyl	0.2–0.3 mcg/kg	0.2 mcg/kg/hour	6 minutes

Table 7.19 Patient-Controlled Analgesia for Sickle Cell Pain in Adult-Sized Patients

Drug	Initial Patient-Administered Dose	Initial Opiate-Naïve Basal Rate	Lockout Interval
Morphine	1 mg	0.5 mg/hour	10 minutes
Hydromorphone	0.2 mg	5–10 mcg/kg/hour	8 minutes
Fentanyl	20 mcg	100 mcg/hour	6 minutes

ACUTE ANEMIA

- Aplastic Crisis
  - Secondary to viral infection (parvovirus B19, EBV, others) causing transient arrest of RBC development in bone marrow
    - Anemia and low reticulocyte count (<1% or < 10,000/mL)
  - Shortened RBC survival in sickle cell patients (~14 days) leads to profound anemia, and may require repeat transfusions during single aplastic crisis
  - Consider transfusion for significant change of Hb from baseline, pallor, tachycardia, fatigue, poor feeding, altered mental status
    - 4 mL/kg PRBC transfusion should raise Hb 1 g/dL
- Splenic Sequestration
  - Marked drop in Hb and splenomegaly, in presence of persistent reticulocytosis
  - Occurs in HbSS patients prior to splenic autolysis, and those with HbSC and sickle cell-thalassemia (who tend to retain their spleens)
  - Treatment: PRBC transfusion (goal Hb 7–9 g/dL) to maintain intravascular volume and maintain adequate delivery of substrate (glucose, oxygen) to tissues (avoid "shock")
  - Generally self-resolves in 1–3 days, with release of RBCs from spleen leading to Hb increase of 2–3 g/dL ("auto-transfusion")
  - Approximate 50% recurrence rate
    - Consider splenectomy after 2nd or 3rd episode
- Hyperhemolytic Crisis
  - Sudden worsening of anemia in presence of adequate reticulocytes
  - May be associated with acute infection, transfusion reaction, or G6PD

DACTYLITIS

- Acute vaso-occlusive crisis in infants and young children
  - Painful swelling of hands with erythema
  - Manage pain as above
  - Intravenous hydration to maintain euvolemia
- Reportedly occurs in ~25% infants by 1 year of age, 40% by 2 years of age
  - May predict more severe SCD complications in the future (more VOC, ACS)

STROKE

- Ischemic (90%) or hemorrhagic (10%) stroke in 10% SCD patient by 10 years of age
- Typical presenting signs include hemiparesis, aphasia, stupor, facial droop
- Evaluation
  - Thorough history, physical and neurologic examination
  - Neuroimaging (CT or MRI), CBC, reticulocyte count, HbS%, type and screen
- Treatment: Goal is rapid reduction in HbS percentage to < 30% total Hb
  - Simple or exchange transfusion (attempt to maintain Hb < 10 g/dL), pheresis
- Prevention
  - Transcranial Doppler (TCD): 1st screen at 2 years of age, then annually if normal, or every 3–6 months if abnormal. 2 consecutive abnormal screens, or history of acute stroke → initiate preventive chronic transfusion therapy
  - Monthly chronic transfusion therapy: Goal is to suppress bone marrow production of native RBCs ("sickle cells") and keep HbS < 30% of total Hb
  - Risk of iron overload, particularly in liver and heart, and alloantibodies

References: *Blood.* 1998;91(1):288–294; *NEJM.* 1998;339(1):5–11.

CHOLELITHIASIS

- Precipitation of bilirubin in gallbladder from rapid RBC turnover
- Prefer laparoscopic removal as decreased pain and postoperative risks (see below)

PRIAPISM

- Sustained erection of ~ 2–4 hours in absence of sexual arousal
- Sickling of cells in erectile tissue (corpora cavernosa), with subsequent sludging, hypoxia. This in turn leads to increased sickling. Generally very painful
- Occurs in ~ 30% males by 15 years of age
- Management: Analgesia, intravenous hydration, urologic drainage of cavernosa
- Preventive: Hydroxyurea, pseudoephedrine, and etilefrine have been suggested for those with recurrent (or stuttering) priapism

IRON OVERLOAD

- Generally occurs when PRBC > 100–120 mL/kg has been transfused
- Monitor heart and liver with yearly MRI and serum ferritin levels
- Consider chelation if ferritin (in non-inflammatory state) > 1000–1500 ng/mL, or liver biopsy shows dry weight liver iron of > 7 mg/g (some chelate at levels > 3 mg/g)
- Chelation options:
  - Deforxamine (*Desferal*): 20–50 mg/kg/day SQ over 8–12 hours (max 2 g/day)
  - Deferasirox (*Exjade*): 20 mg/kg PO daily

Reference: *Pediatrics.* 2011;128(3):484.

SURGERY

- Major surgery can lead to significant complications of sickling, VOC, ACS
  - Perioperative transfusion: Goal HbS < 30% of total, and total Hb ~9–10 g/dL
  - Postoperative incentive spirometry, pain control, fluid management, oxygen therapy are crucial
- Minor/laparoscopic surgery may not require perioperative transfusion

CHAPTER 8 ■ IMMUNOLOGY

IMMUNOSUPPRESSIVE AGENTS

Table 8.1 Immunosuppressive Agents: Dosing and Monitoring Parameters*

Agent	Dose	Monitoring
Antithymocyte Globulin (ATG) (*Thymoglobulin*® = rabbit, *Atgam*® = equine)	Equine: 10–25 mg/kg/day (for aplastic anemia or GVHD) Rabbit: 1.5 mg/kg/day Administer over 6–12 hours through 0.22 micron in-line filter into large vein or central line	Goal: Absolute lymphocyte count of 0.2 ± 0.1 lymphocytes/mL For acute reactions: ↓ infusion rate, administer acetaminophen, diphenhydramine, methylprednisolone
Basiliximab (*Simulect*®)	< 35 kg: 10 mg/kg on days 0 and 4 > 35 kg: 20 mg/kg on days 0 and 4	Goals level > 0.2 mcg/mL (ELISA) Infuse over 20–30 minutes
Daclizumab (*Zenapax*®)	1 mg/kg q 14 days × 5 doses	
Methylprednisolone/Prednisone	0.1–0.3 mg/kg/day maintenance dose after 5–10 mg/kg IV induction dose	
Cyclosporine (*Neoral*® and *SandIMMUNE*®; not bioequivalent)	Maintenance oral dose ~ 3–10 mg/kg/day	Goal levels depend on type of organ and time from transplant. ↑ levels when given with sirolimus or everolimus; give 4 hours apart
Mycophenolate mofetil (*Cellcept*®) and enteric-coated Mycophenolate mofetil (*Myfortic*®)	IV starting dose 0.01–0.05 mg/kg/day Oral maintenance 0.15–0.2 mg/kg/day divided in 2 doses	Measure levels occasionally or if severe side effects (diarrhea, vomiting, leukopenia, anemia, and infections) develop
Azathioprine (*Imuran*®)	25–50 mg/kg/day divided in 2 doses or 1200 mg/m^2/day PO divided in 2 doses	
Tacrolimus (*Prograf*®)	IV starting dose: 0.01–0.05 mg/kg/d Oral maintenance: 0.15–0.2 mg/kg/d divided in 2 doses	Monitor trough levels via high-performance liquid chromatography (HPLC) as immunoassay gives higher levels than HPLC
Sirolimus (*Rapamune*®)	1 mg/m^2/day, often divided q 12 hours	↑ levels when given with CSA; give 4 hours apart HPLC preferred to immunoassay to monitor levels
Everolimus (*Afinitor*®)	0.8–1.5 mg/m^2/day/dose PO bid (max 1.5 mg/dose)	↑ levels when given with CSA; give 4 hours apart HPLC preferred to immunoassay to monitor levels

*All drugs should be used *only* in consultation with transplant surgeon or physician experienced in their use. All drugs have varying regimens, depending on type of transplant and institution.

Table 8.2 Side Effects of Immunosuppressive Agents Commonly Used in Pediatrics

Agent	Side Effects/Notes
Antithymocyte Globulin (ATG) (*Thymoglobulin®, Atgam®*)	Cytokine release syndrome (fever, chills); possible ↑ risk post-transplant lymphoproliferative disorder
Basiliximab (*Simulect®*)	No ↑ risk opportunistic infections; + risk of allergic reaction
Daclizumab (*Zenapax®*)	No ↑ risk opportunistic infections; + risk of allergic reaction
Methylprednisolone/prednisone	↑ blood pressure, hyperglycemia/diabetes mellitus, osteopenia, delayed wound healing, cataracts, behavioral effects/irritability, hyperlipidemia, water retention, Cushing's syndrome, weight gain, hirsutism, acne, ↓ growth, withdrawal, ↑ infections
Cyclosporine (CSA, *Neoral®, SandIMMUNE®*)	Nephrotoxicity, hirsutism, gingival hyperplasia, hypertension, hyperlipidemia, autoimmune hemolytic anemia, leukopenia
Tacrolimus (TAC, *Prograf®*)	Nephrotoxicity, diabetes, tremor, peripheral neuropathy, alopecia, gastrointestinal problems, autoimmune hemolytic anemia, leucopenia; levels ↑ with diarrhea. Erythromycin, clarithromycin, omeprazole can ↑ TAC levels (no effect on TAC levels from azithromycin)
Mycophenolate mofetil (*Cellcept®*), ecMPA (*Myfortic®*)	Gastrointestinal symptoms, leukopenia, lymphopenia,
Azathioprine (AZA, *Imuran®*)	↑ risk of infections and neoplasms, skin cancer (limit sun exposure); pancreatitis, hair loss, hepatotoxicity
Sirolimus (*Rapamune®*)	May ↓ coronary artery vasculopathy in cardiac allografts
Everolimus (*Afinitor®*)	May ↓ coronary artery vasculopathy in cardiac allografts

Table 8.3 Selected Drugs That DECREASE Tacrolimus, Sirolimus, Everolimus, and Cyclosporine Levels

Antacids, carbamazepine, caspofungin, efavirenz, etravirine, fosphenytoin, modafinil, nafcillin, nevirapine, oxcarbazepine, phenobarbital, phenytoin, rifampin, rigabutin, St John's wort

Table 8.4 Selected Drugs (and Foods) That INCREASE Tacrolimus, Sirolimus, Everolimus, and Cyclosporine Levels

Amiodarone, clarithromycin, clotrimazole, diltiazem, erythromycin, fluconazole, grapefruit juice, indinavir, itraconazole, ketoconazole, levofloxacin, lidocaine, metronidazole, nelfinavir, ritonavir, tinidazole, verapamil, voriconazole

Data from: Urschel S. *Pediatr Clin North Am* - 01-APR-2010; 57(2): 433–57.

INDUCTION:
Use of induction and type of induction is highly variable and depends on individual situation

TREATMENT OF ACUTE REJECTION:
- Methylprednisolone 10–20 mg/kg/day IV × 3–5 days
- Mild rejection: prednisone 5 mg/kg/day PO × 3–5 days
- Severe rejection (or heart transplant with altered vital signs): ATG × 3–5 days

TREATMENT OF ANTIBODY-MEDIATED REJECTION:
- Treatment is difficult and controversial. Strategies that have been used: plasmapheresis, plasma exchange, and antigen-specific and nonspecific immunoadsorption columns, as well as immunomodulatory approaches with IV immunoglobulin, rituximab (delayed effect, no effect on plasma cells), bortezomib and eculizumab (early studies in renal transplant)

Abbreviation: ATG: antithymocyte globulin

Reference: *Pediatr Clin North Am.* 2010;57(2)433–457.

ANAPHYLAXIS

Systemic symptoms resulting from the IgE-mediated release of intracellular contents of basophils and mast cells in response to a stimulus (food, medication, infection, etc.).

Systems involved (with signs and symptoms) include:
- Dermatologic: Urticaria, flushing, angioedema, pruritus (oral, perioral, periorbital), edema of tongue, lips, or oropharynx
- Gastrointestinal: Vomiting, nausea, abdominal pain, diarrhea
- Cardiovascular: Hypotension, arrhythmia, syncope/presyncope, dizziness, hypotonia
- Respiratory: Bronchospasm, laryngeal edema (tightness in throat, stridor), sneezing, dyspnea, hypoxemia
- Neurologic: Anxiety, mental status changes
- Reactions can be immediate (stings, IV medications) or delayed (food, PO medication allergies).

■ CLINICAL CRITERIA FOR DIAGNOSING ANAPHYLAXIS[1]
If any of the three following criteria are met, anaphylaxis should be diagnosed and treated:
(1) Two or more of the following occurring rapidly (minutes to hours) after exposure to a likely allergen:
    a. Skin and/or mucous membrane involvement
    b. Respiratory involvement
    c. Reduced SBP (systolic blood pressure) and/or signs of end-organ dysfunction
    d. Significant gastrointestinal symptoms
(2) Cardiovascular involvement (particularly hypotension) after exposure to a known allergen:
    a. Low SBP (< 70 mmHg + [2 × age in years] for children age 1–10, < 90 mmHg for children age ≥ 11)
    b. Greater than 30% decrease in SBP

Table 8.5 Treatment of Anaphylaxis

Secure airway, check breathing and circulation. CPR if indicated. Supplemental oxygen if dyspneic, hypoxemic, or severe reaction. *Call 911.*

Table 8.6 Administer Medications as Indicated by Severity of Reaction

Epinephrine 1:1000: 0.01 mL/kg (max 0.5 mL) SQ or IM as often as q 15 min	
or	
Epinephrine 1:10000: 0.1 mL/kg IV or 10 over 1–2 minutes if ↓ perfusion (max 1 mL/dose, can be repeated as often as q 3–5 min)	
or	
Prefilled epinephrine syringes	*EpiPen Jr:* 1 injection IM for patients < 30 kg
	EpiPen: 1 injection IM for patients > 30 kg

---

1. Adapted from *J All Clin Immun.* 2006;117(2);391–397.

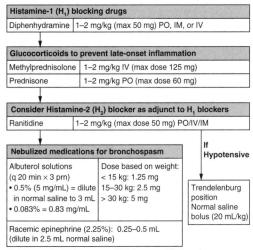

Histamine-1 (H$_1$) blocking drugs	
Diphenhydramine	1–2 mg/kg (max 50 mg) PO, IM, or IV

Glucocorticoids to prevent late-onset inflammation	
Methylprednisolone	1–2 mg/kg IV (max dose 125 mg)
Prednisone	1–2 mg/kg PO (max dose 60 mg)

Consider Histamine-2 (H$_2$) blocker as adjunct to H$_1$ blockers	
Ranitidine	1–2 mg/kg (max dose 50 mg) PO/IV/IM

Nebulized medications for bronchospasm	
Albuterol solutions (q 20 min × 3 prn) • 0.5% (5 mg/mL) = dilute in normal saline to 3 mL • 0.083% = 0.83 mg/mL	Dose based on weight: < 15 kg: 1.25 mg 15–30 kg: 2.5 mg > 30 kg: 5 mg
Racemic epinephrine (2.25%): 0.25–0.5 mL (dilute in 2.5 mL normal saline)	

If Hypotensive

Trendelenburg position
Normal saline bolus (20 mL/kg)

IM: Intramuscular, IO: Intraosseous, IV: Intravenous, NS: Normal
saline, PO: orally, prn: as needed, SQ: Subcutaneous;
SBP: Systolic blood pressure

Figure 8.1

PRIMARY IMMUNODEFICIENCY (PI)[2]

Suspect immunodeficiency when a child has:
- ≥ 8 ear infections, ≥ 2 sinus infections or 2 pneumonias in one year
- Family history of primary immunodeficiency
- Failure of an infant to appropriately gain weight
- Recurrent, deep skin or organ abscesses
- Persistent candidal infection in mouth or elsewhere on skin, after age 1 year old
- Two or more months on antibiotics with little effect or need for intravenous antibiotics to clear infections that normally would not require them

Complete list of identified immunodeficiencies is long.

■ IMMUNODEFICIENCY EVALUATION
Consult with immunologist early in process.
- Growth parameters, CBC with differential, quantitative immunoglobulins, human immunodeficiency virus (HIV) testing
- Consider specific tests depending on type of concerning infection and pathogen:
  ○ Antibody titers after vaccination (*H. influenzae*, *S. pneumoniae*, tetanus)
  ○ CH50 assay (tests complement function)
  ○ Neutrophil oxidative burst (CGD)
  ○ Quantification of T and B cell subsets
  ○ IgG subclass quantification

---

2. Adapted from the Jeffrey Modell Foundation website: http://www.info4pi.org/

■ **TREATMENT**
- May include antibiotic prophylaxis (trimethoprim-sulfamethoxazole for *Pneumocystis* or CGD), subcutaneous or intravenous immunoglobulin (IVIG)* (humoral defects, hyper IgM, Wiskott-Aldrich), thymic transplantation

Table 8.7 Primary Immunodeficiency Disorders

Primary Immune Deficiency	Clinical Presentation
Severe Combined Immunodeficiency (SCID)	Infants present with failure to thrive, chronic diarrhea, recurrent opportunistic infections
Humoral (B-cell) Immune Defects	Sinopulmonary infections with encapsulated bacteria (*S. pneumoniae, H. influenzae*)
Selective IgA Deficiency	Incidence 1:200. Often asymptomatic. May have recurrent sinopulmonary infections, allergic reaction to blood products, autoimmune disorders
Cellular (T-cell) Immune Defects: DiGeorge syndrome, X-linked Hyper-IgM, Wiskott-Aldrich, Ataxia-telangiectasia	Opportunistic infections (cytomegalovirus, *Pneumocystis jiroveci*, mycobacteria)
Neutrophil Defect: Chronic Granulomatous Disease (CGD)	Bacterial (Nocardia, actinomyces, Burkholderia, staph spp.) and fungal (Aspergillus) infections of skin and organs, including deep abscesses, granulomas, osteomyelitis, pneumonia
Terminal Complement Defect	Sinopulmonary infections with encapsulated bacteria and recurrent *Neisseria* infections
Interferon-gamma/Interleukin-12 Pathway Defect	Atypical mycobacterial (include Bacillus Calmette-Guérin) and *Salmonella* infections

DEEP NECK SPACE INFECTIONS (DNSI)

- Includes: Abscess, cellulitis, and phlegmon of the parapharyngeal and retropharyngeal spaces
- Anatomy: Retropharyngeal space is bordered posteriorly by the alar fascia, laterally by the carotid sheaths and parapharyngeal spaces, and anteriorly by the buccal pharyngeal fascia (which envelops the trachea, esophagus, and thyroid gland). It extends inferiorly to tracheal bifurcation
- The "Danger" space, directly behind the retropharyngeal space, extends inferiorly to the diaphragm. Rare complications of DNSI include mediastinitis, carotid or jugular sheath infection (septic thrombophlebitis: Lemierre's disease), rupture into the oropharynx with subsequent aspiration, or compression of the trachea
- Etiology: Polymicrobial: *Strep pyogenes*, *Staph aureus*, anaerobes
- Presentation: Neck stiffness, odynophagia, sore throat, fever, drooling, cervical lymphadenopathy/neck swelling, bulging retropharynx, stridor (rare ~ 1–2%)
- Diagnostic tests:
  - Lateral neck plain radiographs: Limited value due to difficulty getting child's neck into proper extension, leading to increase in prevertebral space width.
    - In good quality films, C2 pre-vertebral soft tissue > 7 mm or retrotracheal width > 14 mm suggestive of DNSI
  - Computed tomography (CT) with intravenous contrast: Low-attenuation (< 20–25 Hounsfield units), occasionally circumscribed area in prevertebral or paratracheal space. Carotid and internal jugular vein may be displaced. CT not reliable at distinguishing phlegmon from frank abscess
- Treatment: Antibiotic therapy alone may be successful in up to 50% cases:
  - Ceftriaxone: 50 mg/kg q 24 hours, *or* cefotaxime: 100–200 mg/kg/day divided q 6–8 hours, *plus*
  - Clindamycin: 40 mg/kg/day IV divided q 6–8 hours, *or* ampicillin + sulbactam (*zosyn*): 100–200 mg ampicillin component/kg/day divided q 6 hours
  - Consider vancomycin: 15 mg/kg/dose IV q 6 hours, depending on local MRSA prevalence and MICs. Check trough prior to fourth or fifth dose
    - MRSA MIC ≥ 1 mcg/mL: Goal trough = 15–20 mcg/mL
    - MRSA MIC < 1 mcg/mL: Goal trough = 10–15 mcg/mL
  - Transition to oral antibiotics if improved (↑ neck range of motion, drinking/eating well, ↓ WBC, ↓ CRP) after several days of parenteral therapy. Outpatient options include:
    - Clindamycin: 10–30 mg/kg/day PO divided q 6–8 hours. Max dose 1.8 g/day, *or* amoxicillin/ clavulanate: 80–100 mg amoxicillin component/kg/day divided q 8 hours (use 600 mg/5 mL suspension)
    - Linezolid (*Zyvox*): 10 mg/kg/dose PO q 8 hours for 10–14 days
  - Consider surgical management for lack of improvement, clinical deterioration, or well-circumscribed abscess on CT

Abbreviations: CRP: C-reactive protein; DNSI: deep neck space infection; MIC: mean inhibitory concentration; MRSA: methicillin-resistant *Staphylococcus aureus*; WBC: white blood cell count

References: *Otolaryngol Head Neck Surg*. 2008;138(3):300–306; *Pediatrics*. 2003;111(6 Pt 1):1394; *Am J Otolaryngol*. 2006;27(4):244–247; *Arch Pediatr*. 2009;16(9):1225–1232; *Am J Health-Syst Pharm*. 2009;66(1):82–98.

INFLUENZA

Influenza A or B cause similar disease. Patients are generally febrile, with some variation of cough, congestion, dyspnea, chills, myalgias, headache, and pharyngitis. Infants and young children may be hypothermic, or only febrile at presentation. Antigenic changes of surface proteins hemagglutinin (HA) and neuraminidase (NA) result in yearly illness variation. Influenza A has avian and other mammalian hosts. Novel (2009 H1N1) and avian strains (H5N1) can cause global pandemics

DIAGNOSIS

- Rapid Influenza Diagnostic Tests (RIDT) have low sensitivity (40–70%), but high specificity (90–95%). Thus, false positives rare, but false negatives common
- If high suspicion of disease and negative RIDT, consider confirmatory test (reverse transcriptase polymerase chain reaction [RT-PCR] test or viral culture)

TREATMENT

- Begin within 48 hours, or as soon as possible for high-risk patients
- High-risk patients include: Hospitalized or those with severe, complicated or progressive disease, or *at risk* for severe disease as follows:
  - Children aged < 2 years
  - Children with chronic pulmonary (including asthma), cardiovascular, renal, hepatic, hematological (including sickle cell disease), metabolic disorders (including diabetes mellitus), or neurologic and neurodevelopment conditions (such as cerebral palsy, epilepsy, stroke, intellectual disability, moderate to severe developmental delay, muscular dystrophy, or spinal cord injury)
  - Immunosuppressed children (HIV, chemotherapy, etc.)
- FDA-approved neuraminidase inhibitors, oseltamivir (*Tamiflu®*) and zanamivir (*Relenza®*), have activity against both influenza A and B viruses. Check current resistance to antivirals and updated guidelines at cdc.gov
- Adamantanes (rimantidine and amantadine) may have activity versus seasonal influenza. Check cdc. gov/flu to determine seasonal sensitivities before prescribing

Table 9.1 Oseltamivir Treatment and Prophylactic Dosing

Age	Treatment	Chemoprophylaxis#
< 1 year old*	3 mg/kg/dose PO bid	3 mg/kg/dose PO daily
≥ 1 yr, < 15 kg	30 mg PO bid	30 mg PO daily
≥1 yr, 15–23 kg	45 mg PO bid	45 mg PO daily
≥ 1 yr, 23.1–40 kg	60 mg PO bid	60 mg PO daily
> 40 kg-adult	75 mg PO bid	75 mg PO daily

*Not FDA approved, but used under emergency use authorization in 2009 pandemic

Table 9.2 Zanamivir Treatment and Prophylactic Dosing

Age	Treatment	Chemoprophylaxis#
≥ 7 years old	10 mg (2 inhalations) twice daily	---
≥ 5 years old	---	10 mg (2 inhalations) once daily

Chemoprophylaxis: 70–90% effective at preventing disease. Should be used as adjunct to yearly influenza vaccination. Duration = 10 days, or 7 days from last known exposure

Table 9.3 Rimantidine and Amantadine Treatment and Prophylactic Dosing

Rimantidine		
Age[¶]	Treatment	Chemoprophylaxis
1–9 years old	6.6 mg/kg/day div bid (max 150 mg/day)	5 mg/kg PO daily (max 150 mg/day)
≥ 10 years old	200 mg PO daily	200 mg PO daily
Amantadine		
Age	Treatment and chemoprophylaxis have same dosing	
1–9 years old	5–8 mg/kg/day PO daily or div bid (max 150 mg/day)	
≥ 10 years old	200 mg/day PO divided bid	

¶ Not FDA approved; however safety and efficacy data have been published

ISOLATION

- Type: Droplet isolation + standard precautions
- Duration: 7 days after onset of illness, or at least 24 hours after symptoms (fever, cough, etc.) resolve, whichever is longer
- Airborne isolation *only* when performing certain procedures (intubation, bronchoscopy, induced sputum collection)

COMPLICATIONS

- Pneumonia (viral hemorrhagic disease or bacterial superinfection with *Strep. pneumoniae* or *Staph. aureus*)
- Otitis media (25%)
- Myositis (post-influenza B, often localizes to calves)
- Reye syndrome (salicylate use in influenza B)
- Myocarditis (rare)

VACCINATION (PREVENTION)

- Indications: All children 6 months–18 years on a yearly basis.
  - If vaccine supply limited, reserve for high-risk patients first

Table 9.4 Influenza Vaccine

Injectable, Inactivated Vaccine[¥]		
Age	Dose	Comment
6–35 months old	0.25 mL IM	2 doses, 1 month apart if first season vaccinated, or < 2 doses influenza vaccine since 7/2010
≥ 3–8 years old	0.5 mL IM	
≥ 9 years old	0.5 mL IM	Single dose/season
Live-Attenuated Influenza Vaccine (*Flumist*)[¥,∞]		
2–8 years old	0.2 mL[∞]	2 doses, 1 month apart if first season vaccinated, or < 2 doses influenza vaccine since 7/2010
≥ 9–49 years old	0.2 mL[∞]	1 dose/season

¥ Contraindicated for: Severe prior reaction to influenza vaccine, severe egg allergy, history of Guillain-Barré syndrome after influenza vaccination, and moderate-severe current illness

∞ Administer as 0.1 mL/spray to each nostril

≠ Not recommended for: Children < 2 years old, 2–4 years old with history of ≥ 1 episode wheezing in past year, close contact with bone marrow transplant patient, any egg allergy, taking long-term aspirin, "weakened" immune system, pregnant women

Data from: http://www.cdc.gov/flu/professionals/antivirals/summary-clinicians.htm (12/5/13); *Clin Infect Dis.* 2009; 48: 1008–1032.; *MMWR.* August 17, 2012 / 61(32); 613–6184; *Pediatrics.* 1987; 80: 275–82.

References: CDC. Influenza Antiviral Medications: Summary for Clinicians. http://www.cdc.gov/flu/professionals/antivirals/summary-clinicians.htm (12/5/13); *Clin Infect Dis.* 2009;48:1008–1032; *MMWR.* 2012;61(32):613–618; *Pediatrics.* 1987;80:275–282.

MENINGITIS

PATHOPHYSIOLOGY

- Hematogenous spread or direct extension to subarachnoid space from local infection (mastoiditis, otitis media, sinusitis, orbital cellulitis, facial cellulitis)
- Inflammatory response leads to neuronal injury and cell death

Table 9.5 Symptoms of Bacterial Meningitis

Neonates	> 1 month old
Poor feeding, irritability, lethargy, apnea, jaundice, hypoglycemia, seizures, hypotonia, fever or hypothermia (62%), bulging fontanelle	Fever (occasionally hypothermia), headache, photophobia, neck pain/nuchal rigidity, irritability, altered mental status, vomiting, bulging fontanelle, seizures, coma, rash/petechiae/purpura, focal neurologic signs (15%)

Table 9.6 Differential Diagnosis of Bacterial Meningitis

Epidural/ subdural abscess	Brain tumor	Brain abscess
CNS leukemia	Lead encephalopathy	Viral syndrome
TB with CNS involvement	Encephalitis	Toxic ingestion

Table 9.7 Bacterial Meningitis Prediction Score Criteria

- Positive CSF Gram stain
- CSF absolute neutrophil count (ANC) ≥ 1000 cells/µL
- CSF protein ≥ 80 mg/dL
- Peripheral blood ANC ≥ 10,000 cells/µL
- History of seizure before or at the time of presentation

Number of criteria fulfilled	0	1	2	3	≥ 4
Likelihood of bacterial meningitis	0.1%	3%	27%	70%	95%

Data from: *JAMA.* 2007;297(1):52–60.

Table 9.8 Common CSF Findings in Different Types of Meningitis*

Bacterial	Opening pressure > 20 cm H_2O, WBC > 1000, glucose < 10, protein > 100. Gram stain + in 90% with pneumococcal disease and 80% with *N. meningitidis*
Viral	Opening pressure < 20 cm H_2O, WBC 5–500, glucose normal, protein 50–100. No organisms on gram stain
Lyme disease	Opening pressure < 20 cm H_2O, WBC 100–500, glucose 10–45, protein 50–150
Tuberculous meningitis	Opening pressure > 20 cm H_2O, WBC 100–500, glucose 10–45, protein > 100

*Rule out mass lesion on clinical grounds (no historical features, focal neurologic findings or evidence of increased ICP) to determine need for CT of brain prior to lumbar puncture (LP)

MOST COMMON ETIOLOGIES OF BACTERIAL MENINGITIS, BY AGE

- Neonatal (< 28 days old)
  - Group B Streptococcus (< 7 days: early onset; ≥ 7 days: late onset)
  - Gram-negative rods: *Escherichia coli*
  - *Listeria monocytogenes*:
    - Can also be seen in immunocompromised children and pregnant ♀
    - Can be misidentified as diptheroid or hemolytic streptococcus
    - Symptoms are often subtle
- Infants and children > 1 month old
  - *Streptococcus pneumoniae:* Gram + lancet-shaped diplococcus, α-hemolytic, person-to-person transmission, 1–7 day incubation, ↑ in winter, up to 30% mortality
  - *Neisseria meningitidis:* Gram-negative intracellular cocci, person-to-person transmission, incubation 1–7 days, up to 10% mortality
  - *Haemophilus influenzae* type b: Uncommon; pleimorphic gram-negative rod, most common in unimmunized children < 3 years, up to 10% mortality

PATHOGENS IN SPECIAL CIRCUMSTANCES IN BACTERIAL MENINGITIS

- Post-neurosurgical procedure/ventriculoperitoneal (VP) shunt present
  - *Staph. epidermidis* and other coagulase-negative staphylococci
  - Remove VP shunt and consider external ventricular drain
- CSF leak: *Strep. pneumoniae* by far most common pathogen
  - Pneumococcal polysaccharade vaccine (Pneumovax) if ≥ 2 years old and fully vaccinated with pneumococcal conjugate vaccine
- Immunocompromised
  - *Pseudomonas, Serratia, Proteus*, diphtheroids, tuberculous meningitis
- Anatomic defects
  - Dermal sinus: *Staph. aureus, Staph. epidermidis*
  - Urinary tract anomalies: *E. coli, Klebsiella*
    - Add aminoglycoside if GNR noted on gram stain

Table 9.9 Poor Prognostic Indicators for *Neisseria meningitidis* Meningitis

Hypotension	Neutropenia	Petechiae < 12 hours into illness
Shock	Acidosis	Very young or older adolescent
Serogroup C	Low ESR or CRP	Disseminated intravascular coagulation

Table 9.10 Treatment of Bacterial Meningitis in Children > 1 Month Old

Empiric therapy	• Vancomycin 80 mg/kg/day divided q 6 hours (goal trough 15–20 mcg/mL; *And, either* • Ceftriaxone 100 mg/kg/day divided q 12 hours (max 4 gm/day), *or* • Cefotaxime 300 mg/kg/day divided q 8 hours (max 8 gm/day)
Neisseria meningitidis (Duration of therapy = 7 days)	• Penicillin G (PCN G) 250,000–300,000 U/kg/day divided q 4–6 hours (max 24 million units/day) • Cefotaxime 300 mg/kg/day divided q 8 hours (max 8 gm/day) • Ceftriaxone 100 mg/kg/day divided q 12 hours (max 4 gm/day) • For patients with anaphylaxis to PCN consider chloramphenicol 75–100 mg/kg/day divided q 6 hours (max 2–4 gm/day)

(Continued)

Table 9.10 Treatment of Bacterial Meningitis in Children > 1 Month Old *(Continued)*

S Pneumo
(Duration of
therapy = 10–14 days)
	• Penicillin G as above if MIC < 0.06 ug/mL
	 ◦ ~20% resistant to penicillin with MIC > 0.12 ug/mL
	• Ceftriaxone or cefotaxime as above if MICs < 0.5 ug/mL
	• Vancomycin if ceftriaxone MIC > 1–2 ug/mL (~7% isolates)
	• Rifampin 20 mg/kg IV divided bid in addition to vancomycin
	 ◦ For isolates with ceftriaxone MIC > 4 ug/mL, poor response to vancomycin,
	   or presence of organisms on repeat LP
	• Beta lactamase inhibitors not useful
	• Levofloxacin has adequate CNS penetration (useful in patients with severe
	  penicillin and vancomycin allergies)

H Influenza
(Duration of
therapy = 7 days)
	• Ampicillin 400 mg/kg/day divided q 6 hours
	  (max 12 gm/day)
	 ◦ 30% of isolates are ampicillin resistant
	• Cefotaxime 300 mg/kg/day divided q 8 hours
	  (max 8 gm/day)
	• Ceftriaxone 100 mg/kg/day divided q 12 hours
	  (max 4 gm/day)
	• For patients with anaphylaxis to PCN consider chloramphenicol 75–100 mg/kg/
	  day divided q 6 hours (max 2–4 gm/day)
	• Dexamethasone 0.15 mg/kg/dose IV q 6 hours × 2–4 days
	 ◦ First dose given before or concurrent with initial antibiotics
	 ◦ Decreased hearing loss
	 ◦ No difference in other neurologic outcomes

Table 9.11 Treatment of Bacterial Meningitis in Neonates

Group B strep (GBS) (Duration of therapy for uncomplicated disease = 14–21 days)	• ≤ 7 days old (full-term) ◦ Penicillin 250,000–450,000 U/kg/day divided q 8 hours, *or* ◦ Ampicillin 150–300 mg/kg/day divided q 8 hours *For synergistic effect, add* ◦ Gentamicin 2.5 mg/kg/dose IV q 12 hours, *or* ◦ Gentamicin 4 mg/kg/dose IV q 24 hours • > 7 days old (full-term) ◦ Penicillin 450,000–500,000 U/kg/day divided q 6 hours, *or* ◦ Ampicillin 200–300 mg/kg/day divided q 6 hours *For synergistic effect, add* ◦ Gentamicin 2.5 mg/kg/dose IV q 8 hours, *or* ◦ Gentamicin 5 mg/kg/dose IV q 24 hours
E coli	• Duration of therapy = 14 days after CSF sterility • Ampicillin susceptible: Ampicillin as dosed by age above • Cefotaxime: • ≤ 7 days old (full-term): 150 mg/kg/day divided q 8 hours • > 7 days old (full-term): 200 mg/kg/day divided q 8 hours
Listeria	• Duration of therapy = 14 days and CSF sterility achieved ◦ Ampicillin and gentamicin as dosed above for GBS

Repeat lumbar puncture and/or neuroimaging if poor response to therapy within 48 hours, persistent fever > 5 days, focal neurologic deficits, highly resistant organism

FLUID MANAGEMENT IN BACTERIAL MENINGITIS

- Bolus with isotonic fluids 20 mL/kg IV if in shock or hypovolemic
- Monitor for syndrome of inappropriate antidiuretic hormone (SIADH)
  - Signs include decreased urine output, decreased serum sodium, positive fluid balance, weight gain, and excessively concentrated urine
  - If serum sodium < 130 mEq/L and child not hypovolemic or in shock, limit initial fluid intake to 1200 mL/m^2/day
  - Once serum sodium > 135 mEq/L, liberalize to maintenance fluids

Table 9.12 Potential Complications of Bacterial Meningitis

- Prolonged fever despite appropriate antimicrobial therapy (*S. Pneumo*)
- Cerebral edema: May lead to uncal herniation, tentorial shifts, CN III or VI palsy (associated with cerebellar impingement), decorticate/decerebrate posturing and respiratory arrest.
- Seizures: In first 3 days no prognostic significance; seizures beyond day 4 associated with higher risk of neurologic sequelae
- Empyema, abscesses: More common with gram negative rod meningitis (neonates); up to 90% of cases of citrobacter meningitis develop abscesses
- Hydrocephalus
- Sensorineural hearing loss (4%): Most common after *S. Pneumo* infection. Risk factors include ↑ ICP, abnormal CT, ↑, low CSF glucose, +nuchal rigidity on exam
- Recurrent meningitis (consider antibiotic tolerance in recurrent *S pneumo*)
- Other neurologic sequelae: Cortical blindness, persistent motor disabilities, hypertonia, ataxia, intellectual impairment, learning disabilities, cerebral atrophy
- Focal neurologic findings: Higher risk for complicated course
- Extremity scarring and amputation from purpura fulminans (*N meningitidis*)
- Subdural effusion (fever and focal neuro signs later in the course)
- Disseminated intravascular coagulation (DIC)/shock (poor prognosis)

Table 9.13 Chemoprophylaxis of Close Contacts* for Meningococcal Meningitis

< 1 month old	Rifampin 5 mg/kg PO/IV q 12 hours × 4 doses
> 1 month—15 years old	Rifampin 10 mg/kg PO/IV q 12 hours × 4 doses (max 600 mg/day), *or* Ceftriaxone 125 mg IM × 1
Adult	Rifampin 600 mg/day PO/IV q 12 hours × 4 doses, *or* Ceftriaxone 250 mg IM × 1, *or* Ciprofloxacin 500 mg PO × 1

* Prolonged (> 8 hours) contact while in close proximity (< 3 feet) to the patient, or directly exposed to the patient's oral secretions (mouth—mouth resuscitation, deep suctioning, endotracheal intubation) between 1 week before the onset of the symptoms until 24 hours after initiation of appropriate antibiotic therapy

Data from: *MMWR*. 2005; 54(RR-7):1.

Table 9.14 Chemoprophylaxis of Close Contacts* for Haemophilus Meningitis

< 1 month old	Rifampin 10 mg/kg PO/IV q 24 hours × 4 days
> 1 month old	Rifampin 20 mg/kg PO/IV q 24 hours × 4 days (max 600 mg/day)

* > 4 hours/day in same household/daycare or close contact for 5 of the last 7 days prior to diagnosis, or household with < 4-year-old not up-to-date on Hib vaccine, or household with immunocompromised child

Data from: *AMA*. 2007;297(1):52–60; *Clin Inf Dis.* 2004; 39: 1267–1284; *Lancet Infect Dis.* 2010; 10(1): 32–42; AAP Redbook. Report from Committee on Infectious Disease, 2012; *MMWR* CDC. 2005; 54(RR-7):1.

References: *Clin Inf Dis*. 2004; 39: 1267–1284; *Lancet Infect Dis*. 2010; 10(1): 32–42;

AAP Redbook. Report from Committee on Infectious Disease, 2012 (http://aapredbook.aappublications.org/).

OSTEOMYELITIS

OVERVIEW

- Osteomyelitis in children tends to be spread hematogenously
- Most commonly affects long bone metaphyses (~10% cases vertebral or pelvic)
- Direct inoculation of the bone via trauma or overlying skin infection occasionally is the source

CLINICAL FINDINGS

- Indolent onset common, with initial malaise and low-grade fever
- Appendicular skeleton infections generally associated with decreased use of extremity (pain with diaper changes in lower extremities of neonates)
- Refusal to ambulate, swollen extremity, and localized tenderness common
- Adjacent joint swelling, erythema, and warmth common (especially if infected bone within joint capsule)

LAB FINDINGS VARIABLE

- CRP, ESR, WBC often elevated
  - Sensitivity and specificity of each marker is variable

IMAGING

- Plain radiographs often normal early (< 7 days) in course of AHO
  - Useful to rule out oncologic causes and fractures
  - Eventually show periosteal new bone formation and lytic lesions
- MRI: Useful in cases where plain radiographs normal but clinical suspicion high
  - Accurately identifies pus collections that could be drained
  - Not affected by previous surgery
  - Frequently requires sedation to accomplish
- Scintigraphy (3-Phase technetium 99m [99mTc] bone scan):
  - Useful if high suspicion but no localizing signs or multiple sites suspected
- Ultrasound: Can identify fluid collections and elevations of periosteum
  - Useful for guiding needle aspiration of identified fluid collections

DIFFERENTIAL DIAGNOSIS

- Fracture
- Tumor: Osteosarcoma, osteoid osteoma, Ewing's sarcoma, leukemia, neuroblastoma
- Inflammatory/autoimmune: Chronic recurrent multifocal osteomyelitis
  - Children and adolescents (3–17, median 9.6 years old)
  - Multiple sites (often long bones), occasionally isolated to mandible
  - Associated with family or past history of autoimmunity
  - Radiologic appearance differs from AHO
    - Lack of fluid collections, acute inflammation, raised periosteum
  - Responds to glucocorticoids, TNF-α inhibitors, methotrexate

PATHOGENS IDENTIFIED AND TREATMENT

Isolation of pathogen important to narrowing treatment: Obtain blood culture, and fluid from identified soft tissue/sub periosteal/intra-articular collections

See section on Bacterial (Septic) Arthritis for common pathogens by age, empiric antibiotics, and antibiotic options for transitioning to oral therapy

Abbreviations: AHO: acute hematogenous osteomyelitis; CRP: C-reactive protein; ESR: erythrocyte sedimentation rate; MRI: magnetic resonance imaging; WBC: white blood cell

References: *J Pediatr Orthop.* 1995;15(2):144; *Pediatrics.* 2012;130(5):e1190; *BMC Infect Dis.* 2002;2:16; *Pediatrics.* 2009;123(2):636.

SEPTIC ARTHRITIS

Table 9.15 Limp

Cause of Limp	Presentation	Workup/ Treatment
Toxic Synovitis *(peak age 2–6 years, male > female)*	Afebrile or low-grade fevers; nontoxic; limited range of motion of involved joint; ½ follow viral infection	CBC, ESR, CRP usually normal. X-rays normal; supportive care, pain control, and close follow-up
Septic Arthritis *(usually < 5 years old, peak < 1 year old)*	Refusal to bear weight; usually febrile; ± toxic appearance; hip held flexed/ externally rotated; ± warmth/swelling at joint	Elevated WBC count, ESR and CRP; synovial fluid analysis indicated; blood culture + in 40–50%. Treated by surgical drainage
Osteomyelitis *(usually < 5 years old, pelvic ~ 8 years old; also consider vertebral osteo)*	Pain, fever, ± swelling/erythema	↑ WBC, ESR, CRP; blood culture positive in 50%; ± x-rays (may see soft-tissue swelling at metaphysis early; more reliable after 7–21 days); bone scan/MRI diagnostic; admit
Discitis *(toddlers)*	Refusal to walk or sit; decreased range of motion spine; ± fevers	Usually increased WBC, ESR, CRP; x-ray may show disc space narrowing; MRI diagnostic; admit
Psoas Muscle Abscess *(variable age)*	Fever, back pain, limp; may see abdominal or genitourinary pain; hip held flexed and child has pain when extended surgical drainage (positive "psoas sign"); may be idiopathic, hematogenous spread, or associated with pyelonephritis, Crohn's disease, appendicitis	Usually increased WBC, ESR, CRP; CT is diagnostic; usually caused by *S. aureus;* treated by surgical drainage

Data from: *J Bone Joint Surg.* 2006; 88A:1254.

Table 9.16 Predictors of Septic Hip

ESR > 40 mm/hour
WBC > 12,000/mm^3
T > 38.5°C (101.5°F)
Refusal to bear weight
CRP > 2 mg/dL

Data from: *CMAJ.* 2006;174(7):924. *Orthop Clin North Am.* 2006;37(2):133–140. *Infect Dis Clin North Am.* 2006;20(4):789–825. *Am Fam Physician.* 2005; 71(10):1949–1954. *Am Fam Physician.* 2005;72(2): 297–330.

- Clinical features of septic arthritis: Lower extremity (~80%), single joint (< 10% polyarticular) infections most common

Table 9.17 Pathogens and Clinical Findings in Septic Arthritis

Age	Pathogen	Clinical Signs/Symptoms
< 3 months old	*S. aureus*, Group B streptococcus, Gram-negative rods	Fever, irritability, sepsis, poor appetite, malaise, crying with diaper change (hip)
3 months to ≤ 5 years	*S. aureus, H. influenzae, Kingela kingae[1], strep pyogenes, strep pneumoniae*	Fever, restricted movement of extremity, irritability, poor appetite
> 5 years old	*S. aureus, strep pyogenes,* Gonorrhea (adolescents)	Hip held abducted in external rotation

Table 9.18 Lab Findings in Synovial Fluid Analysis

Bacterial arthritis	Yellow–green fluid, > 50,000 WBC/mm^3, > 75% PMNs, gram stain +. Consider PCR testing for Kingela kingae[1], especially if preschool aged, afebrile, or culture does not yield pathogen
Transient synovitis	Clear fluid, small volume, usually < 2000 WBC/mm^3, gram stain negative
Lyme arthritis	Yellowish fluid, average 25,000 WBC/mm^3 (variable), < 50% PMNs, gram stain and culture usually negative. PCR testing + in 85% cases
Gonococcal arthritis	Yellowish fluid, 25–65,000 WBC/mm^3, > 75% PMNs, gram stain and culture often negative. PCR testing + in 75% cases

Table 9.19 Nonsynovial Fluid Predictors of Septic Hip

Clinical Predictors	ESR > 40 mm/hour, serum WBC > 12,000/mm^3, temp > 38.5°C, refusal to bear weight, CRP > 2 mg/dL					
# Predictors Present	0	1	2	3	4	5
Likelihood Septic Hip	16.9%	36.7%	62.4%	82.6%	93.1%	97.5%

J Bone Joint Surg. 2004;88A:1629–1635.

MANAGEMENT: ANTIBIOTICS + EITHER JOINT ASPIRATION OR SURGICAL ARTHROTOMY

- Antibiotics
  - Empiric → pathogen and susceptibility-specific once culture results known
  - Duration 3–4 weeks of IV + PO
  - Transition from IV → PO based on resolution of fever and local signs of inflammation, improved use of extremity, normalized serum WBC, CRP decrease by > 50%, ESR decreased by > 20%
- Joint aspiration (often need repeated aspirations) *or* surgical arthrotomy
  - If possible, obtain fluid prior to initiation of antibiotics to maximize likelihood of isolating pathogen

Table 9.20 Empiric Intravenous Treatment of Bacterial Arthritis, By Age

Age	Empiric Intravenous Treatment
< 3 months old (Full term *and* > 2 kg)	Nafcillin*: 100 mg/kg/day div a 6 hr, *or* Vancomcin: 30 mg/kg/day div q 12 hr, *or* Clindamycin: 20–30 mg/kg/day div q 8 hr *And* Cefotaxime: 100–150 mg/kg/day div q 8 hr, *or* Gentamicin: 5–7.5 mg/kg/day div q 8 hr
> 3 months old to ≤ adolescent	Nafcillin*: 150 mg/kg/day div q 6 hr (max 12 g/day), *or* Vancomycin: 60 mg/kg/day div q 6–8 hr, *or* Clindamycin: 30–40 mg/kg/day div q 8 hr (max 1.8 g/day), *And* Cefotaxime: 100–150 mg/kg/day div q 6–8 hr (max 12 g/day), *or* Cefuroxime: 150 mg/kg/day div q 8 hr (max 1 g/day), *or* Ceftriaxone: 50 mg/kg daily (max 4 g/day)
Adolescents	Treat as above, but consider adding coverage for gonococcus (with third-generation cephalosporin) if gram stain negative

*Used only when community MRSA rate < 10%

Table 9.21 Oral Antibiotics for Bacterial (Septic) Arthritis

Use antibiotic with similar spectrum to those used for intravenous therapy
Higher doses than generally prescribed may be necessary to reach adequate intra-articular concentrations

- Clindamycin: 30–40 mg/kg/day div q 8 hours (max 1.8 g/day)
- Cephalexin*: 150 mg/kg/day div q 6 hours (max 4 g/day)
- Dicloxacillin*: 100 mg/kg/day div q 6 hours (max 2 g/day)
- Cefixime: 8 mg/kg/day daily or div q 12 hours (max 400 mg/day)
- Penicllin V*: 150 mg/kg/day div q 6 hours (max 3 g/day)
- Linezolid: 30 mg/kg/day div q 8 hours (max 1.8 g/day)
  - TMP-SMX (> 2 months old): 8–12 mg/kg/day div q 6 hours (doses as high as 20 mg/kg/d used in some studies)
    TMP-SMX generally not recommended due to lack of prospective data. Single retrospective study suggests efficacious and safe

*Beta-lactam drugs dosed up to 200 mg/kg/day likely safe and may provide better antibiotic levels in desired joint/bone
Data from: *J Clin Microbiol.* 2009; 47:1837—41; *J Bone Joint Surg.* 2004; 88A: 1629—1635; *Pediatrics.* 2012; Oct 130(4): e821—8; *Pediatr Infect Dis J.* 2011;30(12):1019

CRP: C-reactive protein; ESR: erythrocyte sedimentation rate; GBS: group B streptococcus; GNR: gram-negative rod; MRSA: methicillin-resistant *Staphylococcus aureus*; *S. aureus: Staphylococcus aureus*; PMN: polymorphonuclear cells

References: *J Clin Microbiol.* 2009;47:1837–1841; *Pediatrics.* 2012;130(4):e821–e828; *Pediatr Infect Dis J.* 2011;30(12):1019.

BRONCHIOLITIS[1]

■ **PATHOPHYSIOLOGY:** Acute, self limited, inflammatory disease of lower respiratory tract leading to obstruction of small airways from edema, mucous, and cellular debris.
  • Air trapping is a result of ↑ resistance during exhalation.
  • Atelectasis occurs when obstruction complete.
  • Ventilation/perfusion (V/Q) mismatch leads to hypoxemia and tachypnea.
  • Hypercapnia occurs in severely affected infants with respiratory rates > 60–70 breaths/minute, often just prior to decompensation.

■ **EPIDEMIOLOGY:** Winter outbreaks, universal infection by age 2, reinfection common. 11–12% of all infants develop bronchiolitis. 1–2% of infected infants are hospitalized. Accounts for 17% of infant hospitalizations and 200–500 deaths/year.

■ **ETIOLOGY:** Respiratory syncytial virus (*RSV*) > 50% cases. Other viruses include parainfluenza type 3, mycoplasma, adenovirus, human metapneumovirus (hMPV), influenza.

■ **RSV:** Transmission by direct or close contact with contaminated secretions.
  • Persists on countertops ~6 hours, rubber gloves ~90 minutes, hands ~30 minutes
  • Incubation period: 2–8 days.
  • Viral shedding: Usually 3–8 days, though up to 3–4 weeks in infants.

■ **DIAGNOSIS:** Clinical diagnosis based on history and physical exam.
  • General symptoms: Fever (100–104°F), malaise, copious rhinorrhea.
  • Lower respiratory symptoms: Wheezing (obstructive > bronchospasm), retractions, grunting, nasal flaring, tachypnea, hypoxia.
  • Exam varies: Migratory wheeze, rhonchi, and crackles as infant mobilizes secretions.

■ **LABS/RADIOLOGY (not necessary to confirm diagnosis or initiate treatment)**
  • RSV nasal wash: Not necessary to confirm diagnosis. Useful in rooming hospitalized patients together (cohorting) and disease surveillance.
  • Chest x-ray: Wandering atelectasis common: Often misinterpreted as lobar infiltrate. Hyperinflation, peribronchial cuffing, and streaky perihilar infiltrates common. Often leads to unnecessary antibiotics for perceived bacterial pneumonia.
  • Complete blood count: Leukocytosis and bandemia common with RSV. Not sensitive or specific for presence of bacterial superinfection during bronchiolitis.
  • Chemistry panel: Not necessary. Clinically assess hydration and PO capability.
  • Blood gas: Use as clinically indicated to determine risk of respiratory compromise.

Table 9.22 Differential Diagnosis of Bronchiolitis

• Asthma: Plus family history, no URI symptoms, repeat episode, eosinophilia
• Bacterial pneumonia: Fixed crackles, limited upper respiratory sounds, infiltrate on CXR
• Cystic fibrosis: Failure to thrive, clubbing of digits
• Congestive heart failure: Grunting, muffled heart tones, murmur
• Pertussis: Staccato, paroxysmal cough with cyanosis +/− inspiratory "whoop"
• Foreign body: Fixed exam, stridor, wheezing or crackles depending on location

CXR=Chest radiograph, URI=upper respiratory infection

■ **ADMISSION CRITERIA FOR BRONCHIOLITIS**
Severe dyspnea, dehydration (poor feeding), room air SpO$_2$ < 90–93%. Consider admission for infant ≤ 28 days in first 48–72 hours of illness (↑ apnea risk), poor social situation, or underlying condition (congenital heart disease, chronic lung disease, etc).

---

[1] *Pediatrics*. 2006;118(4):1774–1793.

Table 9.23 Treatment of Bronchiolitis

Hydration	• Consider nasogastric feeds or intravenous fluids if breathing > 60–80/minutes and/or unable to maintain hydration.
Nasal Bulb Suction	• Before feeds, before respiratory treatments and as needed. • No controlled studies of efficacy or morbidity.
Supplemental O_2	• For persistent SpO_2 < 90–92% or significant distress.
SpO_2 Monitors	• No change in outcome. ↑ hospital length of stay due to prolonged O_2 therapy. Consider spot SpO_2 checks instead.
Hypertonic Saline	• Variable results to studies on efficacy of varying concentrations (*Cochrane Rev* Jan 2008(4):CD006458, *Arch Ped Adol Med* 2009;163(11):1007–1112). • 4 ml of 3% saline nebulized at 6 liters/min shown safe without bronchodilator (*Pediatrics* 2010;126(3):e520–552).
Racemic Epinephrine	• 0.05 mL/kg/dose (max 0.5 mL) of 2.25% solution mixed with normal saline to make 3 mL, nebulized over 10–15 minutes; may nebulize standard epinephrine solution 1:1000, 0.25 mL in 2.5 mL normal saline. • Probable efficacy from ↓ in airway edema. • May also have some bronchodilation effect.
β_2-adrenergic Agonists	• ~25% of patients respond, though evidence shows little effect on clinical scores or hospital admission/length of stay. • Pre/post β_2-agonists evaluation essential. • Responders may be future asthmatics, and may be effective if subsequently readmitted with bronchiolitis.
Antibiotics	• Not generally indicated. Consider coexisting serious bacterial infection (UTI) in infants < 2 months old with fever. • 75% of OM associated with bronchiolitis is from RSV
Corticosteroids	• Not in hospitalization, length of stay, or respiratory distress assessment instrument (*Pediatrics* 1987;87:939–945.) score vs placebo (*NEJM* 2007(26);357:331–339.) • Used in adenovirus bronchiolitis to ↓ bronchiolitis obliterans.
Ribavirin	• In vitro activity vs. RSV, but NOT recommended except in select population (immunocompromised, hemodynamically significant cardiac disease). Not to be used as rescue medication. • No evidence of benefit (no change in mechanical ventilation rate, duration of PICU/hospital stay). • Potential teratogen.
• No evidence of efficacy for *antihistamines, decongestants, nasal vasoconstrictors, chest physiotherapy,* or *cool mist.*	

RSV=respiratory syncytial virus; OM=otitis media; SpO_2=Peripheral oxygen saturation; O_2=oxygen
Cochrane Database Syst Rev 2007 Jan 24;(1):CD004881; Arch Ped Adoles Med 2004;158;127–137.

■ PREVENTION

Contact isolation: Gown and glove with good hand washing and/or alcohol rub.

Encourage breast feeding and secondhand smoke avoidance.

Table 9.24 Criteria for High Risk Infants to Receive Passive RSV Passive Immunization

Palivizumab (*Synagis*): 15 mg/kg/ dose IM monthly during RSV season (November– April in northern hemisphere) = ~ five injections	• Ex-32 week or less premature infant < 2 years old with chronic lung disease (O_2, chronic steroids, bronchodilators, *and/or* diuretic requirement) • Ex-29–32 week premature infant < 6 months old at *start* of RSV season • Ex-28 week or less premature infant during first RSV season • < 12 months old with hemodynamically significant congenital heart disease

Data from: *Pediatrics* 2014;134;415–420.

■ PROGNOSIS: Most recover without sequelae.

- Apnea can occur in neonates, generally age < 1 month old (or premature infants), in first 48 hours of illness. May precede respiratory symptoms.
- Case fatality < 1% (causes: Prolonged apnea, respiratory acidosis, dehydration).
- Average duration of illness in children age < 24 months old is 12 days (18% ill at 3 weeks).

URINARY TRACT INFECTION (UTI)

■ EPIDEMIOLOGY

UTI more common in females, uncircumcised males, any male < 1 year old, Caucasians, patients with dysfunctional voiding, vesicoureteral reflux, obstruction, family history of UTI, indwelling catheter, and/or recent sexual intercourse.

■ PATHOGENS

Escherichia coli (80%), *Klebsiella, Proteus, Enterococcus*. Resistance to amoxicillin and ampicillin widespread with E. coli. Know local resistance patterns of E. coli to determine optimal presumptive outpatient therapy. Recent antibiotics, long-term prophylaxis, and complicated anatomy ↑ risk of non-E. coli and resistant pathogen.

Table 9.25 Urinalysis (UA)

Nitrites	• High specificity (98%) for Gram-negative rods. Low sensitivity (53%): Gram positive-bugs (enterococcus) and frequent urination (infants)
Leukocyte Esterase	• Breakdown product of WBC = indirect evidence of UTI
Microscopy	• Suspicious if > 8 WBC/hpf or large amount of bacteria

Table 9.26 Culture: Number Bacteria Indicative of True Urine Pathogen by Collection Method (Clean Catch not recommended collection technique)

Clean Catch not recommended Good sensitivity, poor specificity	Catheterization > 50,000 CFU/ml	Suprapubic Aspiration > 50,000 CFU/ml

CFU=Colony forming units, hpf=high-powered field, WBC=White blood cell

Table 9.27 Treatment of Acute UTI Patient Based on Age at Presentation

< 30 Days	• IV ampicillin plus either gentamicin or cefotaxime X 10–14 days (Some recommend entire course IV given possible hematogenous origin, others transition to PO once well-appearing)	
30 Days–2 Months	• IV cefotaxime, gentamicin, or cefepime until afebrile, no emesis, culture and sensitivity (C and S) known; then PO to complete 10–14 days	
2 Months–2 Years*	**Non-toxic, no emesis:** Treatment 7-14 days • AM/CL: 25–45 mg/kg/day po div tid • TMP/SMX: 8–10 mg TMP/kg/d po div bid • cefixime: 8 mg/kg po daily x 7–14 days. Max daily dose 400 mg.	**Toxic or vomiting:** • IV ceftriaxone or gentamicin initially. • Switch to PO when afebrile, no emesis, culture and sensitivities known. Complete 7–14-day course
> 2 Years Old*	• TMP/SMX or AM/CL PO x 3–5 d	

- **Complicated UTI**: Indwelling catheter, structural anomalies (reconstructed bladder), or functional defect (neurogenic bladder) leading to difficult to clear infection and/or unusual pathogens.
  - *Ciprofloxacin (> 1 year old): 20–30 mg/kg/day po div q 12 hr. Max daily dose 1.5 gm.*

AM/CL=Amoxicillin/ clavulanate, TMP/SMX=trimethoprim/ sulfamethoxazole
*Choose antibiotic based on local sensitivity patterns

■ **IMAGING**

See *Pediatrics* 2011; 128(3):595–610 & www.nice.org/uk/CG54.

- *Renal ultrasound (US)*: Identifies structural abnormalities (Hydronephrosis, perinephric abscess, calculi). Indicated for 1st febrile UTI in < 24 month olds, poor follow up, abnormal voiding pattern, abdominal mass, or symptoms > 48–72 hours despite antibiotics.
- *Contrast voiding cystourethrogram (VCUG)*: Most sensitive test for VUR. Moderate radiation dose to pelvis. Perform *after* acute infection resolved *and* voiding normal (often within 3 days of treatment). See Topic on VUR.
- *Radionucleotide cystography (RNC)*: Used for follow up of known VUR or for screening with familial VUR. RNC = one-tenth radiation dose of VCUG, but ↓ sensitivity and less accurate at grading VUR.
- *DMSA (99mTc Dimercaptosuccinic acid) scan*: Sensitive for renal scars; only necessary if will change management.

VESICOURETERAL REFLUX (VUR)

■ **EPIDEMIOLOGY**

30–40% young children with febrile urinary tract infection (UTI) and ~1% all newborns have VUR. May predispose to recurrent infection, renal scarring, hypertension, glomerular dysfunction, and end-stage renal disease.

■ **SCREENING RECOMMENDATIONS**

Various screening protocols exist

- *Renal ultrasound*: Used to screen for hydronephrosis, anomalies, scarring.
- *VCUG/RNC*: Perform for evidence of hydronephrosis or scarring. Value of knowing presence of low-grade VUR unclear. Depends on efficacy of continuous antibiotic prophylaxis. Radiation dose: RNC < VCUG.
- *DMSA*: Very sensitive to renal scarring. Presence of scarring may be more useful than presence of VUR in determining who deserves prophylaxis.

N Engl J Med. 2003;348(3):195–202.
Pediatrics 2011;128(3):595–610
nice.org.uk/CG54.
J Urol 2010;184:1134.

Table 9.28 Grading of Vesicoureteral Reflux

- *Grade I*: Reflux of urine into ureter; no dilation of ureter.
- *Grade II*: Reflux into ureter and renal pelvis without dilation.
- *Grade III*: Mildly dilated ureter, collecting system and blunting of calyces.
- *Grade IV*: Grossly dilated ureter and collecting system. Half of calyces blunted.
- *Grade V*: Tortuously dilated ureter, all calyces blunted, possible cortical thinning.

Table 9.29 Management of VUR (By Grade)

Resolution in first 5 years of life common. Depends on age, laterality, and grade of VUR. Resolution calculator at deflux.com)

Grade I–II	• Antibiotic prophylaxis an option, though controversial. • Repeat VCUG or RNC in 12–24 months. • If bilateral VUR or scarring, refer to pediatric urologist.
Grade III–V	• Consider antibiotic prophylaxis and refer to pediatric urologist for evaluation. • < 2 years old, often watch and wait with repeat VCUG/RNC every 12–24 months. • > 2 years old, failed prophylaxis, poor social situation or high-grade renal scarring: Consider reimplantation (open/laparoscopic/robotic) vs. endoscopic peri-ureteral hyaluronidase injection (Deflux®).

Table 9.30 Options for Continuous Antibiotic Prophylaxis by Age

< 2 months old	Cephalexin: 10 mg/kg PO nightly
> 2 months old	TMP/SMX: 2 mg TMP/kg po *or* nitrofurantoin 1–2 mg/kg po nightly

■ CONTINUOUS ANTIBIOTIC PROPHYLAXIS

Goal is ***prevention of renal scarring*** though data mixed on efficacy. 2010 AUA guidelines recommend prophylaxis for recurrent febrile UTI, renal scarring, child age < 1 (with any grade VUR and a history of febrile UTI, or Grade III–V VUR in the absence of UTI), presence of bowel/bladder dysfunction, or obstruction. Observation with prompt initiation of antibiotics for UTI is option in all other patients.

J Urol. 2010;184(3):1145–1151.
auanet.org/content/guidelines.

■ SCREENING OF SIBLINGS

~25% of sibling concurrence of VUR. Clinical significance of asymptomatic VUR (no previous febrile UTI) in sibling unclear, and screening is an "option" in AUA VUR guidelines. Cost of screening to prevent future UTI high, and concern exists regarding unnecessary exposure to radiation.

Pediatrics. 2010;126:865–871.

CONGENITAL HEART DISEASE SCREENING

TECHNIQUE

- Place pulse oximetry probe on right hand *and* either foot
- High specificity (unlikely to have false negatives), moderate sensitivity
- Measurements more successful when infant calm and awake
- Consider screening for CCHD at same time as hearing screen

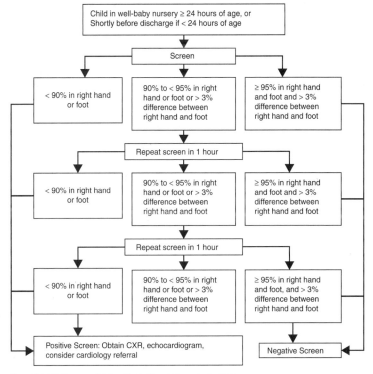

Figure 10.1 CDC-Recommended Algorithm for Neonatal Screening for CCHD

Reprodeuced from http://www.cdc.gov/ncbddd/pediatricgenetics/pulse.html (accessed 12/7/12).

IMPLICATIONS OF POSITIVE SCREEN

- In European study of > 38,000 newborns, 87 positive screens
  - 18/87 (20.6%) newborns with + screens had CCHD:
    - Tetralogy of Fallot, total anomalous pulmonary venous return, truncus arteriosus, tricuspid atresia, transposition of great vessels, hypoplastic left heart syndrome, pulmonary atresia with intact septum
  - Of the remaining 69 + screens, 35% were normal (false +) and 65% had another problem:
    - Persistent pulmonary hypertension of the newborn, transitional circulation, other congenital heart defects, infections, pulmonary causes

References: *BMJ.* 2009;338:a3037; CDC: http://www.cdc.gov/ncbddd/pediatricgenetics/pulse.html (accessed 12/7/12); *Pediatrics.* 2011;128:e000; *Pediatrics.* 2012;129(1):190–192.

GBS PROPHYLAXIS

Table 10.1   Indications and Non-indications for Intrapartum Antibiotic Prophylaxis to Prevent Early-Onset Group B Streptococcal (GBS) Disease

Intrapartum GBS Prophylaxis Indicated	Intrapartum GBS Prophylaxis Not Indicated

• Previous infant with invasive GBS disease
• GBS bacteriuria during any trimester of the current pregnancy*
• Positive GBS vaginal–rectal screening culture in late gestation[†] during current pregnancy*
• Unknown GBS status at the onset of labor (culture not done, incomplete, or results unknown) and any of the following:
  – Delivery at < 37 weeks' gestation[§]
  – Amniotic membrane rupture ≥ 18 hours
  – Intrapartum temperature ≥ 100.4°F (≥ 38.0°C)[¶]
  – Intrapartum NAAT** positive for GBS
	• Colonization with GBS during a previous pregnancy (unless an indication for GBS prophylaxis is present for current pregnancy)
	• GBS bacteriuria during previous pregnancy (unless an indication for GBS prophylaxis is present for current pregnancy)
	• Negative vaginal and rectal GBS screening culture in late gestation[†] during the current pregnancy, regardless of intrapartum risk factors
	• Cesarean delivery performed before onset of labor on a woman with intact amniotic membranes, regardless of GBS colonization status or gestational age

* Intrapartum antibiotic prophylaxis is not indicated in this circumstance if a cesarean delivery is performed before onset of labor on a woman with intact amniotic membranes

† Optimal timing for prenatal GBS screening is at 35–37 weeks' gestation

§ Recommendations for the use of intrapartum antibiotics for prevention of early-onset GBS disease in the setting of threatened preterm delivery are presented in Figures 10.5 and 10.6

¶ If amnionitis is suspected, broad-spectrum antibiotic therapy that includes an agent known to be active against GBS should replace GBS prophylaxis

** NAAT testing for GBS is optional and might not be available in all settings. If intrapartum NAAT is negative for GBS but any other intrapartum risk factor (delivery at < 37 weeks' gestation, amniotic membrane rupture at ≥ 18 hours, or temperature ≥ 100.4°F [≥ 38.0°C]) is present, then intrapartum antibiotic prophylaxis is indicated

Abbreviation: GBS: Group B Streptococcus; NAAT: Nucleic acid amplification tests

Data from: Prevention of Perinatal Group B Streptococcal Disease. *MMWR.* November 19, 2010, Vol. 59, No. RR-10. www.cdc.gov/mmwr

HYPERTENSION

All medications should be used in conjunction with specialist familiar with treating neonatal hypertension (neonatologist, pediatric nephrologist)

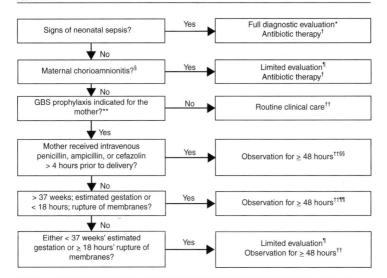

* Full diagnostic evaluation includes a blood culture, a complete blood count (CBC) including white blood cell differential and platelet counts, chest radiograph (if respiratory abnormalities are present), and lumbar puncture (if patient is stable enough to tolerate procedure and sepsis is suspected)
† Antibiotic therapy should be directed toward the most common causes of neonatal sepsis, including intravenous ampicillin for GBS and coverage for other organisms (including *Escherichia coli* and other gram-negative pathogens) and should take into account local antibiotic resistance patterns
§ Consultation with obstetric providers is important to determine the level of clinical suspicion for chorioamnionitis. Chorioamnionitis is diagnosed clinically and some of the signs are nonspecific
¶ Limited evaluation includes blood culture (at birth) and CBC with differential and platelets (at birth and/or at 6–12 hours of life)
** See Table 10.1 for indications for intrapartum GBS prophylaxis
†† If signs of sepsis develop, a full diagnostic evaluation should be conducted and antibiotic therapy initiated
§§ If ≥ 37 weeks' gestation, observation may occur at home after 24 hours if other discharge criteria have been met, access to medical care is readily available, and a person who is able to comply fully with instructions for home observation will be present. If any of these conditions is not met, the infant should be observed in the hospital for at least 48 hours and until discharge criteria are achieved
¶¶ Some experts recommend a CBC with differential and platelets at age 6–12 hours

Data from: *MMWR*. November 19, 2010, Vol. 59, No. RR-10. www.cdc.gov/mmwr; *Pediatrics*. 2011;128(3):611–616; *Pediatrics*. 2012;129:1006.

Figure 10.2 Algorithm for secondary prevention of early-onset group B streptococcal (GBS) disease among newborns

Table 10.2 Treatment Options for Neonatal Hypertension

	Class	Administration	Comments
Captopril (*Capoten®*)	ACE inhibitor	0.01–0.5 mg/kg tid (max 6 mg/kg QD)	Drug of choice monitor Cr/K⁺
Clonidine (*Catapres®*)	Central α agonist	0.05–0.1 mg bid–tid	Side effects: dry mouth, sedation, rebound hypertension
Hydralazine (*Apresoline®*)	Vasodilator (arteriolar)	0.25–1.0 mg/kg tid–qid (max 7.5 mg/kg qd)	Suspension stable up to 1 week Tachycardia and fluid retention common Lupus-like syndrome in slow acetylators

(Continued)

Table 10.2   Treatment Options for Neonatal Hypertension *(Continued)*

	Class	Administration	Comments
Minoxidil *(Loniten®)*	Vasodilator (arteriolar)	0.1–0.2 mg/kg per dose bid–tid	Most potent oral vasodilator—excellent for refractory HTN
Isradipine *(Prescal®)*	Ca²⁺ channel blocker	0.05–0.15 mg/kg qid (max 0.8 mg/kg qd)	Suspension may be compounded Useful for both acute and chronic HTN
Amlodipine *(Norvasc®)*	Ca²⁺ channel blocker	0.1–0.3 mg/kg bid (max 0.6 mg/kg per day)	Less likely to cause sudden hypotension than isradipine
Propranolol *(Inderal®)*	β blocker	0.5–1.0 mg/kg tid (max 8–10 mg/kg qd)	Maximal dose depends on heart rate. Avoid in infants with BPD
Labetalol *(Normodyne®, Trandate®)*	α and β blocker	1.0 mg/kg bid–tid (max.10 mg/kg qd)	Monitor heart rate Avoid in infants with BPD
Spironolactone *(Aldactone®)*	Aldosterone antagonist	0.5–1.5 mg/kg bid	Potassium "sparing" Monitor electrolytes Takes several days to see maximum effectiveness
Hydrochlorothiazide *(Hydrodiuril®)*	Thiazide	1–3 mg/kg qid	Monitor electrolytes
Chlorothiazide *(Diuril®)*	Thiazide	5–15 mg/kg bid	Monitor electrolytes
Diazoxide *(Hyperstat®)*	Vasodilator (arteriolar)	2–5 mg/kg per dose Rapid bolus injection	Slow injection ineffective Duration unpredictable Use with caution—may cause rapid hypotension
Enalaprilat *(Vasotec®)*	ACE inhibitor	15 ± 5 mg/kg per dose over 5–10 min	Repeat q 8–24 hr May cause prolonged hypotension and acute renal insufficiency
Esmolol *(Brevibloc®)*	β1 blocker	100–300 mg/kg/min	Short-acting—constant infusion necessary
Hydralazine *(Apresoline®)*	Vasodilator (arteriolar)	0.15–0.6 mg/kg/dose 0.75–5.0 mg/kg/min	Tachycardia frequent side effect Administer q 4 hr when given as an IV bolus
Labetalol *(Trandate®)*	α and β blocker	0.20–1.0 mg/kg/dose 0.25–3.0 mg/kg/hr	Heart failure and BPD relative contraindications
Nicardipine *(Cardene®)*	Ca⁺² channel blocker	1–3 mg/kg/min	May cause reflex tachycardia
Sodium nitroprusside *(Nitropress®)*	Vasodilator (arteriolar and venous)	0.5–10 mg/kg/min	Thiocyanate toxicity can occur with prolonged (> 72 hr) use or in renal failure

INFANT OF DIABETIC MOTHER

CONDITIONS ASSOCIATED WITH INFANTS OF DIABETIC MOTHERS (IDM)
- Increased risk of congenital malformations, including:
  - Cardiac: TGA, truncus arteriosus, tricuspid atresia, HLHS

- Recommend fetal echo or level II US in second trimester
- If ventricular septal hypertrophy noted, check postnatal echo to document cardiac function, as at risk for CHF
  - ○ Neural tube defects: Meningomyelocele, encephalocele
  - ○ Skeletal defects: Caudal regression, syringomyelia
  - ○ Gastrointestinal: Duodenal atresia, small left colon syndrome
  - ○ Genitourinary: Hydronephrosis, renal agenesis, cystic kidneys
- 1% of all pregnancies occur in mothers with preexisting type I or II diabetes
  - ○ Preconceptional HbA1c and predicted risk of congenital anomaly
    - HbA1c < 7%: no increased risk over general population (2% risk)
    - HbA1c ~9%: 6% risk of congenital anomaly
    - HbA1c ~11.8%: 12% risk of congenital anomaly
    - HbA1c > 13.9%: 20% risk of congenital anomaly

CONDITIONS COMMON IN IDMs REQUIRING POSTNATAL MONITORING

- Macrosomia: Seen in 15–45% of IDMs; increased risk shoulder dystocia
- Hypoglycemia: Due to in utero hyperinsulism needed to maintain euglycemia
- Polycythemia: Increased metabolism from hyperglycemia leads to relative fetal hypoxia → increased RBCs to increase O_2-carrying capacity
- Hyperbilirubinemia: Due to increased RBC load and delayed liver function
- Respiratory distress due to delayed lung maturation/decreased surfactant

Abbreviations: CCHD: Congenital coronary heart disease; CHF: Congestive heart failure; HLHS: Hypoplastic left heart syndrome; RBC: Red blood cell; TGA: Transposition of the great arteries; US: Ultrasound.

References: *Diabetes Care.* 2007;30(7):1920–1925. *Arch Dis Child.* 1979;54(8):635–637.

NEONATAL ABSTINENCE/WITHDRAWAL

Prenatal exposure to illicit drugs (cocaine, opiates, marijuana, hallucinogens, nonmedical use of prescription drugs, methamphetamine) can lead to multiple adverse outcomes: Intrauterine growth restriction (IUGR), prematurity, postnatal withdrawal, postnatal neurodevelopmental/behavior problems

PREVALENCE

Data from 2009 suggest pregnant women between 15–44 years of age, 4.5% used illicit drugs, 11.9% drank alcohol ("binge or heavy drinking") in first trimester, 15.3% continued tobacco use

CNS DEPRESSANTS

Classic "neonatal abstinence syndrome" (NAS) validated on infants exposed to opiates. Benzodiazepines and barbiturates may cause similar symptoms in withdrawing infants

CNS STIMULANTS

Cocaine, methamphetamine, etc., do not have a defined abstinence syndrome. May see hyperactivity, high-pitched cry, excessive sucking, poor coordination of feeds. Often note symptoms in first few postnatal days

MARIJUANA

Not associated with an overt withdrawal syndrome, but may have effect on long-term neurobehavioral development

ONSET OF WITHDRAWAL SYMPTOMS

Depends on type of drug, dose, duration, frequency, proximity to delivery, neonatal metabolism

Table 10.3   Onset of Withdrawal Symptoms in Neonatal Abstinence Syndromes

Drug	Typical Onset	Range
Heroin	< 24 hours	1–7 days
Methadone	24–72 hours	1–7 days
Buprenorphine	24–48 hours	1–5 days
Barbiturate	4–7 days	1–14 days
Ethanol	3–12 hours	

COMPONENTS OF NEONATAL ABSTINENCE SCORING (SCORE IN BRACKETS)

- Central Nervous System Disturbances
  - Cry quality and duration: Excessive [2], continuous [3]
  - Sleep duration after feeding: < 1 hour [3], < 2 hours [2], < 3 hours [1]
  - Moro reflex: Hyperactive [2], markedly hyperactive [3]
  - Tremors when disturbed: mild [1], moderate [2]
  - Tremors at rest: mild [3], moderate–severe [4]
  - Muscle tone: Increased [1]
  - Excoriations on chin, knees, elbows, toes, nose [1]
  - Myoclonic jerks [3]
  - Generalized seizure activity [5]
- Metabolic/Vasomotor Disturbances
  - Sweating [1]
  - Temperature of 38.0–38.3°C [1]
  - Temperature of > 38.3°C [2]
  - Yawning > 3–4 times per scoring interval [1]
  - Mottling of skin [1]
  - Nasal stuffiness [1]
  - Sneezing > 3–4 times per scoring interval [1]
- Respiratory Disturbances
  - Nasal flaring [2]
  - Respiratory rate > 60 breaths/minute [10]
  - Respiratory rate > 60 breaths/minute + retractions [2]
- Gastrointestinal Disturbances
  - Excessive sucking [1]
  - Poor feeding (infrequent/uncoordinated suck) [2]
  - Regurgitation (≥ 2 times during/post-feeding) [2]
  - Projectile vomiting [3]
  - Loose stools [2]
  - Watery stools [3]

FREQUENCY OF SCORING:

- First score ~ 2 hours after birth
- If any score ≥ 8, then subsequent scores q 2 hours until 24 hours from last score ≥ 8
- If initial score < 8, then subsequent scores every 4 hours
- Discontinue scoring when scores persistently < 8 without pharmacologic therapy, taking into account usual time frame of onset of symptoms (generally at least 3 days, longer for methadone)

TREATMENT:

- Consider initiation of pharmacologic therapy if 3 consecutive scores ≥ 8, and not responding to nonpharmacologic interventions
- Nonpharmacologic interventions:
  - Minimize excessive light, sound, and other external stimulation
  - Swaddle to avoid "auto-stimulation"
  - Comforting techniques (swaying, rocking)
  - Small-volume, frequent feeding
  - Hypercaloric formula (or augmented breast milk) to reach 150–250 kcal/kg/day (due to increased energy expenditure, regurgitation, loose stools)
- Opiate Pharmacologic Interventions:
  - Methadone: 0.05–0.2 mg/kg q 6–12 hours. Increase by 0.05–0.1 mg/kg/dose q 6–12 hours to effect (withdrawal score < 8). Wean by 10% of dose q 48–72 hours depending on abstinence scores.
  - Morphine: Initial: 0.04 mg/kg PO q 3–4 hours. Increase by 0.04 mg/kg dose to max 0.2 mg/kg/dose
- Adjuvant/Nonopiate Pharmacologic Interventions:
  - Clonidine: 0.5–1 mcg/kg PO q 3–6 hours as needed (max 1 mcg/kg/dose)
  - Lorazepam: 0.05–0.1 mg/kg/dose PO or IV as needed
  - Phenobarbital: 4–5 mg/kg/day PO or IV divided q 12–24 hours (usual dose 2–8 mg/kg/day)

References: *Pediatrics*. 2012;129:e540-e560; 2009 National Survey on Drug Use and Health: Substance Abuse and Mental Health Services Administration; *Current Therapy In Neonatal-Perinatal Medicine*, 2d ed. Ontario: BC Decker; 1990; *Acta Paediatr*. 2008;97(10):1358–1361; *Neoreviews*. 2009;10(5):222–229.

NEONATAL RESUSCITATION

- Birth
  - Immediately assess gestation, respirations, and tone
    - Normal:
      - Warm, dry, clear airway, standard physical examination
      - Stay with mother and provide routine care
    - Abnormal: Premature, impaired respirations, poor tone
      - Clear airway, stimulate, warm, dry
      - Re evaluate at 30 seconds of life (see next section)
- 30 seconds of life
  - Assess heart rate (HR goal > 100 bpm) and respirations
    - HR < 100 beats per minute (bpm), apnea *or* gasping:
      - Initiate positive pressure ventilation (PPV) and check SpO_2
        - See table below for goal SpO_2 by minute of life
      - Reevaluate at 60 seconds of life (see next section)
    - HR > 100 bpm *but* cyanotic or labored breathing:
      - Clear airway, check SpO_2, consider CPAP
      - Reevaluate at 60 seconds of life (see next section)
    - HR > 100, unlabored breathing → Routine care
      - Warm, dry, clear airway, standard physical examination
      - Routine care
- 60 seconds of life and beyond for the ill neonate
  - Assess heart rate (HR goal > 100 bpm)
    - HR > 100 bpm → post-resuscitation care (see below)
    - HR < 100 bpm despite PPV/BVM

- Ensure adequate ventilation/initiate corrective steps
  - Corrective steps: Readjust mask, reposition airway, suction mouth and nose, open mouth slightly
- HR < 60 bpm
  - Consider endotracheal intubation
    - Laryngeal mask airway (LMA) is option in infants > 1500 g where intubation not feasible
  - Initiate chest compressions (coordinated with PPV)
    - 2-thumb technique encircling chest
    - 2-finger technique: tips of 1st/2nd fingers on sternum
      - Apply pressure on lower 1/3 of sternum and perpendicular to sternum
      - Depth of compressions 1/3 of AP diameter of chest
      - Rate: 3 compressions: 1 breath
        - 90 compressions/minute: 30 breaths per minute
- Reassess after 30 seconds of appropriate PPV and chest compressions
  - HR > 100 bpm, spontaneous respirations → post-resuscitative care
  - HR 60–100 bpm: Reassess ventilation with corrective steps as above
  - HR < 60 bpm: Continue CPR and PPV (Reassess ventilation with corrective steps as above). Consider:
    - Epinephrine (1:10,000 solution)
      - IV [first-line] 0.01–0.03 mg/kg (0.1–0.3 mL/kg) q 3–5 min
        - Endotracheal (only if no IV access): 0.03–0.1 mg/kg q 3–5 min = 0.3–1 mL/kg of 1:10,000 soln
    - Hypovolemia: 0.9% saline 10 mL/kg over 5–10 minutes
    - Sodium bicarbonate: 1 mEq/kg over at least 1 minute

Table 10.4 Goal SpO$_2$ by Minute of Life

Minutes	1 min	2 min	3 min	4 min	5 min	10 min
Goal SpO$_2$	60–65%	65–70%	70–75%	75–80%	80–85%	85–95%

Data from: AHA Guidelines for CPR, 2010. *Circulation* 2010; 122:S909–919.

POSITIVE PRESSURE VENTILATION (PPV)

- Self-inflating bag: Does not require compressed gas source
  - With oxygen reservoir and O$_2$ source: Delivers FiO$_2$ ~90–100%
  - Without O$_2$ reservoir: FiO$_2$ depends on flow of attached O$_2$ source
    - FiO$_2$ likely 30–60% at flows of 1–2 L/min 100% O$_2$
  - Release valve can be set to determine tidal volumes and pressures
    - Initial breath in term infants may require high pressures (30–40 cm H$_2$O)
    - Subsequent breaths: goal tidal volume 4–5 mL/kg^2
- Flow-inflating bag (anesthesia bag): Requires compressed gas source
  - Requires "tight" face-mask seal to inflate bag
  - Requires manometer to monitor pressures, as no built-in "pop-off" valve
- T-piece resuscitator (Neopuff™)
  - Simple ventilator circuit that can be used in delivery room
  - Connect to gas sources (oxygen and air, with blender)

   ○ Set max inspiratory pressure and PEEP, then attach t-piece to ETT
   ○ Covering PEEP valve delivers controlled positive-pressure breath for duration that PEEP valve is covered
   ○ Uncover valve to allow exhalation

POSSIBLE CAUSES OF LACK OF RESPONSE TO RESUSCITATION

- Impaired lung function:
  ○ Pneumothorax, pleural effusion, congenital diaphragmatic hernia
- Mechanical obstruction of airways:
  ○ Laryngeal web, meconium or mucous plug
- Cardiac abnormalities:
  ○ Congenital cyanotic heart disease or heart block
- Neurologic abnormalities:
  ○ Neuromuscular disorder, hypoxic–ischemic injury, maternal opioids
  ○ Maternal opioids
    – Naloxone: No longer recommended, as adequate oxygenation and ventilation usually sufficient to resuscitate opioid-affected infants

NONINITIATION AND WITHHOLDING RESUSCITATION

- Parental involvement:
  ○ Discussion with parents should preferably occur prior to birth of infant
  ○ Parents should be full participants in resuscitation decision making
  ○ If prognosis unclear, but likely poor or associated with significant morbidity, parental wishes should determine resuscitative efforts
- Noninitiation (know local laws and outcomes data relevant to resuscitation):
  ○ Appropriate if infant likely to die or survive with very high morbidity
  ○ Appropriate if prenatal diagnosis confirms anencephaly, certain chromosomal anomalies generally not compatible with life (trisomy 13, trisomy 18, etc.), gestational age < 23 weeks, or estimated birth weight < 400 g

DISCONTINUATION OF RESUSCITATION

- No signs of life (no heart beat or respiratory effort for > 10 minutes) after at least 10 minutes of resuscitation, *or*
- If outcome likely death or high morbidity as determined by information gained during resuscitation
  ○ Should confer with parents before discontinuing resuscitation efforts

Abbreviations: bpm: beats per minute; BVM: bag-valve mask ventilation; CPAP: continuous positive airway pressure; HR: heart rate; PPV: positive pressure ventilation; SpO_2: oxygen saturation

References: *Circulation*. 2010;122:S909–S919; *J Pediatr*. 2008;153(6):741–745; *Cochrane Database Syst Rev*. 2005; Apr 18(2):CD003314; *Pediatrics*. 2007;119:401–403.

FLUIDS AND ELECTROLYTES IN NEONATES

Full-term total body water (TBW) = 75% (35% ICF + 40% ECF)
   Pre-term TBW = 90% (30% ICF + 60% ECF)

Table 10.5   Fluid Requirements for Newborns

	Total Fluids	Glucose	Na	K	Ca†
Term Infant DOL 1	D10W 60–80 mL/kg/day	6–7 mg/kg/min	0	0	calcium gluconate 200–400 mg/kg/d***
Term Infant DOL 2–7	D10W 80–120 mL/kg/day (↑ 10–20 mL/kg/day from baseline if tolerated)	↑ by 10–15%/day if tolerated	2–4 meq/kg/day (adjust to keep serum sodium 135–145 meq/L)	1–3 meq/kg/day (document urine output first)	
Preterm Infant DOL 1–3	< 800 g: D5W 120–140 mL/kg/day; 800–1000 g: D7.5W 80–100 mL/kg/day;	5–6 mg/kg/min	2–4 meq/kg/day (adjust to keep serum sodium 135–145 meq/L)	1–3 meq/kg/day (document urine output first)	
Preterm Infant DOL 3–7	May begin to approach term rec's; adjust as tolerated.	↑ by 10–15%/day if tolerated	2–4 meq/kg/day (adjust to keep serum sodium 135–145 meq/L)	1–3 meq/kg/day (document urine output first)	

* ↑ fluid rate if weight loss is > expected, ↓ urine output (urine output should be > 1 mL/kg/hr after DOL 1), ↑ urine specific gravity, and/or ↑ serum sodium. Fluid restriction recommended for infants with: RDS, BPD, PDA, HIE
** If fluid rate is changed, glucose concentration must be adjusted to keep glucose delivery stable
*** Ca should not be infused by peripheral line but intermittent doses of calcium gluconate 50–100 mg/kg IV q 6 hr can be used with close monitoring for extravasation. Can continuously infuse in central line after position confirmed
† Ca supplementation most important in preterm, SGA, asphyxiated, septic, postoperative, infants of a diabetic mother

Table 10.6   Laboratory Monitoring for Young Infant on IV Fluids in First Week of Life

Birth Weight	Frequency of Electrolyte and Ca++ Measurement
< 750 g	q 8–12 hr × 3–4d, then daily
750–1,500 g	q 12 hr × 3–4 days, then daily
> 1,500 g	Daily

Table 10.7   Neonatal Nutritional Requirements

Nutritional Component	Daily Requirement
Total daily caloric requirements (cal/kg/day)	**Term:** 100–120 kcal/kg/day (goal 15–30g/day wt gain) **Preterm:** 110–150 kcal/kg/day (goal 15 g/day/day) **BPD, CHD, other illness:** may require 160–180 kca/kg/day
Carbohydrate requirements	11–15 g/kg/day (30–60% total calories)
Protein Requirements	2–4 g/kg/day (max 4 g/kg/day; 7–16% total calories)
Fats	4–6 g/kg/day (< 55% total calories to avoid ketosis); 2–5% linoleic acid, 0.6% linolenic acid

(Continued)

Table 10.7   Neonatal Nutritional Requirements *(Continued)*

Nutritional Component	Daily Requirement
Vitamin A	Term: 500 IU; Preterm: 1400 IU
Vitamin D	Term: 400 IU; Preterm: 600 IU
Vitamin E	Term: 5 IU; Preterm: 5–25 IU
Vitamin C	Term: 20 mg; Preterm: 60 mg
Vitamin K	15 mcg (same for term and preterm)
Thiamine	0.2 mg (same for term and preterm)
Riboflavin	0.4 mg (same for term and preterm)
Niacin	5 mg (same for term and preterm)
Vitamin B_6	0.4 mg (same for term and preterm)
Vitamin B_{12}	1.5 mcg (same for term and preterm)
Folic acid	50 mcg (same for term and preterm)
Biotin	6 mcg (same for term and preterm)
Calcium	Term: 60 mg/kg; Preterm: 200 mg/kg
Phosphorous	Term: 40 mg/kg; Preterm: 100 mg/kg
Magnesium	8 mg/kg (same for term and preterm)
Sodium	Term: 1–2 meq/kg; preterm: 2–3.5 meq/kg; 1500 g: 4–8 meq/kg
Potassium	2–3 meq/kg (same for term and preterm)
Iron	Term: 6–10 mg; preterm 2 mg/kg after 8 wks of age
Copper	Term: 35 mcg/kg; Preterm: 110 mcg/kg
Zinc	Term: 500 mcg/kg; Preterm: 1300 mcg/kg

Table 10.8   Total Parenteral Nutrition in Neonates

Total fluid volume (mL/kg/day)	See above
Total daily caloric requirements (cal/kg/day)	**Term:** 100–120 kcal/kg/day (goal 15–30 g/day wt gain) **Preterm:** 110–150 kcal/kg/day (goal 15 g/kg/day) **BPD, CHD, other illness:** may require 160–180 kca/kg/day
Dextrose concentration and glucose infusion rate (mg/kg/min)	Usually start D10 at 6–8 mg/kg/min*; ↑ by 1–2 mg/kg/min/day to max ~ 15 mg/kg/min (Max dextrose through peripheral catheter is D12.5; central may go up to D25). Follow urine to assess for glucosuria
Protein (g/kg/day)/amino acids**	Start after infant is getting at least 40 g/kg/day glucose. **< 1500 g:** start at 0.5 g/kg/day, max in premature infants 1.5 g/kg/day. **Term infants:** start at 1.5 g/kg/day to max 3 g/kg/day.
Lipid (g/kg/day) *Start at 24–30 hr life	< 1000 g: 0.5 g/kg/day 1000–2000 g: 1–2 g/kg/day >2000 g: 2–3 g/kg/day Goal 3 g/kg/d, follow TG levels

(Continued)

Table 10.8   Total Parenteral Nutrition in Neonates *(Continued)*

Electrolytes	Only added electrolyte in first 2–3 days should be Ca. -Start Na at ~2 days -Start K once voiding and serum K < 3.5 -Ca, Mg, Phos, Cl, Acetate depending on labs
Trace elements	Zn (term: 100 mcg, preterm 500 mcg), Cu (term/preterm 20 mcg), Mn (2–10 mch term/preterm), Cr (0.15–0.2 mcg), Mo, I (3–5 mcg)
Vitamins	Neonatal or pediatric MVI

*Glucose requirement (mg/kg/min) = (% glucose × Rate (cc/hr) × 0.167)/wt (kg)
OR Glucose requirement = (glucose/mL of fluid × total fluids)/wt (kg)
** 1 g/kg/day protein = 100 mL/kg/day of 1% AA solution; 3 g/kg/day = 100 mL/kg/day of 3% AA solution

Table 10.9   Monitoring of Infants on TPN

Daily	Weight, OFC, Glucose, Electrolytes (qd initially then 2–3 ×/week); qod BUN/creatinine; urine specific gravity and glucose each void initially then bid.
Weekly	Length, Mg, bilirubin, ammonia, total protein, albumin, ALT/AST, Tg

Table 10.10   Glucose and Energy Content of Dextrose Solutions

D5W (5%)	50 mg/mL (0.17 kcal/ml)
D10W (10%)	100 mg/mL (0.34 kcal/mL)
D12.5W (12.5%)	125 mg/mL (0.425 kcal/mL)
D15W (15%)	150 mg/mL (0.51 kcal/mL)
D25W (25%)	250 mg/mL (0.85 kcal/mL)

*Please see also **Chapter 13: Nutrition** for more information about infant formulas and infant nutrition.

Table 10.11   Enteral Feeds of newborns in NICU

< 1250 g	Start non-nutritive feeds within 12 hr (2 cc/kg sterile water first feed); 10–15 cc/kg/d in q 4 hr bolus; if tolerates then may advance to formula as tolerated
1250–1750 g	Start within 12 hr; 20 mL/kg/day (i.e., 4–5 mL/kg/feed q 2–3 hr)
> 1750 g or term	Start feeds within 6 hr; q 1–4 hr or ad lib

* For preemies, advance by 10–20 cc/kg/d to reach goal by 2 weeks of life. Monitor for abdominal distension, emesis, residuals

INTRAUTERINE GROWTH RETARDATION

Table 10.12   Causes of Intrauterine Growth Retardation (IUGR)

Fetal	Placental	Maternal
• Chromosomal anomalies • TORCH infection • Congenital syndromes • Multiple gestation • Insulin deficiency • Insulin-like growth factor type I deficiency	• ↓ Placental weight, surface area, or cellularity • Placental infection • Placental infarction • Placental separation • Twin–twin transfusion	• Hypertension • Hypoxemia • Malnutrition • Sickle cell anemia • Drugs (tobacco, alcohol, cocaine, methamphetamine)

(Continued)

Table 10.12 Causes of Intrauterine Growth Retardation (IUGR) *(Continued)*

- Symmetric IUGR (involves head, length, and weight): Often due to early gestational insult/infection (TORCH) or chromosomal anomaly. Generally worse prognosis, with frequent neurologic problems
- Asymmetric IUGR: More likely late gestational event, such as placental insufficiency. Generally good prognosis

- Prolonged in-hospital newborn observation as ↑ risk for hypoglycemia, polycythemia, hyperbilirubinemia, and temperature instability

TORCH: Toxoplasma, "other" (such as syphilis), rubella, cytomegalovirus, hepatitis, HIV
Reprinted with permission Elsevier publishing. Originally printed in *J Pediatrics*. 1991;119:417–423.

Table 10.13 Characterization of Fetal Growth

Appropriate for gestational age (AGA)	Birth weight 10th and 90th percentile for given gestational age (GA)
Small for gestational age (SGA)	Birth weight > 90th percentile for GA
Large for gestational age (LGA)	Birth weight < 3–10th percentile or −2 standard deviations below mean weight for GA
IUGR	↓ Expected fetal growth pattern

Table 10.14 Workup/Management of Infants with IUGR

Physical exam, look closely for dysmorphic features (this will determine further workup)
Labs (CBCD, serum electrolytes, and Ca++)
May have increased total fluid and calorie requirements

NEONATAL MECHANICAL VENTILATION

Table 10.15 Indications for Mechanical Ventilation of Neonates

Hypercarbia: arterial pH < 7.20 and $PaCO_2$ > 60 mm Hg
Hypoxemia: arterial PaO_2 < 50 mm Hg despite oxygen ≥ 70% on nasal CPAP
Severe apnea
Decrease metabolic demand for very ill infants or congenital heart disease

Table 10.16 Endotracheal Tube (ETT) Guidelines

Preterm infant	2.0–3.0 F, 8–9 cm deep
Full-term infant	3–3.5 F, 10 cm deep

- ↑ Oxygenation by ↑ FiO_2 or ↑ mean airway pressure (affected by I:E ratio, PIP, and PEEP)
- ↓ $PaCO_2$ by increasing minute ventilation (affected by PIP and RR)
- If RR > 80/min and PCO_2 < 50 mmHg, consider sedation. If RR > 80/min and PCO_2 normal, consider ↑ Tidal Volume

I:E ratio: inspiratory to expiratory ratio; PCO_2: partial pressure of CO_2 in blood; $PaCO_2$: partial pressure of CO_2 in alveoli; PEEP: positive end-expiratory pressure; PIP: peak inspiratory pressure; RR: respiratory rate; TV: tidal volume.

Table 10.17   Continuous Flow, Time-Cycled Pressure-Limited (TCPL) Ventilator

Settings to Consider	
PIP	15–25 cm of H_2O
Inspiratory Time	0.35–0.45 seconds
Respiratory Rate	30–40/min
PEEP	3–5 cm H_2O
FiO_2	0.21–0.6
SIMV	When patient initiates breath, machine will deliver breath according to settings at set rate. Prevent fighting the ventilator. May be preferable for infants < 28 wks. May ↑ oxygenation stability, ↓ variations in BP, be more comfortable, and ↓ duration of ventilator support. Adjust PIP to keep TV approximately 3–6 mL/kg
Assist/Control	Every breath initiated by baby will result in positive pressure breath, and baby can breathe over set minimum rate
Pressure Support	May add to IMV ventilation; counteracts resistance of endotracheal tube and ventilator circuit and maximizes inspiratory time; initial settings: FiO_2: 0.21–0.6 TV: 4–5 mL/Kg PEEP: 3–6 cm Rate: 30–50/min Set Ti at 0.4 sec for infants < 1000 g Set PIP 1–2 cm > PIP needed for target TV Often used for babies with BPD requiring long-term ventilation or difficulty weaning from SIMV. Contraindicated if need IT > 0.2, atelectasis.
Volume-Controlled Ventilation*	Tidal volume is set at 4–6 mL/kg; RR and inspiration time limit also set. Flow rate, PIP, and inspiratory time vary.
Volume-Guarantee Ventilation (VG)*	Set expiratory tidal volume (4–5 mL/kg), inspiratory time (0.3–0.4), and max PIP value (1–2 cm > average PIP needed to get the target TV); should be < 30 cm H_2O). *Use for infants treated with surfactant*. Contraindicated if air leak > 30%

* Volume-targeted methods may be preferable for infants at risk for BPD and receiving surfactant

Table 10.18   High-Frequency Oscillating Ventilation (consider if PIP ≥ 30 cm H_2O or MAP > 10–12 cm H_2O on conventional ventilator)

High-frequency oscillator ventilator (HFOV)	Set **amplitude** (10–30 cm H_2O, controls ventilation: ↑ amplitude → ↓ CO_2), **frequency** (1 Hz = 60 breaths/min; BW < 1000 grams: start with 15 Hz; BW 1000–2000 grams: start with 12 Hz; BW > 2000 grams: start with 10 Hz; Term infant meconium aspiration: start at 6–10 Hz) **MAP** (use conventional ventilator MAP, ↑ 1–4 cm H_2O for diffuse alveolar disease, ↓ for PIE), **Inspiratory time, and FiO_2**. Active expiration. Check CXR 1 hr after initiating, after significant MAP change to ensure inflation to ≥ 8–9 posterior ribs
High-frequency jet ventilator (HFJV)	Set PIP (for jet and conventional), PEEP, frequency of jet breaths (~ 420 breaths/ minute), the inspiratory jet valve on-time (usually 0.02 seconds), and FiO_2. Passive expiration
High-frequency flow interrupter (HFFI)	Flow of gas interrupted by valve on conventional ventilator; not commonly used

- Overall high frequency ventilation does not appear to significantly reduce mortality or BPD in preterm babies with RDS

Table 10.19 Trouble-Shooting HFOV

Patient has ↑ CO_2	Check for pneumothorax, mechanical obstruction, ET placement, atelectasis, need for sedation?
Patient has ↓ O_2	Check for pneumothorax, mechanical obstruction (suction?), ET placement, atelectasis/hypotension, need sedation?

Table 10.20 Less invasive forms of respiratory support in neonates

CPAP (continuous positive airway pressure)	Apnea of prematurity, mild RDS
NIPPV (nasal intermittent positive pressure ventilation)	Apnea of prematurity, post extubation (superior to CPAP), infants with RDS

Data from: *Nelson Textbook of Pediatrics, 19th ed.*; Chapter 65; UTDOL Mechanical ventilation in neonates.

Nitric oxide: pulmonary vasodilator, may increase pulmonary blood flow; useful for PPHN, decreased pulmonary flow

Helium-oxygen mix (Heliox): decreases turbulence of flow; useful in subglottic stenosis, vascular ring, large airway obstruction

UMBILICAL CATHETERIZATION

Umbilical Vein Catheter Placement:
- Often successful in infants up to 2 weeks of age
- Length of insertion: Measure shoulder to umbilicus length (cm) × 0.6
- 3.5-French or 5-French catheter diameter
- Infant in warmer, frog-leg position and restrained, monitor in place, sterile surgical attire including gloves, hat, and mask
- Attach 3-way stopcock to catheter
- Flush with heparin 1 unit/mL or sterile 0.9% saline (2 ports and catheter)
- Scrub abdomen and umbilical stump with antiseptic (2% chlorhexidine, 70% alcohol, or povidone–iodine solution), then drape in sterile fashion
- Place purse-string suture or umbilical tape loosely at base of umbilicus
- Cut top of umbilicus horizontally with scalpel, 1–2 cm from base
- Attach hemostats at 3:00 and 9:00 positions to evert edges of umbilicus
- Remove any clot from umbilical vein, then insert flushed catheter into vein
  - In emergency, advance catheter 2–5 cm, or until blood return obtained, then use as IV access
  - In non-emergencies, goal is catheter to traverse ductus venosus, with tip located above diaphragm where IVC and right atrium join
  - Stop if resistance felt: Stop, reposition baby, try again
  - Do not infuse through catheter if suspected to be coiled in the liver
  - Do not advance if sterile technique broken
- Secure catheter with suture to cord, then taped to abdomen
- Check placement with CXR
- Run low-flow fluid continuously to avoid clot

Abbreviations: CXR: chest X-ray; IVC: inferior vena cava

Umbilical Artery Catheterization:
- Catheter size: infant < 2 kg: use 3.5- or 4-French; Infant > 2 kg: use 5-French
- Depth of insertion (various techniques to calculate):

- ○ Distance from xiphoid to pubic symphysis + ½ distance of umbilicus to pubic symphysis
  - ○ ½ of gestation age in cm is approximate quick reference
  - ○ Birth weight (kg) × 3 + 9
- Follow steps for umbilical vein catheter except identify umbilical *arteries*
- Dilate artery gently for 15 seconds using curved forceps to depth of 1 cm
- Direct catheter caudally toward feet: If resistance is felt when inserting catheter, consider possible false tract. At ~ 5 cm insertion, easy blood return should be noted
- X-ray to determine placement
  - ○ Ideal "high" placement between T6–T9 vertebrae
  - ○ Ideal "low" placement between L3–L4 vertebrae
- Attach blood pressure manometer an initiate fluids to maintain patency
  - ○ 0.45% NS + 0.5–1 unit heparin/mL to run at 1 mL/hour

MANAGEMENT OF THE TERM NEWBORN

Table 10.21 Apgar Score*

	Heart Rate	Respiratory Effort	Muscle Tone	Response to Stimuli (catheter in nose)	Color
0	Absent	Absent	Limp	No response	Blue or pale
1	< 100	Slow or irregular	Some flexion	Grimace	Body pink, acrocyanosis
2	> 100	Crying	Active	Cough/sneeze	Completely pink

*Performed at 1 and 5 minutes after birth
Apgar V. A proposal for a new method of evaluation of the newborn infant. *Curr Res Anesth Analg.* 1953 Jul–Aug;32(4):260–267. Reprinted by permission of Lippincott Williams & Wilkins.

Table 10.22 Common Newborn Interventions

Intervention*	Medical Reasoning
Vitamin K (0.5–1 mg IM) within 1 Hour of Birth	• Prevents early (birth–2 weeks) and late (2–12 weeks) vitamin K deficiency bleeding (VKDB) • PO vitamin K not recommended: Prevents early, but not late, VKDB (exclusive breastfeeding ↑ risk of vitamin K deficiency) • No evidence that IM vitamin K contributes to future cancers
Gonococcal Ophthalmia Prophylaxis	• 1-cm ribbon erythromycin 0.5% (tetracycline 1% acceptable alternative) instilled in each eye within 1 hour of birth • 1 gtt 1% silver nitrate solution other acceptable alternative • Occasionally causes chemical conjunctivitis
Hepatitis B Single-Antigen Vaccination	• If mom HbsAg+ or unknown, give within 12 hours of birth • HBIG 0.5 mL IM at site separate from vaccine if HbsAg+ mom or high-risk and unknown status
Newborn Screen	• Early discovery of treatable genetic, metabolic, hematologic, and endocrine diseases • Provide pamphlet describing tests to new parents • Some states only allow refusal on religious grounds
Hearing Screen	• Early diagnosis and intervention of congenital hearing loss has improved outcomes. Refer "failed" tests and infants with ear anomalies for follow-up outpatient audiologic evaluation

* Check local laws regarding indications and paperwork required for parental refusal of above interventions.
Data from: *Pediatrics.* 2003;12(1):191–192.

HYPOGLYCEMIA

- *Definition:* Level at which symptoms become noted. Some experts recommend keeping glucose > 40–45 mg/dL in first 24 hours of life, and > 45–50 mg/dL after 24 hours of life. No evidence or nomograms to support these expert recommendations
- *Symptoms:* Often asymptomatic. May have jitters, poor feeding, transient cyanosis, apnea, lethargy, convulsions, pallor, high-pitched cry, tachypnea
- *At risk:* Prematurity, maternal diabetes, hypothermia, hypoxia, sepsis; SGA (term < 2500 g) and LGA (term > 4000 g) infants
- *Screen:* At-risk infants at 30–60 minutes of life. If normal value but risk factors, repeat at 30 minutes intervals until age 2 hours. Follow abnormal levels after intervention
- *Treatment:* Early breast or formula feeding. Goal glucose > 45 mg/dL. If symptomatic and unable to feed, transfer to intensive care unit for IV glucose infusion 4–8 mg/kg/minute
- Severe or prolonged hypoglycemia may lead to neuro-developmental problems

References: *Pediatrics.* 2000;105(5):1141–1145; *J Pediatr.* 2009;155(5):612–617; *Pediatrics.* 2008;122:65–74.

POLYCYTHEMIA (VENOUS-DRAWN HEMATOCRIT [HCT] > 65%)

- More common at high altitude (5%), in post-term (2–3%), SGA (8%), LGA (3%), infants of diabetic mothers, delayed cord clamping, hypothyroidism, and numerous syndromes
- *Presents:* Often asymptomatic, but may present with plethora (red/purple, ruddy skin color) and signs of hyperviscosity: Feeding problems, lethargy, cyanosis, tachypnea, jitteriness, hyperbilirubinemia, hypoglycemia, thrombocytopenia (if DIC developing)
- *Treatment:* Consider partial exchange transfusion (with normal saline) for symptomatic infants (generally Hct at least 70–75%). Controversial, as may increase risk of NEC without significant improvement in short- or long-term outcomes. No defined hematocrit criteria for treatment of asymptomatic infants
- Volume of exchange (mL) = Blood volume (85 mL/kg) × (Observed/desired Hct)/(Observed Hct)^2. Desired Hct = 55%

Abbreviations: DIC: disseminated intravascular coagulation; Hct: hematocrit; LGA: large for gestational age; NEC: necrotizing enterocolitis; SGA: small for gestational age

References: *Pediatrics.* 1986;78(1):26–30; *Cochrane Rev.* 2005; (1):CD005089; *Pediatrics.* 1981;68:168–174.

CLAVICLE AND HUMERUS FRACTURES

- Heal remarkably well within 1–4 weeks. Look for brachial plexus injury
- Immobilization of arm by strapping/pinning sleeve to chest at 90° angle is generally sufficient

BRACHIAL PLEXUS INJURY

- *Definition:* Varying degree of paralysis of arm from lateral traction on head and neck, often seen in macrosomic infants with shoulder dystocia
- *Exam:* Arm held adducted, internally rotated, forearm in pronation. Lack of Moro and biceps reflex in affected arm. Severe cases have flaccid paralysis
- *Evaluation:* Radiographs to rule out fracture. Consider orthopedic, neurology, and occupational therapy (OT) assessment
- *Treatment:* Range of motion exercises prevent contracture: Passive external rotation in adduction and supination with elbow flexed at 90°, to the point where tension can be felt. Timing of microsurgical intervention unclear (may help severe cases of flaccid paralysis)

- *Natural history:* Usually resolves in 2–6 months. 5–15% may require microsurgery
- Bad prognostic indicators for long-term recovery of function include Horner's syndrome (ipsilateral ptosis and miosis), ipsilateral diaphragm paralysis, and complete flaccid paralysis of arm

TRANSIENT TACHYPNEA OF THE NEWBORN

- *Signs:* Tachypnea, with occasional signs of distress (grunting, retracting) in the first day (or two) of life. Rarely require oxygen. Lungs clear. Thought to be from slow absorption of fetal lung fluid. Possible ↑ incidence in planned C-sections
- *Radiographs:* Normal or show hyperinflation with small amount of fluid in fissures
- *Differential diagnosis:* Respiratory distress syndrome, meconium aspiration, pneumothorax, persistent pulmonary hypertension of the newborn, choanal atresia

Table 10.23   Ophthalmia Neonatorum

Causative Agents	Exam Findings	Associated Symptoms	Treatment
Chlamydia, N. Gonorrhea*, Staph, strep, Haemophilus influenzae, herpes simplex virus	• *Chlamydia:* First 10 days of life • *Gonorrhea:* First 3–5 days; copious purulent discharge; usually bilateral; • *Complications:* Keratitis, loss of vision, corneal perforation	• *Chlamydia:* Evaluate for pulmonary involvement • *Gonorrhea* can be associated with arthritis, bacteremia, and/or meningitis	*Chlamydia:* Erythromycin 30–50 mg/kg/d PO div qid *Gonorrhea:* • Hospitalize • Blood, eye, CSF cultures • Ceftriaxone† 25–50 mg/kg IM/IV × 1 • Test for other STIs, treat mother/partner

CSF: Cerebrospinal fluid, STI: Sexually transmitted infections
†Cefotaxime is alternative especially if hyperbilirubinemia.
*Infants born to mothers with known untreated gonorrhea infection should get ceftriaxone 25–50 mg/kg IM × 1 (or cefotaxime).

No topical treatment necessary

DISCHARGE CRITERIA FOR HEALTHY TERM NEWBORNS (37–41 WEEKS' GESTATION)

- No exam anomalies requiring continued hospitalization
- Normal vital signs (RR < 60, HR 100–160, temp 36.5–37.4°C [open crib])
- Social risk factors (drug use, teen mother) have been evaluated
- Parents/caregivers educated in basic newborn care
- Evaluated and monitored for sepsis based on maternal risk factors for GBS
- Assessment of hyperbilirubinemia risk with appropriate management and follow-up scheduled
- Infant blood tests have been reviewed (cord type and Coombs if indicated)
- If circumcised, minimal bleeding > 2 hours after
- Physician follow-up assured
- Regular urination and stooled × 1 spontaneously
- Minimum two successful consecutive feeds with assessment of ability to suck, swallow, and breathe
- Maternal hepatitis B, syphilis, and HIV (depending on state regulations) status known/reviewed
- For infants discharged age < 48 hours old, scheduled follow-up within 48 hours
- Hearing and metabolic screen performed (as mandated by local law)

References: AAP, ACOG. *Guidelines for Perinatal Care,* ed. 5. 2002; *Pediatrics.* 2010;125:405–409.

NEONATAL VOMITING

- Regurgitation common. Often mucoid or even bloody. Apt test differentiates swallowed maternal blood from blood originating from the infant.
- If bilious, consider intestinal obstruction. Make infant NPO (nothing by mouth), obtain urgent upper gastrointestinal series and surgical consultation to evaluate for malrotation, midgut volvulus, sepsis, intestinal atresia, Hirschsprung's disease, or meconium ileus.
- If emesis persists, consider obstruction, ↑ sepsis, intracranial pressure, metabolic disorders.

DEVELOPMENTAL DYSPLASIA OF THE HIP (DDH)

Screening Controversies: American Academy of Pediatrics recommendations (2002) are summarized below. US Preventive Services Task Force (USPSTF) 2006 statement does not recommend screening exams, noting spontaneous resolution in many cases and unclear risks to treatment options.

Table 10.24   Risk Factors for DDH
Family history, female sex, oligohydramnios, breech position, possibly swaddling (very low incidence in Asian, African countries where children in slings, not swaddled)

Ortolani	Newborn supine, fingers on greater trochanter and thumb on inner thigh; hip flexed and abducted while lifting anteriorly. "Clunk" is positive sign
Barlow	Newborn supine, legs adducted and posterior pressure placed on knee; clunk or noted movement/feeling of looseness is positive sign

- *High-pitched clicks are very common and usually inconsequential if no red flags (asymmetry of thigh/gluteal folds, leg length/knee height discrepancy, restricted hip abduction), no evidence of looseness, and neg Ortolani and Barlow test*

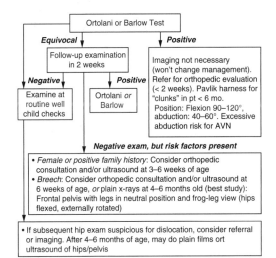

Figure 10.3 Neonatal Hip Evaluation

AVN: Avascular necrosis of the hip

Data from: *Pediatrics*. 2010;125(3):e577–583; *J Bone Joint Surg*. 2009;91(7):1705–1718; USPSTF Mar 2006.

ASSESSING NEUROMUSCULAR AND PHYSICAL MATURITY OF THE NEWBORN

NEUROMUSCULAR MATURITY

NEUROMUSCULAR MATURITY SIGN	SCORE							RECORD SCORE HERE
	−1	0	1	2	3	4	5	
POSTURE								
SQUARE WINDOW (Wrist)	> 90°	90°	60°	45°	30°	0°		
ARM RECOIL		180°	140°–180°	110°–140°	90°–110°	< 90°		
POPLITEAL ANGLE	180°	160°	140°	120°	100°	90°	< 90°	
SCARF SIGN								
HEEL TO EAR								

TOTAL NEUROMUSCULAR MATURITY SCORE

SCORE

Neuromuscular____
Physical_____
Total_____

MATURITY RATING

SCORE	WEEKS
−10	20
−5	22
0	24
5	26
10	28
15	30
20	22
25	34
30	36
35	38
40	40
45	42
50	44

PHYSICAL MATURITY

PHYSICAL MATURITY SIGN	SCORE							RECORD SCORE HERE
	−1	0	1	2	3	4	5	
SKIN	Sticky friable transparent	Gelatinous red translucent	Smooth pink visible veins	Superficial peeling and/ or rash, few veins	Cracking pale areas rare veins	Parchment deep cracking no vessels	Leathery cracked wrinkled	
LANUGO	None	Sparse	Abundant	Thinning	Bald areas	Mostly bald		
PLANTAR SURFACE	Heel-toe 40–50 mm: −1 < 40 mm: −2	> 50 mm no crease	Faint red marks	Anterior transverse crease only	Creases ant. 2/3	Creases over entire sole		
BREAST	Imperceptible	Barely perceptible	Flat areola no bud	Stippled areola 1–2 mm bud	Raised areola 3–4 mm bud	Full areola 5–10 mm bud		
EYE/EAR	Lids fused loosely: −1 tightly: −2	Lids open pinna flat stays folded	Sl. curved pinna; soft; slow recoil	Well-curved pinna; soft but ready recoil	Formed and firm instant recoil	Thick cartilage ear stiff		
GENITALS (Male)	Scrotum flat, smooth	Scrotum empty faint rugae	Testes in upper canal rare rugae	Testes descending few rugae	Testes down good rugae	Testes pendulous deep rugae		
GENITALS (Female)	Clitoris prominent and labia flat	Prominent clitoris and small labia minora	Prominent clitoris and enlarging minora	Majora and minora equally prominent	Majora large minora small	Majora cover clitoris and minora		

TOTAL PHYSICAL MATURITY SCORE

GESTATIONAL AGE (weeks)

By dates_____
By ultrasound_____
By exam_____

Figure 10.4 New Ballard Score for Estimating Gestational Age

Reprinted with permission Elsevier publishing. Originally printed in *J pediatrics* 1991;119:417–423.

Score each neuromuscular and physical maturity category, sum the total score, and plot on the "maturity rating" table to determine approximate gestational age.

References: *N Engl J Med.* 2005;353(15):1574–1584; *BMC Pediatrics.* 2007;7:30–33; *Clin Perinatol.* 2009;36(4):881–900.

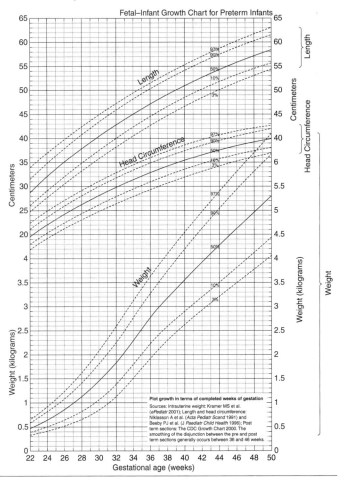

Fetal–Infant Growth Chart for Preterm Infants

Plot growth in terms of completed weeks of gestation
Sources: Intrauterine weight: Kramer MS et al. (ePediatr 2001); Length and head circumference: Niklasson A et al. (*Acta Pediatr Scand* 1991) and Beeby PJ et al. (*J Paediatr Child Health* 1996); Post term sections: The CDC Growth Chart 2000. The smoothing of the disjunction between the pre and post term sections generally occurs between 36 and 46 weeks.

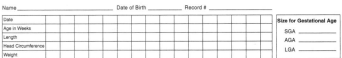

Figure 10.5 Fetal–Infant Growth Chart for Preterm Infants

Table 10.25 Newborn Screen

Newborn screen is different in every state. Common disorders included are:

Disorder	Follow-up to Positive Screen	Overview of Care of Child
Congenital Hypothyroidism	• Thyroid-stimulating hormone (TSH), free thyroxine (FT4) • Consider ultrasound or uptake scan of thyroid • Thyrotropin-binding inhibitor immunoglobulin if evidence of maternal autoimmune thyroid disease • May need to re-screen premature infants at 2–6 weeks	• L-thyroxine 10–15 mcg/kg/d • Goal thyroxine 10–16 mcg/dL and TSH < 6 mU/L • Follow-up labs (TSH & FT4) 2–4 weeks after start treatment • First year of life: Check TSH and FT4 every 1–2 months • 1–3 years old: Check labs every 3–4 months or 2–4 weeks after dose change
Galactosemia	• Examine in office for signs of lethargy, hepatic failure • Quantitative galactose 1-phosphate uridyltransferase (GALT), red blood cell galactose-1–phosphate	• Galactose restriction via galactose-free formula (soy-based formula) • No breast-feeding
Cystic Fibrosis (CF)	• Immunoreactive trypsinogen, CF mutation analysis • Newborn sweat chloride (> 40 mmol/L is positive; > 30 mmol/L needs follow-up)	• Nutrition: pancreatic enzyme and fat-soluble vitamin (ADEK) supplements • Pulmonary support • May check fecal elastase
Phenylketonuria	• Quantitative phenylalanine and tyrosine	• Phenylalanine-restricted diet • Monitor phenylalanine levels
Sickle Cell Disease (see section on sickle cell)	• Confirm with hemoglobin electrophoresis, isoelectric focusing, or DNA-based methods by 2 months of age • Genetic counseling	• PCN prophylaxis (by 2 months old) • Immunize: Pneumococcal, meningococcal • Monitor for complications
Medium-chain acyl-CoA Dehydrogenase Deficiency (MCAD)	• If octanoylcarnitine > 1.0 μmol/L, then check: – Plasma acylcarnitine profile – Urine organic acid analysis	• Avoid fasting • Prompt evaluation if vomiting, lethargic • Low-fat diet • L-carnitine: (100 mg/mL soln) 50–100 mg/kg/day

Other disorders commonly screened for: biotinidase deficiency, congenital adrenal hyperplasia, homocystinuria, fatty acid oxidation disorders, maple syrup urine disease, and tyrosinemia.

FT4: free thyroxine, PCN: penicillin, TSH: thyroid stimulating hormone

Data from: Newborn Screening Fact Sheet. *Pediatrics*. 2006;118:934–963.

Early VCUG for moderate to severe hydronephrosis to evaluate for VUR (10–40% incidence) or posterior urethral valves (especially if bilateral hydronephrosis in male). Consider antibiotic prophylaxis while awaiting studies:

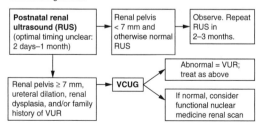

Figure 10.6 Prenatal Hydronephrosis

Data from: *Pediatr Neurol*. 2008;39:77–79; *Seizure*. 2010;19(3):185–189; *N Engl J Med*. 2005;353(15):1574–1584;BMC Pediatrics.

Table 10.26 Neonatal Seizures

Presentation		May be tonic (sustained posturing), clonic (rhythmic jerking), myoclonic (isolated jerks), or subtle (tongue/mouth movements, pedaling, swimming, eye movements/sustained eye deviation)
Differential Diagnosis		Sandifer syndrome (arching with gastroesophageal reflux), jittery (flexion and extension duration are the same; in seizure one is longer than the other), benign neonatal sleep myoclonus (sleep only), apnea, startle response
Causes	Metabolic	Hypoglycemia, electrolyte anomalies (hypo/hypernatremia, hypocalcemia, hypomagnesemia), pyridoxine dependent, hypermetabolic state from exposure to maternal drug use
	Vascular	Hypoxic-ischemic encephalopathy, hemorrhage (intraventricular, subdural, cortical, subarachnoid), arterio-venous malformation, infarction (arterial or venous)
	Infectious	Meningitis (bacterial, HSV), TORCH infection
	Genetic	Cerebral dysgenesis, migrational defects
	Other	Benign neonatal seizures
Evaluation		EEG, Cranial US, MRI. Rule out acute infection and metabolic derangement (glucose, electrolytes, CBC, CSF)
Treatment	Hypoglycemia	D10W: 2 mL/kg IV bolus, then dextrose infusion at 5–8 mg/kg/minutes
	Hypocalcemia	Calcium gluconate (50 mg/mL): 1–2 mL/kg = 100–200 mg/kg/dose, over 15–30 minutes
	Persistent Seizures: first line	Phenobarbital: 20 mg/kg IV load over 15 minutes, then 3–5 mg/kg/day PO div qd–bid Phenytoin or fosphenytoin: 15–20 mg/kg IV load (max rate: 1 mg/kg/minutes), then 5–8 mg/kg/d PO div bid–tid
	second line	Pyridoxine: 25–50 mg/day IV for pyridoxine-dependent seizure Lorazepam (second line): 0.05–0.1 mg/kg/dose IV
	Off-label use	Levetiracetam (10 mg/kg/dose) and topiramate (10 mg/kg/dose) recommended by some neurologists as second- or third-line therapy. Both currently lack safety/ pharmacologic data.

CBC: Complete blood count, CSF: Cerebrospinal fluid, EEG: Electroencephalogram, HIE: Hypoxic–ischemic encephalopathy, HSV: Herpes simplex virus, TORCH: Toxoplasma, rubella, cytomegalovirus, herpes virus; US: ultrasound

Data from: *Pediatr Neurol.* 2008;39:77–79; *Seizure.* 2010;19(3):185–189; *N Engl J Med.* 2005;353(15):1574–1584; BMC Pediatrics. 2007;7:30–33; *Clin Perinatol.* 2009;36(4):881–900.

UNCONJUGATED HYPERBILIRUBINEMIA IN TERM AND NEAR-TERM INFANTS

- Elevated total serum bilirubin (TSB) with conjugated (dbili) < 20% of TSB.

PATHOPHYSIOLOGY

- Heme from red blood cells (RBCs) and myoglobin converted to unconjugated bilirubin, travels to liver bound to albumin. Glucuronyl transferase conjugates to dbili, secreted in bile, eliminated via stool. If infant is not stooling well, dbili is hydrolyzed in the colon and reabsorbed back into the circulation.

RISK FACTORS FOR DEVELOPMENT OF SEVERE HYPERBILIRUBINEMIA

- Previous sibling required phototherapy, jaundiced in the first 24 hours of life, polycythemia, blood group incompatibility and Coombs+, cephalohematoma, significant bruising, prematurity (particularly < 37 weeks EGA), small for gestational age, East Asian or Native American ethnicity, hypothyroidism, sepsis, asphyxia, significant weight loss, exclusive breastfeeding, macrosomic infant of diabetic mother.

Table 10.27   Etiology of Unconjugated Hyperbilirubinemia

Decreased Conjugation
• **Physiologic jaundice:** Diagnosis of exclusion for infants 24 hours–14 days old. Rise < 5 mg/dL/day, peak TSB usually < 13 mg/dL. Presumed causes: Immature hepatic enzymes, ↑ RBC volume, ↓ RBC survival, recirculation from colon
• **Breastfeeding:** Unconjugated, peaks late (1–2 weeks), TSB 12–20 mg/dL, possibly from inhibition of liver enzymes. Resolves with switch to formula for 2 days
• **Glucuronyl transferase defect** (Crigler-Najjar I and II): Jaundiced often by 24 hours, rapid rise, may require exchange transfusion
• **Decreased liver function:** Sepsis, hypothyroidism, hepatitis, galactosemia, glycogen storage disease

Overproduction of Heme
• **Antibody-mediated hemolysis:** ABO or Rh incompatibility. Direct Coombs positive
• **Red blood cell membrane defects:** Spherocytosis, elliptocytosis
• **RBC enzyme deficiencies:** Glucose-6-Phosphate dehydrogenase (G6PD) deficiency, pyruvate kinase deficiency (PKD), others
• **Extravascular blood collection:** Cephalohematoma, intracranial bleed, hematoma at humerus or clavicle fracture

Abnormal Excretion or Reabsorption of Bilirubin
• **Obstruction:** Biliary atresia, choledochal cyst, cystic fibrosis, alagille syndrome
• **Abnormal bilirubin transport mechanism:** Dubin-Johnson and rotor syndrome

Data from: *JPed Gastro Nutr.* 2004;39:115–128.

EVALUATION

Every infant should be assessed for jaundice and risk factors prior to discharge. (Check TSB in any jaundiced infant age < 36 hours old.)

- *Ill-appearing:* Consider sepsis, admit to hospital, IV antibiotics. Measure albumin.
- *Well-appearing:* Besides TSB, consider dbili, complete blood count (with differential and pathology review of peripheral smear), reticulocyte count, blood type, direct Coombs test and catheterized urine specimen for culture. G6PD if poor response to phototherapy or ethnicity suggestive (11–13% African Americans have G6PD).
- *Jaundice present age ≥ 3 weeks:* TSB and dbili, check results of newborn thyroid and galactosemia screen. If dbili elevated, evaluate for cholestasis.
- *Transcutaneous bilirubin monitors* (TcB): Unclear if ↓ costs, limits serum TSB measurement, or ↓ readmissions; ↓ accuracy in dark-skinned infants, and if previously exposed to sunlight or phototherapy.[2]
- Universal screening (TcB or TSB) may ↓ severely elevated TSB (> 25 mg/dL).[1,2]

TREATMENT

- Use *hour-specific* tables on subsequent pages to determine need for intensive phototherapy.
- *Ensure hydration:* Continue breastfeeding q 2–3 hours. Supplement with formula or intravenous fluid if significantly dehydrated or limited maternal milk supply.
- *Intensive phototherapy:* Blue–green spectrum (430–490 nm), 30 μW/cm^2, maximize skin exposure (diaper and eye protection only). If approaching exchange transfusion levels, line incubator with aluminum foil or white material.

MATERNAL–FETAL ABO INCOMPATIBILITY

- Occurs in 20–25% of pregnancies. However, only 10% cases result in significant immune-mediated hemolysis.
- Phototherapy required in 10–20% of Coombs+ infants.
- Severe anemia requiring transfusion (hemoglobin 6–7 g/dL or symptomatic [poor feeding, tachypnea]) rarely occurs and may respond to IVIG. Once deemed stable for discharge, outpatient follow-up of hemoglobin and reticulocyte count crucial.

---

[1] *Pediatrics.* 2010;125:e1143–1148.
[2] *NACB Guideline.* 2006, pp. 5–12.

CHOLESTASIS (DIRECT BILIRUBIN > 2 MG/DL OR > 20% OF TSB)[1]

- Differential diagnosis includes: Biliary atresia, neonatal hepatitis, sepsis (particularly urinary tract infection), choledochal cyst, Alagille syndrome, inspissated bile, alpha-1 antitrypsin deficiency, hypothyroidism, cystic fibrosis, total parenteral nutrition.
- If signs of sepsis or specific metabolic/genetic disease, treat appropriately.
- If otherwise well, obtain abdominal ultrasound to evaluate for extrahepatic bile ducts (absence implies biliary atresia) and choledochal cyst.
- If abdominal ultrasound normal, consider scintigraphy, alpha-1 antitrypsin assay, and liver function testing. Refer to gastroenterologist or pediatric surgeon for liver biopsy.

Table 10.28   Prediction of Future Hyperbilirubinemia

(Future likelihood of bilirubin level [in mg/dL] exceeding 95th percentile)

		Low Risk Zone (0%)	Low–Intermediate Risk Zone (2.2%)	High–Intermediate Risk Zone (12.9%)	High Risk Zone (39.5%)
	12	< 4	4–5.1	5.2–7	> 7
	18	< 4.7	4.7–5.8	5.9–7.3	> 7.3
	24	< 5	5–6	6.1–7.8	> 7.8
	30	< 6	6–7.5	7.6–9.5	> 9.5
	36	< 7	7–9	9.1–11	> 11
	42	< 8	8–10	10.1–12.3	> 12.3
	48	< 8.5	8.5–10.9	11–13.1	> 13.1
	54	< 9	9–11.7	11.8–14	> 14
	60	< 9.6	9.6–12.6	12.7–15.1	> 15.1
	66	< 10.3	10.3–13	13.1–15.5	> 15.5
Hour of Life	72	< 11.1	11.1–13.4	13.5–16	> 16
	78	< 11.4	11.4–14	14.1–16.3	> 16.3
	84	< 11.7	11.7–14.6	14.7–16.8	> 16.8
	90	< 12	12–15	15.1–17.1	> 17.1
	96	< 12.3	12.3–15.2	15.3–17.3	> 17.3
	102	< 12.6	12.6–15.3	15.4–17.3	> 17.3
	108	< 12.9	12.9–15.4	15.5–17.5	> 17.5
	114	< 13.1	13.1–15.6	15.7–17.6	> 17.6
	120	< 13.2	13.2–15.8	15.9–17.7	> 17.7
	126	< 13.2	13.2–15.7	15.8–17.6	> 17.6
	132	< 13.2	13.2–15.6	15.7–17.5	> 17.5
	138	< 13.2	13.2–15.5	15.6–17.4	> 17.4
	144	< 13.2	13.2–15.4	15.5–17.3	> 17.3

Data from: *Pediatrics*. 2004; 114:297–316.

[1] *jPed Gastro Nutr.* 2004;39:115–128.

Table 10.29   Follow-up Based on Risk Zone

Risk Zone	Schedule Follow-up Within
Low Risk	72 hours
Low Intermediate	48–72 hours
High Intermediate	24–48 hours
High Risk	24 hours

Data from: *Pediatrics*. 1999;103(6).

Table 10.30   Phototherapy

Approximate hour-specific levels at which phototherapy should be considered based on neurotoxicity risk zone

	Hour of Life	Neurotoxicity Risk Zone		
		Low Risk ≥ 38 weeks EGA *and* well	**Medium Risk** ≥ 38 weeks EGA + neurotoxicity risk factor, *or* 35–37 6/7 weeks EGA and well	**High Risk** < 38 weeks EGA *and* neurotoxicity risk factor
	18	10.4 mg/dL	8.8 mg/dL	7 mg/dL
	24	11.7 mg/dL	9.9 mg/dL	8 mg/dL
	30	12.7 mg/dL	10.8 mg/dL	8.8 mg/dL
	36	13.6 mg/dL	11.7 mg/dL	9.6 mg/dL
	42	14.5 mg/dL	12.4 mg/dL	10.5 mg/dL
	48	15.3 mg/dL	13.1 mg/dL	11.4 mg/dL
	54	16 mg/dL	13.9 mg/dL	12 mg/dL
	60	16.6 mg/dL	14.6 mg/dL	12.5 mg/dL
	66	17.2 mg/dL	15.1 mg/dL	13.1 mg/dL
	72	17.7 mg/dL	15.5 mg/dL	13.6 mg/dL
	78	18.3 mg/dL	16.1 mg/dL	13.9 mg/dL
	84	18.9 mg/dL	16.6 mg/dL	14.1 mg/dL
	90	19.4 mg/dL	16.9 mg/dL	14.3 mg/dL
	96	19.9 mg/dL	17.2 mg/dL	14.5 mg/dL
	102	20.3 mg/dL	17.6 mg/dL	14.7 mg/dL
	108	20.6 mg/dL	17.9 mg/dL	14.9 mg/dL
	114	20.8 mg/dL	18 mg/dL	15 mg/dL
	≥ 120	21 mg/dL	18 mg/dL	15 mg/dL

Neurotoxicity Risk Factors: Isoimmune hemolytic disease, G6PD deficiency, asphyxia, lethargy, temperature instability, sepsis, acidosis, albumin < 3.0 g/dL

Data from: Adapted from *Pediatrics*. 2004;114:297–316.

Table 10.31   Exchange Transfusion

Hour-specific levels at which exchange transfusion should be considered based on neurotoxicity risk zone

		Neurotoxicity Risk Zone		
		Low Risk ≥ 38 weeks EGA *and* well	*Medium Risk* ≥ 38 weeks EGA + neurotoxicity risk factor, *OR* 35–37 6/7 weeks EGA and well	*High Risk* < 38 weeks EGA *and* neurotoxicity risk factor
Hour of Life	24	19 mg/dL	16.6 mg/dL	15 mg/dL
	30	20 mg/dL	17.3 mg/dL	15.5 mg/dL
	36	20.9 mg/dL	18 mg/dL	16 mg/dL
	42	21.6 mg/dL	18.5 mg/dL	16.6 mg/dL
	48	22.2 mg/dL	19.1 mg/dL	17.1 mg/dL
	54	22.6 mg/dL	19.6 mg/dL	17.5 mg/dL
	60	23 mg/dL	20.2 mg/dL	18 mg/dL
	66	23.5 mg/dL	20.8 mg/dL	18.2 mg/dL
	72	24 mg/dL	21.3 mg/dL	18.5 mg/dL
	78	24.3 mg/dL	21.7 mg/dL	18.7 mg/dL
	84	24.5 mg/dL	22 mg/dL	18.8 mg/dL
	90	24.7 mg/dL	22.2 mg/dL	18.9 mg/dL
	96	25 mg/dL	22.5 mg/dL	19 mg/dL
	102	25 mg/dL	22.5 mg/dL	19 mg/dL
	108	25 mg/dL	22.5 mg/dL	19 mg/dL
	114	25 mg/dL	22.5 mg/dL	19 mg/dL
	≥ 120	25 mg/dL	22.5 mg/dL	19 mg/dL

Neurotoxicity Risk Factors: Isoimmune hemolytic disease, G6PD deficiency, asphyxia, lethargy, temperature instability, sepsis, acidosis, albumin < 3.0 g/dL

Data from: *Pediatrics*. 2004;114:297–316.

CHAPTER 11 ■ NEPHROLOGY

HYPERTENSION

↑ systolic blood pressure (SBP) and/or diastolic blood pressure (DBP) > 95% for age, gender, and height on ≥ three occasions. Check BP at every visit in children age ≥ 3 years

Table 11.1 Pearls for Checking Blood Pressure

BP Technique: Child should be seated and calm for 5 minutes (and off caffeine and other stimulants). Cuff bladder around ≥ 80% circumference of the extremity
***Manual BP with auscultation preferred:** Stethoscope bell on brachial artery, listen for onset of Korotkoff sounds (SBP) and muffling/disappearance (DBP)
***Too small cuff falsely elevates BP.** Too large cuff, minimal effect
***Ambulatory Blood Pressure Monitoring (ABPM):** Portable outpatient BP device, useful in: "White coat" HTN, severe HTN (with risk of end organ damage), drug resistant HTN, hypotensive symptoms while on therapy

Table 11.2 Symptoms of Hypertension

Patients are often asymptomatic, but may present with irritability, headache, epistaxis, fatigue, shortness of breath, impaired exercise tolerance, or impaired academic performance

Table 11.3 Indications to Check Blood Pressure in a Child < 3 Years Old

Prematurity, neonatal intensive care unit stay, history of umbilical lines, congenital heart disease, urinary tract infection, hematuria, proteinuria, renal disease, urologic malformations, organ transplant, bone marrow transplant, malignancy, illnesses associated with hypertension (neurofibromatosis, tuberous sclerosis), use of drugs known to ↑ blood pressure (pseudoephedrine), or family history of congenital renal disease

Table 11.4 Differential Diagnosis by Age of Patient

< 1 year	Renal artery or vein thrombosis, congenital renal anomalies, coarctation of the aorta, bronchopulmonary dysplasia, central causes (increased intracranial pressure), endocrinopathies (pheochromocytoma, thyroid disease, congenital adrenal hyperplasia [11-hydroxylase deficiency produces aldosterone receptor agonist → hypertension])
1–6 years	Renal parenchymal disease, renal artery stenosis, coarctation of the aorta, Wilms tumor, neuroblastoma, endocrine causes
6–12 years	Renal parenchymal disease, renovascular anomalies, endocrine causes (hyperthyroidism), essential HTN
> 12 years	Metabolic syndrome, renal parenchymal disease, endocrine causes, essential HTN

Table 11.5 Categories of Hypertension

Pre hypertension	SBP or DBP 90–95% for age, gender, and height, or > 120/80
Stage I HTN	SBP or DBP 5 mmHg > 95% for age, gender, and height
Stage II HTN	SBP or DBP 5 mmHg > 99% for age, gender, and height
HTN Emergency	HTN + acute end-organ dysfunction (severe irritability, seizures, altered mental status, encephalopathy). Immediate referral to intensive care unit

Table 11.6   95th Percentile BP Measurements for *BOYS* by Age and Height Percentile

Age	SBP, mmHg per height percentile			DBP, mmHg per height percentile		
	5th	50th	95th	5th	50th	95th
1	98	103	106	54	56	58
2	101	106	110	59	61	63
3	104	109	113	63	65	67
4	106	111	115	66	69	71
5	108	112	116	69	72	74
6	109	114	117	72	74	76
8	111	116	120	75	78	80
10	115	119	123	78	80	82
12	119	123	127	78	81	83
14	124	128	132	80	82	84
16	129	134	137	82	84	87

Data from: NHCB, 4th report on high blood pressure in children, *Pediatrics* 2004;114(2) Suppl.

Table 11.7   95th Percentile BP Measurements for *GIRLS* by Age and Height Percentile

Age	SBP, mmHg per height percentile			DBP, mmHg per height percentile		
	5th	50th	95th	5th	50th	95th
1	100	104	107	56	58	60
2	102	105	109	61	63	65
3	104	107	110	65	67	69
4	105	108	112	68	70	72
5	107	110	113	70	72	74
6	108	111	115	72	74	76
8	112	115	118	75	76	78
10	116	119	122	77	78	80
12	119	123	126	79	80	82
14	123	126	129	81	82	84
16	125	128	132	82	84	86

Data from: NHCB, 4th report on high blood pressure in children, *Pediatrics* 2004;114(2) Suppl.

Table 11.8   Three-Phase Approach to the Evaluation of Hypertension

Phase 1	BUN, creatinine, electrolytes, urinalysis, complete blood count, lipid panel, calcium, uric acid, renal ultrasound with Doppler flow, echocardiography, polysomnography, urine toxicology
Phase 2	Nuclear medicine renal scan with angiotensin converting enzyme inhibitor, magnetic resonance angiography of the renal vessels, renin profiling, urine catecholamines, plasma, and urinary steroids
Phase 3	Renal angiogram/venogram, renal vein renin, nuclear med scan of adrenal, caval catecholamines sampling, aortic angiography

Table 11.9 Common Oral Medications for Hypertension Based on Comorbid Condition

Condition	Drug
Renal parenchymal disease; Any degree of proteinuria	Angiotensin Converting Enzyme Inhibitor (ACEi)[Δφ] *Infants:* Captopril (*Capoten*®): 0.15–0.3 mg/kg/dose tid (max 6 mg/kg/day) *Children > 1 year old:* Can use captopril dosed as above, *or* Enalapril (*Vasotec*®): Initial: 0.08 mg/kg PO daily (max 0.58 mg/kg/d or 20 mg daily), *or* Lisinopril (*Prinivil*®): Initial: 0.07 mg/kg/day, up to 5 mg/dose (max 0.6 mg/kg/day or 40 mg/day, increase weekly) Once ACEi max dose, add angiotensin II receptor blocker[Δ] (not approved for children < 6 years old) Losaratan (*Cozaar*®): Initial: 0.7 mg/kg/day, max initial dose 50 mg (max daily dose 1.4 mg/kg/day or 100 mg/day), *or* Irbesartan (*Avapro*®): 6–12 years old: 75–150 mg/day, ≥ 13 years old: 150–300 mg/day (max 300 mg/day). Single daily dose Valsartan (*Diovan*®): 0.4 mg/kg or 5–10 mg daily (max 3.4 mg/kg or 80 mg daily)
Concomitant migraine	Beta-blocker*: Metoprolol ER* (*Toprol*®, *Lopressor*®): Children > 6 years old: 1 mg/kg/day PO div bid (max 2 mg/kg/day or 200 mg/d), *or* Propranolol* (*Inderal*®): Initial: 1–2 mg/kg/day div bid–tid (max 4 mg/kg/day or 640 g/day), or Atenolol* (*Tenormin*®): Initial 0.5–1 mg/kg/day div daily–bid (max 2 mg/kg/day or 100 mg/day), or Calcium Channel Blocker: Isradipine (*Prescal*®): 0.05–0.15 mg/kg dose div qid (max 0.8 mg/kg/day up to 20 mg/day) Nifedipine XL (*Procardia XL*®): Initial: 0.25–0.5 mg/kg per day div daily–bid (max 3 mg/kg/day or 120 mg/day) Amlodipine (*Norvasc*®): Children 6–17 years old: 2.5–5 mg/daily
Vasculitis; Vasoconstriction	Vasodilators: Hydralazine (*Apresoline*®): 0.75–1 mg/kg/day PO div q 6–12 hours (max 7.5 mg/kg/day up to 200 mg/day) Minoxidil (*Loniten*®): Start 0.2 mg/kg/day div daily–tid. Increase every 3 days prn up to 0.25–1 mg/kg/day (max 50 mg/day)
Sodium retention; Fluid overload; Edema; (PSGN, CHF)	Diuretics: Hydrochlorothiazide (*Hydrodiuril*®, *Microzide*®): Initial: 1 mg/kg/day (max 3 mg/kg/day or 50 mg/day) Chlorthiazide (*Diuril*®): Neonate: 10–30 mg/kg/day div daily–bid; > 6 months old: 10–20 mg/kg/day div daily–bid (max 375 mg/day in children < 2 years old, 1000 mg/day 2–12 years old, 2000 mg/day adolescents) Chlorthalidone (*Thalitone*®): Initial: 0.3 mg/kg daily (max 2 mg/kg or 50 mg daily) Spironolactone (*Aldactone*®): Initial: 1 mg/kg/day div daily–bid (max 3.3 mg/kg/day or 100 mg/day)
Centrally mediated hypertension	Central alpha-agonist: (For children ≥ 12 years old) Clonidine (*Catapres*®): 0.2 mg/day div bid (max 2.4 mg/day). Side effects include sedation, dry mouth, rebound hypertension Peripheral alpha-antagonist: (beware of first-dose hypotension) Doxazosin (*Cardura*®): Initial: 1 mg daily (max 4 mg daily) Prazosin (*Minipress*®): Initial: 0.05–0.1 mg/kg/day div tid (max 0.5 mg/kg/day div tid) Terazosin (*Hytrin*®): Initial: 1 mg daily (max 20 mg daily)
If BP uncontrolled with max dose of single agent, add drug with different mechanism of action (e.g., ACE inhibitor + diuretic, or vasodilator + beta-blocker)	

\# Contraindicated in headache, intracranial hemorrhage or tumor, pulmonary pathology

*Contraindicated in asthma, bronchopulmonary dysplasia, congestive heart failure, infants < 1 year old. May mask hypoglycemic symptoms (do not use in insulin-dependent diabetics). Heart rate is dose limiting. May impair athletic performance

Δ Contraindicated in pregnancy. Use with caution in renal artery stenosis, renal impairment, hyperkalemia, volume depletion. Only to be used if GFR ≥ 30 mL/min/1.73 m^2

φ Adjust dose to 75% for GFR 10–50 mL/min/1.73 m^2, and 50% for GFR < 10 mL/min/1.73 m^2

ACEi: angiotensin converting enzyme inhibitor; bpm: beats per minute; BP: blood pressure; GFR: glomerular filtration rate; IV: intravenous; Na+: sodium; PO: oral

Data from: NHLBI Expert Panel on Integrated Guidelines for Cardiovascular Health and Risk Reduction in Children and Adolescents, NIH Publication No. 12-7486, October 2012; National High Blood Pressure Education Program (NHBPEP) Working Group on High Blood Pressure in Children and Adolescents. *Pediatrics*, 2004, 114 (Suppl 4th Report):555–76.

HYPERTENSIVE EMERGENCY

Systolic or diastolic blood pressure > 99% and signs/symptoms of end organ involvement. Goal is to reduce BP by ~25% in fist 8 hours, normalized in 24–48 hours

Table 11.10   Treatment Options for Hypertensive Emergency

	Drug	Dose	Comments
1st-Line Therapy	Hydralazine	0.2–0.5 mg/kg/dose IV q 4–6 hours	Tachycardia, Na+ retention
	Labetalol*	0.2 mg/kg IV push over 2 minutes. ↑ to 0.4 mg/kg/dose if still HTN in 5–10 minutes	Max 40–60 mg/dose Hold for pulse < 60 bpm
2nd-Line Therapy	Nicardipine#	0.5–5 mcg/kg/min IV drip	
	Labetalol*	0.25–1 mg/kg/hr IV drip	Max 3 mg/kg/hr Hold for pulse < 60 bpm
3rd-Line Therapy	Esmolol*	100–500 mcg/kg loading dose, then 100–500 mcg/kg/min	Hold for pulse < 60 bpm
	Nitroprusside	0.5–10 mcg/kg/min	Cyanide toxicity with prolonged (> 72 hr) use
Other	Diazoxide	1–3 mg/kg/dose IV push. Repeat PRN in 5–10 min	Max 10 mg/kg/day Vasodilator
	Clonidine	5–25 mcg/kg/day PO div q 8–12 hours	Quick, effective oral med
	Enalaprilat	5–10 mcg/kg/dose IV q 18–24 hours	ACE-inhibitor
	Phentolamine	0.05–0.1 mg/kg/dose IV bolus; max 5 mg/dose	Useful in patients with pheochromocytoma; α-adrenergic blocker

Contraindicated in headache, intracranial hemorrhage or tumor, pulmonary pathology
*Contraindicated in asthma, bronchopulmonary dysplasia, congestive heart failure, infants < 1 year old. May mask hypoglycemic symptoms (do not use in insulin-dependent diabetics). Heart rate is dose limiting. May impair athletic performance

ACUTE RENAL FAILURE

Table 11.11   Classification of Renal Failure

Acute Kidney Injury Network (AKIN)		Pediatric Modified RIFLE Criteria (critically ill children)		
	↑ Serum Cr		Estimated CrCl	Urine Output
Stage I	150% (× 1.5)	Risk	↓ by 25%	< 0.5 mL/kg/hr × 8 hours
Stage II	200% (× 2)	Injury	↓ by 50%	< 0.5 mL/kg/hr × 16 hours
Stage III	300% (× 3)	Failure	↓ by 75%	< 0.3 mL/kg/hour × 24 hours or no UOP × 12 hours
		Loss	Failure × > 4 weeks	
		End Stage	Failure × > 3 months	

CrCl: Creatinine Clearance
Data from: *Nelson Textbook of Pediatrics 19th edition* chapter 529.

Table 11.12 Creatinine Clearance Estimation

Estimated creatinine clearance = k × L/ PCr (L = length in cm)			
	k Values	*Creatinine Clearance Normal Values: (mL/min/1.73 m²)*	*Normal Creatinine (mg/dL)*
Preterm to < 1 yr old	k = 0.33	< 2 weeks old: 11–28 > 2 weeks old: 15–65	< 2 weeks old: 0.7–1.4 > 2 weeks old: 0.7–0.9
Term to < 1 yr old	k = 0.45	< 2 weeks old: 17–68 2 weeks–1 month old: 26–68 > 1 month old: 70–100	< 2 weeks old: 0.4–1 > 2 weeks old: 0.3–0.5
Girls	k = 0.55	100–120	0.2–1.0 (0.6–1.2 in teens)
Boys	k = 0.7	100–120	0.2–1.0 (0.6–1.2 in teens)

Data from: *Nelson Textbook of Pediatrics 19th edition* chapter 529.

Table 11.13 Causes of Acute Renal Failure (ARF) in Children

Pre-renal (↓ kidney perfusion, ↓ GFR)	Intrinsic (renal parenchymal damage)	Post-renal (obstruction of urinary tract)
Cardiogenic shock Septic shock Hypovolemic shock (dehydration, burns hemorrhage) Hypotension	Post-strep glomerulonephritis (PSGN) Lupus nephritis Henoch-Schönlein Purpura (HSP) Hemolytic uremic syndrome (HUS) Tumor lysis syndrome Acute tubular necrosis Drugs/ toxic exposure	Posterior urethral valves Ureteropelvic junction obstruction (UPJ) Neurogenic bladder Tumor Kidney stone

Data from: *Nelson Textbook of Pediatrics 19th edition* chapter 529.

Table 11.14 Workup of Acute Renal Failure

Serum Chemistries	↑ BUN, creatinine, uric acid, potassium, phosphate; ↓ serum sodium, ↓ Ca⁺⁺, ↓ bicarbonate (HCO₃) Acidosis
Complete Blood Count	+/– anemia, WBC ↓ or ↑, ↓ platelets in HUS
Complement (C3)	↓ in SLE, PSGN
Antistreptolysin O	↑ in PSGN
ANA, anti-DS DNA	+ in SLE (see section on rheumatology for more)
Urinalysis	RBC casts: usually glomerulonephritis; WBC casts: usually tubulointerstitial disease
Fractional Excretion of sodium (FENa)*	< 1%: most likely to be prerenal renal failure
Imaging	Renal ultrasound
Biopsy	Often required to make definitive diagnosis of etiology

* FENa = (Urine Na/Plasma Na) / (urine creatinine/plasma creatinine) × 100

ANA: Antinuclear antibodies; anti-DS DNA: anti-double stranded DNA; BUN: Blood urea nitrogen; HUS: Hemolytic uremic syndrome; PSGN: Post-strep glomerulonephritis; SLE: Systemic lupus erythematosus; RBC: Red blood cell; WBC: White blood cell
Data from: *Nelson Textbook of Pediatrics 19th edition* chapter 529.

Table 11.15   Treatment of Acute Renal Failure

Fluids	Volume repletion if no signs of volume overload or heart failure. Consider blood products if history of blood loss. Patients in shock may require vasopressors
Diuretics (after volume resuscitation)	**Mannitol** 0.5 g/kg IV or **furosemide** 2–4 mg/kg IV. Continuous IV infusion may be considered. Low-dose dopamine (2–3 mcg/kg/min) may be considered
Fluid Restriction	If no response to diuretics, limit fluid intake to 400 mL/m^2/24 hr (insensible losses) plus urine replacement. Replace extrarenal losses (emesis) cc per cc
Monitoring	Daily monitoring of fluid intake, urine and stool output, body weight, serum chemistries
Acid–Base and Electrolyte Correction	See section on electrolyte and acid–base disturbances
Hypertension	See section on hypertension/hypertensive emergency
Anemia	Transfusion of PRBCs if Hgb < 7 g/dL; 10 cc/kg over 4–6 hours to avoid potential for volume overload (if dialyzing, give during dialysis)
Diet	Restrict sodium, potassium, phosphorus, and protein

Data from: *Nelson Textbook of Pediatrics 19th edition* chapter 529.

Table 11.16   Indications for Dialysis

Refractory volume overload Refractory hyperkalemia Symptomatic hypocalcemia	Neurologic symptoms BUN > 100 mg/dL or rapid increase

Data from: *Nelson Textbook of Pediatrics 19th edition* chapter 529.

Table 11.17   Types of Dialysis

Intermittent hemodialysis	Takes 3–4 hour sessions, up to 7 days/week; for patients with stable hemodynamics
Peritoneal dialysis	Dialysis performed through catheter in peritoneum, most commonly used in infants
Continuous renal replacement therapy (CRRT)	Continuous: For use in children with unstable hemodynamic or multi-organ failure

Data from: *Nelson Textbook of Pediatrics 19th edition* chapter 529.

CHRONIC KIDNEY DISEASE

Table 11.18   Staging of Chronic Kidney Disease in Children

Stage I	Glomerular filtration rate (GFR) > 90 mL/min/1.73 m^2
Stage II	GFR 60–89 mL/min/1.73 m^2
Stage III	GFR 30–59 mL/min/1.73 m^2
Stage IV	GFR 5–29 mL/min/1.73 m^2
Stage V	GFR < 15 mL/min/1.73 m^2

Table 11.19   Treatment of Chronic Renal Disease in Children

Electrolytes and Acid–Base Disturbances	Restriction of potassium, phosphorus, and sodium may be necessary Fluid restriction if ESRD Most develop acidosis and require 1 mEq sodium citrate/mL (Bicitra™) or sodium bicarbonate tablets (650 mg = 8 mEq of base)
Nutrition	Protein intake 2.5 g/kg/24 hr Supplement with water-soluble vitamins routine and, if deficient, zinc and/or iron
Growth	Consider endocrinology and growth hormone (GH) supplementation for persistent growth failure
Renal Osteodystrophy	If ↓ 25(OH)D (25-hydroxy-vitamin D) levels (< 30 ng/mL) treat with ergocalciferol. Dose varies 2000–8000 IU/day depending on severity of deficiency If normal 25(OH)D level (> 30 ng/mL) but elevated PTH level treat with 0.01–0.05 mcg/kg/24 hr of calcitriol (Rocaltrol®, 0.25-mcg capsules or 1 mcg/mL suspension)
Anemia	Erythropoeitin if Hgb < 10 g/dL (50–150 mg/kg/dose SQ 1–3 ×/week). Goal Hgb ~ 11 g/dL
Hypertension	See section on hypertension
Medication dose	Adjust medication dose or interval for all drugs metabolized by kidney

Data from: *Nelson's Textbook of Pediatrics*: 529.2.

HEMATURIA

MICROSCOPIC HEMATURIA

(no vaginal, GI, urethral prolapse, hematologic disease, or UTI source)

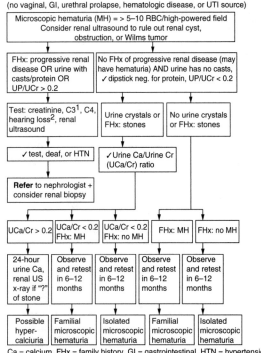

Ca = calcium, FHx = family history, GI = gastrointestinal, HTN = hypertension,
UCa = urine calcium, UCr = urine creatinine, UP = urine protein,
US = ultrasound, UTI = urinary tract infection

[1]Depressed C3 and/or C4 associated with postinfectious
glomerulonephritis, SLE, membrano-proliferative
glomerulonephritis, endocarditis, shunt nephritis, Hep B, HIV
[2]e.g., Alport's syndrome

Figure 11.1 Evaluation of Atraumatic Microscopic Hematuria Without Source

Data from: *Pediatrics* 1998; 102:e42.

GROSS/ MACROSCOPIC HEMATURIA

Table 11.20   Causes of Gross Hematuria in Children

Glomerular origin: Brown, cola-colored, tea-colored, painless	Bladder/urethra origin: Pink or red colored, often painful
Glomerulonephritis: Usually associated with edema, hypertension, proteinuria, RBC casts Most commonly post-streptococcal glomerulonephritis and IgA nephropathy	Trauma UTI Stones (may be positive family history, colicky pain) Tumor Structural anomalies Schistosoma hematobium Hypercalciuria

Table 11.21   Evaluation of Macroscopic (Gross) Hematuria

Reasonable for all patients with gross hematuria	• Vitals including HR, BP; stabilize patient first! • Full history and physical • Urinalysis (look for RBCs, WBCs, casts, protein) • Consider 24-hour urine collection • Basic metabolic panel, renal function • Urine calcium/creatinine ratio • Strongly consider renal ultrasound
Suspect glomerulonephritis	• Basic metabolic panel • Complete blood count • Complement C3, albumin, antistreptolysin titer (ASO) and streptozyme • 24-hour urine protein (if urine protein excretion of < 25 mg/dL in 24 hours, unlikely to be glomerulonephritis)
Suspect trauma	Computed tomography (CT) of abdomen/pelvis
Suspect UTI	Urinalysis, urine culture, renal ultrasound
Suspect stones	• Renal ultrasound • 24-hour urine collection for stone profile • If there is an obstruction by a stone, urgent urology referral warranted
Unclear etiology based on history and physical	• Renal ultrasound • Urine culture • Test parents for hematuria • Hemoglobin electophoresis • Urine calcium/creatinine ratio

Table 11.22   Other Causes of Red or Pink Urine

Myoglobin Desferoxamine (chelation of iron) Porphyrins Chloroquine (antimalarial drug) Urates	Phenazopyridine (Pyridium) Beets, blackberries Benzene Phenolphthalein (acid–base indicator) Red dyes in foods/food colorings

Table 11.23   Other Causes of Dark Brown Urine

Methemoglobinemia	Bile pigments
Melanin	Homogentisic acid
Thymol (flavoring/preservative)	Alkaptonuria
Alanine (amino acid)	Resorcinol (used in ointments
Cascara (laxative)	for psoriasis, hair dyes, other
Tyrosinosis	compounds)

Table 11.24   Treatment of Macroscopic Hematuria

Stabilize patient, treat individual symptoms as needed (hypertension, anemia, hypovolemia, pain, infection, etc.)
For glomerular causes of hematuria, consult pediatric nephrologist
For tumors or urinary tract abnormalities, consult pediatric urologist

Data from: *Urol Clin N Am.* 2004;31:559–573.

KIDNEY TRANSPLANT

Table 11.25   Indications for Kidney Transplant/Underlying Disease

Most children with ESRD are candidates for kidney transplant, unless they have multiple medical problems that make recovery unlikely

Obstructive uropathy (posterior urethral valves)	Hemolytic uremic syndrome (HUS)
Renal dysplasia	Membranoproliferative glomerulonephritis (MPGN)
Focal segmental glomerulosclerosis (FSGS)	Infantile polycystic kidney disease (PKD)
Prune belly syndrome	Vesicoureteral reflux (VUR)

Table 11.26   Recipient Pretransplant Workup

History and physical
Electrocardogram (ECG)
Chest X-ray (CXR)
Comprehensive metabolic panel including liver function tests, Ca, Mg, Phos
Viral studies, including cytomegalovirus (CMV), Epstein-Barr virus (EBV), human immunodeficiency virus (HIV)
Urinalysis, Urine culture
Urologic studies if indicated (VCUG, post-void residuals, urodynamic studies)

Table 11.27   Post Kidney Transplant Management Issues

Desensitization	Highly sensitized individuals (PRA* > 80%) may benefit from desensitization with high- or low-dose immune globulin (IVIG), rituximab, +/− plasmapheresis, +/− splenectomy May ↓ chances of rejection
Maintenance of systolic BP	Typically > 130 mmHg
Diuresis	Mannitol 1 g/kg and furosemide 1 mg/kg often given intraoperatively
Postoperative fluids determined by UOP	1% glucose solution in ½ NS plus 1 amp NaHCO$_3$ to replace urine output 1 mL to 1 mL if UOP < 300 mL/hr; 0.8 mL/1 mL if UOP > 300 mL/hr

(Continued)

Table 11.27 Post Kidney Transplant Management Issues *(Continued)*

Monitor for anatomic or physiologic complications	Arterial: thrombosis, stenosis Venous: thrombosis Ureter: leak, stenosis, reflux Other: hematoma, seroma, lymphocele
Monitor for early graft dysfunction	Defined as need for dialysis in first week after transplant. ↑ risk with ↑ cold ischemia time. May result from nephrotoxicity due to immunosuppressive agents (tacrolimus, cyclosporine) and may reverse with dose decrease
Monitor for acute rejection	Mild rejection may be treated with oral course of prednisone (5 mg/kg/day); Moderate rejection: Pulse of IV methylprednisolone (10–20 mg/kg/day for 3–5 days) or 3–5 days of ATG

PRA: panel reactive antibody; ATG: antithymocyte globulin

Data from: *Pediatr Clin North Am.* 2010;57(2):393–400.

NEPHROLITHIASIS

Table 11.28 Symptoms of Nephrolithiasis in Children

UTI	Renal colic
Hematuria	Dysuria
Irritability	Sterile pyuria

Table 11.29 Evaluation of Nephrolithiasis

Laboratory Analysis	Imaging
Urinalysis (check: pH, blood? crystals?)	Renal and bladder US
24-hour urine for calcium, cysteine, citrate, oxalate, uric acid	**Non-contrast** CT scan (most sensitive)
Serum chemistries, Ca^{++}, Mg, Phos, Uric acid	
Intact parathyroid hormone (iPTH) level	

Table 11.30 Treatment of Nephrolithiasis

1. Extracorporeal shock wave lithotripsy (ESWL): success 50–100%, often requires general anesthesia in children 2. Endoscopic surgery: Ureteroscope or nephroscope 3. Open surgery (rarely required)

Data from: *Comprehensive Pediatric Hospital Medicine.* St. Louis, MO: Mosby, 2007; 943–945.

BRAIN DEATH

DEFINITION:

Brain death is the loss of cerebral and brain stem functions, to the point where the brain is no longer capable of coordinating the complex interplay of organs necessary for the body to function as a whole

DETERMINATION OF BRAIN DEATH:

Brain death cannot be declared if a child is:

- < 37 weeks estimated gestational age, *or*
- < 24 hours from latest cardiopulmonary resuscitation attempt, *or*
- < 24 hours from brain injury event, *or*
- if there are differences of opinion regarding the neurologic examination, *or*
- if reversible causes of coma (including medication effect, metabolic disturbances, etc.) have not been reliably excluded

CLINICAL EXAMINATION:

- Child must have 2 exams (including apnea testing with each exam)
  - performed by different physicians
  - separated by either 12 hours (for children > 30 days–18 years old) or 24 hours (term newborns to 30 days of age)
- Coma: Child must lack any evidence of responsiveness (eye opening either spontaneously or to noxious stimuli, purposeful movements to noxious stimuli)
- Loss of brain stem reflexes:
  - Absent gag, cough, suck, rooting, and corneal reflexes
  - Fixed, dilated, midposition pupils
  - Flaccid bulbar musculature
  - Absent oculovestibular reflexes
    - No eye movement for at least 1 min after 10–50 mL ice water irrigated into external auditory canal with head elevated 30°
- Flaccidity: No spontaneous or induced movements other than spinal reflexes/myoclonus

APNEA TESTING:

Should be performed twice, at age-based intervals listed above, but may be performed by same physician.

- Preparation:
  - Core body temperature > 35°C, normal pH, $PaCO_2$, and mean arterial pressure
  - Pre-oxygenate for 5–10 minutes with 100% FiO_2
  - Continuous monitoring of pulse, respirations, and oxygen saturation
- Test: Disconnect child from mechanical ventilation
  - Any spontaneous respirations indicate some level of brain function and are inconsistent with brain death
  - Arterial blood gas (assuming patient remains hemodynamically stable and SpO_2 remains ≥ 85%): $PaCO_2$ ≥ 60 mmHg *and* ≥ 20 mmHg above baseline level without evidence of respirations *is* consistent with brain death
  - Discontinue apnea testing if child develops hemodynamic instability, SpO_2 < 85%, or if $PaCO_2$ ≥ 60 mmHg cannot be achieved
  - Repeat testing can be done at later time once child is stabilized. If unable to stabilize child, ancillary testing is indicated (see below)

ANCILLARY BRAIN DEATH TESTS

- **Not a substitute for neurologic examination**
- To be used in lieu of initial apnea testing if testing unable to be completed as above, uncertainty in neurologic examination, or concern that medication effect may interfere with evaluation of patient
  - ○ Electroencephalogram
  - ○ Radionuclide cerebral blood flow testing
- If ancillary studies consistent with brain death, second neurologic exam and apnea testing can be performed at age-specific intervals as noted above
  - ○ Repeat ancillary studies used to assist in determination of brain death should be done > 24 hours after the first study

References: *CMAJ.* 2006;174(6):S1; *Crit Care Med.* 2011;39(9):2139–2155.

FEBRILE SEIZURES

INCIDENCE

- In children ages 6 months to 5 years, ~2–5% have febrile seizures

DEFINITION

- Seizure associated with fever
- Not associated with intracranial infection, metabolic disorder, or other identifiable cause
- Usually occurs within the first 24 hours of a fever or illness
- Most common between age 6 and 60 months old

Reference: *N Eng J Med.* 1993;329:79–84.

Table 12.1   Classification of Febrile Seizures

Seizure Type	Age	Duration	Seizure Type	Episodes
Simple (~75%)	6 months to 5 years	< 15 min	Generalized tonic-clonic	1 in 24 hours
Complex (~25%)	Any	> 15 min	Focal	> 1 in 24 hours

All criteria under "simple" category must be present for seizure to be classified as a "simple febrile seizure." If any characteristic listed under "complex" category is present, then seizure should be classified as "complex febrile seizure"

Table 12.2   Management of Febrile Seizures

Simple	Workup	Treatment
	• Identify source of fever • Rule out electrolyte disturbances, hypoglycemia, ingestions • If mental status returns to baseline, normal neuro exam, and no signs of intracranial infection or head trauma, no specific workup needed • Consider lumbar puncture in children < 6 months old, altered mental status or failure to return to baseline	• Reassurance • Antipyretics do not ↓ risk of febrile seizure • Rectal diazepam if prolonged seizure • Daily prophylaxis with phenobarbital, valproic acid, or primidone, as well as oral diazepam at fever onset, ↓ seizure risk • Risks of prophylaxis likely outweigh benefits, as long-term outcome generally good regardless of treatment
Complex	• More in depth workup warranted • Identify source of fever • Consider lumbar puncture • Consider electroencephalogram and neuroimaging studies	

Table 12.3   Prognosis of Febrile Seizures

Simple	Age at First Seizure	Recurrence Risk	Epilepsy Risk
	< 12 months	30–50%	1–2.4% (with more seizures)
	> 12 months	30%	1% (slightly > general population)
Complex	Higher risk of underlying pathology and developing epilepsy (2–4%)		

Data from: *N Eng J Med.* 1993;329:79–84; *Neurology.* 2000;55:616–623; *Pediatrics.* 2008;121(6):1281–1286; *Pediatrics.* 2009;123(1):6–12.

GUILLAIN-BARRÉ SYNDROME

DEFINITION/PATHOPHYSIOLOGY

- Acute, autoimmune demyelinating polyneuropathy (AIDP) affecting the peripheral nervous system usually resulting in symmetric, ascending paralysis
- Two out of three are post-infectious (respiratory or gastrointestinal symptoms)
  - Identified pathogens include *Campylobacter*, CMV, EBV

SYMPTOMS/EXAM FINDINGS

- Gait disturbance, neuropathic pain (79%), loss of deep tendon reflexes, generally intact sensation. During course of illness, 50% have cranial nerve involvement and autonomic dysfunction, 60% unable to ambulate, 25% unable to use arms
- Diaphragmatic involvement can cause respiratory failure
- Miller-Fisher variant involves cranial nerves/facial muscles (ophthalmoplegia, ataxia, areflexia) prior to extremities (descending paralysis)

LABORATORY FINDINGS

- EMG: Abnormal F response (dispersed, impersistent, prolonged, or absent), ↑ distal latencies, conduction block or temporal dispersion of compound muscle action potential (CMAP), ↓ conduction velocity of motor and sensory nerves
- CSF analysis ↑ protein with either normal, or slightly ↑ WBC count

TREATMENT

- Transfer to intensive care (PICU) for impending respiratory failure (vital capacity < 20 mL/kg), rapid progression, bulbar paralysis (loss of gag), autonomic instability
- Intravenous immunoglobulin (IVIG): 400 mg/kg IV daily × 5 days, or 2 g/kg IV × 1.
  - Unclear if beneficial, but most children are treated
- Plasmapheresis: 40–50 mL/kg body weight plasma exchange
  - Complications include hypocalcemia, bleeding (decreased clotting factors), urticaria, infection (depletion of immunoglobulins), hypotension
- Physical and occupational therapy to help regain lost function
- Mechanical ventilation for respiratory failure

PROGNOSIS

- Better than adults; > 85% will have full recovery
  - Children with slower onset of symptoms have faster, more complete recoveries
  - At least half walking by 6 months, 70% by 1 year
- Mortality 3–4%; due to cardiac or pulmonary complications during intensive care
- Recurrence (chronic inflammatory demyelinating polyneuropathy): 3–4%

Abbreviations: CMV: cytomegalovirus; EBV: Epstein-Barr virus

References: *Cochrane Database Syst Rev.* 2010 Jun 16;(6):CD002063; Korinthenberg R, et al. *Pediatrics.* Jul 2005;116(1):8–14; *Am J of Kidney Diseases.* 2008; 52(6):1180–1196; Korinthenberg R, et al. *Neuropediatrics.* 2007;38(1):10; Vajsar, et al. *J Pediatr.* 2003;142(3):305; Agarwal S, et al. *Arch Dis Child Educ.*

HEADACHE

Table 12.4   Classification of Headaches

Type	Description	Differential Diagnosis
Acute	First episode of headache	Systemic or CNS infection (viral or bacterial), elevated intracranial pressure (bleed, mass), migraine, tension headache, medication effect
Acute Recurrent	Episodic, with symptom free interval	Migraine, tension-type headaches
Chronic Progressive	Increasing headache without remission	Elevated intracranial pressure (bleed, mass)
Chronic Non-progressive	Daily (or near-daily) non-worsening headache	Chronic migraine or tension-type (more common in adolescents)
Mixed pattern	Daily headache with superimposed attacks	

RED FLAGS FOR UNDERLYING PATHOLOGY IN PATIENTS WITH HEADACHE

- Associated head injury
- Headache with onset in middle of night or early morning, particularly if associated with vomiting
- Seizure or recent neurologic changes (balance, speech, school performance, gait, vision, handedness, other behavior)
- Children < 3 years old
- Associated with straining/Valsalva
- Explosive onset, first headache, or steadily progressive headache
- Absence of family history of migraine/headache syndrome

MEDICATIONS ASSOCIATED WITH HEADACHE

- Decongestants, antihistamines, clonidine, antibiotics (tetracycline, doxycycline), oral contraceptives, glucocorticoids, levothyroxine, caffeine (withdrawal), SSRIs
- "Overuse" headache associated with most medications used to treat headache: Triptans, ibuprofen, acetaminophen, aspirin

EVALUATION OF PATIENTS WITH HEADACHE

- Electroencephalogram (EEG) and lab testing not routinely recommended
- Computed tomography (CT) should be considered for:
  - ○ Recent onset (< 1 month) of severe headache
  - ○ Progressively worsening headache
  - ○ Associated neurologic dysfunction
  - ○ Change in type of headache
  - ○ Associated seizure disorder

MIGRAINE

Table 12.5 Treatment of Migraine

Drug	Route	Dose
Ibuprofen	PO	10 mg/kg/dose q 6 hours (max 400 mg/dose)
Acetaminophen	PO	10–15 mg/kg/dose q 4–6 hours (max 1000 mg/dose, 75 mg/kg/day up to 4 g/day)
Naproxen	PO	250 mg PO q 8 hours for children > 12 years old
Sumatriptan*§	PO	Efficacy not established
	IN	5, 10, or 20 mg × 1 as soon as possible after onset
	SQ	3 or 6 mg × 1 as soon as possible after onset
Rizatriptan*	PO	5–10 mg × 1 as soon as possible after onset
Almotriptan*	PO	6.25–12.5 mg × 1, can repeat in 2 hours if needed (max 2 doses/day or 25 mg/day)

*Contraindicated in patients with CVA (stroke, TIA), basilar, and hemiplegic migraine
§ Use in patients < 18 years old not recommended by manufacturer as "safety and efficacy have not been established"
CVA: cerebrovascular accident; IN: intranasal; PO: oral; SQ: subcutaneous; TIA: transient ischemic attack

Table 12.6 Treatment of Refractory Migraine/Status Migrainosus

Drug	Dose
Ketorolac€	0.5 mg/kg/dose IV q 6 hours (max 30 mg/dose) × maximum of 5 days; monitor renal function
Prochlorperazine¶€	0.1–0.15 mg/kg IV (max 10 mg/dose)
Promethazine¶€	0.25–0.5 mg/kg/dose (max 25 mg/dose) PO, IM, or PR
Sumatriptan/Naproxen€	10 mg/60 mg, 30 mg/180 mg, 85 mg/500 mg PO × 1. Use smaller doses in children < 12 years
Dihydroergotamine¶	1 mg IV over 3 min q 8 hours. Premed 30 minutes prior with prochlorperazine, metoclopramide, or ondansetron

¶ Beware extrapyramidal reaction (oculogyric crisis)
€ See FDA.gov/drugs for black-box warning

MEDICINES COMMONLY USED FOR PROPHYLAXIS OF MIGRAINES

- Cyproheptadine, propranolol, valproate, topiramate, amitriptyline, trazodone, gabapentin, levetiracetam all occasionally used; however, American Academy of Neurology (AAN) practice parameter notes "insufficient evidence to make recommendations regarding their use"
- Flunarizine: 5–10 mg PO daily. Not available in U.S.

References: American Academy of Neurology Practice Parameter: evaluation of children and adolescents with recurrent headache. *Neurology*. 2002;59(4):490–498; American Academy of Neurology Practice Parameter: treatment of migraine headache in children and adolescents: report of the American Academy of Neurology. *Neurology*. 2004;63:2215–2224; Medina LS, Kuntz KM, Pomeroy SL. Children with headache suspected of having a brain tumor: a cost-effectiveness analysis of diagnostic strategies. *Pediatrics*. 2001;108:255–263; Hamalainen ML, et al. Ibuprofen or acetaminophen for the acute treatment of migraine in children: a double-blind, randomized, placebo-controlled, crossover study. *Neurology*. 1997;48(1):103–107; The use of triptans for pediatric migraine. *Paediatr Drugs*. 2010;12(6):379–389; *Pediatr Emerg Care*. 2008 May;24(5):321–330; Kabbouche, et al. *Pediatrics*.2001;107:e62; Kabbouche, et al. *Headache*. 2009;49(1):106.

INFANTILE WEAKNESS

Table 12.7   Hypotonia or Weakness in an Infant

Diagnosis	Clinical Presentation	Treatment
Nerve		
Spinal Muscular Atrophy	• Infantile type (Werdnig-Hoffman) caused by motor neuron apoptosis in anterior horn • Muscle atrophy secondary to denervation • Classically presents < 3 months of life • Progressive weakness, proximal → distal, loss of reflexes, no gain of motor milestones • Spares facial and oculomotor muscles = "Alert facies" • SMN1 gene +	• Supportive care
Guillain-Barré Syndrome/CIDP	• Ascending demyelinating paralysis • Areflexia common • LP may show elevated protein without WBCs • Slowed nerve conduction on EMG	• Consider IVIG • Alt: Steroids, plasmapheresis
Neuromuscular Junction		
Infantile Botulism	• Constipation • Difficulty feeding (poor suck/latch, trouble swallowing, impaired gag) • Descending flaccid paralysis • Bulbar involvement prominent: Ptosis, sluggish pupils, weak or absent gag, dysphagia, difficulty handling secretions, weak cry • Sensation intact • Decreased facial expressions • Decreased reflexes	• Botulism anti-toxin (BabyBIG®) • Call: 510-231-7600 to reach CDPH clinical specialist • infantbotulism.org • Supportive care • Beware rapid decompensation requiring intensive care
Myasthenia Syndromes	• Autoimmune (maternal ant-AChR antibody), or genetic defect in various components of NMJ • Bulbar, respiratory muscle weakness, ptosis (in congenital) • Arthrogryposis at birth common	• Neostigmine prior to feedings for autoimmune • Consider anticholinesterase inhibitor for congenital myasthenias as well
Muscle		
Congenital Myopathies	• Impaired development from birth • May present with arthrogryposis	• Physical and occupational therapy
Electrolyte Disorders	• Hypokalemia, hypophosphatemia, hypocalcemia, hypermagnesemia	• Replete K+, Ca++, Phos+ if deficient • Supportive care until magnesium normalizes
Metabolic Disorders (many exist, 2 listed below as examples)		
Acid Maltase Deficiency	• Accumulation of glycogen in tissues • Hypotonia within first weeks of life	• Enzyme replacement therapy
Cytochrome Oxidase Deficiency	• Respiratory chain disorder = impaired energy production • Weakness, hypotonia, poor feeding, lactic acidosis	• Supportive care • Infants can be profoundly ill, improve in childhood

CDPH: California Department of Public Health; CIDP: Chronic Inflammatory Demyelinating Polyneuropathy; Ca++: Calcium; K+: Potassium; Mg+: Magnesium; Phos+: Phosphorous

SEIZURES

Table 12.8 Classification/Nomenclature of Seizures

Partial: One cerebral hemisphere
Generalized: Both hemispheres involved
Simple: Consciousness unaffected; **Complex**: Consciousness impaired
Motor: Tonic, clonic, or tonic-clonic; **Absence**: Blinking/staring
Status Epilepticus: Prolonged (> 20–30 minutes) or multiple seizures

DIFFERENTIAL DIAGNOSIS

- Syncope (+/− convulsive movements)
- Breath-holding spells
- Atypical migraine
- Benign myoclonus (sleep or neonatal)
- Tic disorders
- Reflux/Sandifer syndrome
- Pseudoseizures
- Acute dystonic reaction (medication side effect)
- Night terrors, panic attacks

Table 12.9 Causes of Seizures in Children and Adolescents

Infectious	Febrile, meningitis, encephalitis, abscess, neurocysticercosis
Toxic	Cocaine/other street drugs, lead, isoniazid, lithium, tricyclic antidepressants, hypoglycemic agents
Withdrawal	Alcohol, anticonvulsants
Electrolytes	↓ calcium, ↓ sodium, ↓ glucose, ↓ magnesium, hyperosmolality
Vascular	Stroke, arteriovenous malformation, hypertensive encephalopathy, traumatic hemorrhage
Structural	Brain tumor (primary or metastases), congenital anomalies
Endocrine	Adrenal insufficiency, hypo- or hyperthyroidism
Metabolic	Inborn errors of metabolism

Table 12.10 Evaluation of First Afebrile Seizure

Lab	• Glucose, CBC, metabolic panel, and consider toxicology screen • Lumbar puncture: For altered mental status and/or meningeal signs. Value in otherwise well children < 6 months old debated.
EEG	• OK to do as outpatient; helps to determine type and recurrence risk
Imaging	• *Emergent imaging*: Studies suggest that 25–33% of patients will have abnormal acute non-contrast CT scan, and that 3–9% of patients will have findings that require acute intervention. Consider for trauma (known or suspected), delay in return to baseline, significant cognitive or motor impairment, abnormal neurologic examination, focal seizure (+/− generalization), child < 1 year old, or abnormal EEG

Data from: *J Pediatr.* 2008;153:140–2; *Neurology.* 2000;55:616–23; *Neurology.* 2007;69:1772–80; *Neurology.* 2010;74:150–56.

Table 12.11   Treatment of Seizures by Type (second-line or adjunctive treatment in parenthesis)

Partial seizures	Carbamazepine, valproic acid, oxcarbazepine, lamotrigine, topiramate, levetiracetam
Generalized tonic-clonic	Topiramate, oxcarbazepine, phenytoin, valproic acid, carbamazepine
Juvenile myoclonic epilepsy	Valproic acid (lamotrigine, topiramate, levetiracetam)
Absence seizures	Ethosuximide, valproic acid (lamotrigine)
Rolandic epilepsy	Gabapentin, carbamazepine, or observation without meds
Lennox-Gastaut syndrome	Topiramate (lamotrigine [may ↑ myoclonic seizures in some patients], valproic acid, rufinamide)
Infantile spasms	Corticotropin = ACTH, *Acthargel* (vigabatrin [if patient has tuberous sclerosis], valproic acid)
Neonatal seizures	Phenobarbital, phenytoin (pyridoxine as adjunct)
Febrile seizures	Rectal diazepam for prolonged seizure

Data from: *Neurology* 2004; 63(4).

Table 12.12   Possible Side Effects of Anti-epileptic Drugs

Carbamazepine	Weight gain, sedation, neutropenia/agranulocytosis, ↑ liver enzymes, ↑ cholesterol
Ethosuximide	Aplastic anemia, hiccups, sedation, rash
Gabapentin	Weight gain, emotional lability, leukopenia
Lamotrigine	Rash, dizziness, sedation, Stevens-Johnson syndrome
Levetiracetam	Somnolence, mood changes/agitation/aggression
Oxcarbazepine	Hyponatremia, leukopenia, nausea, sedation, rashes
Phenobarbital	↓ Cognitive performance, ↓ attention, ↑ cholesterol, sedation
Phenytoin	Hirsutism, gingival hyperplasia, drowsiness, cardiac
Topiramate	Somnolence, weight loss, nephrolithiasis
Valproic acid	Weight gain, thrombocytopenia, ↑ liver function tests

Table 12.13   Dosing of Common Anti-epileptic Drugs[¶]

Drug	Initial Daily Dose (mg/kg/day)	Maintenance Daily Dose[§] (mg/kg/day)	Number Doses/Day
Carbamazepine	10–20; or 100 mg bid	20–35; or 1000 mg/day	2–3 (tablet) 4 (susp)
Clobazam	0.25–1 or 5 mg/day	0.5–1; or 40 mg/day	1–3
Clonazepam	0.01–0.05; or 1.5 mg/day	0.1–0.2; or 20 mg/day	2–3
Ethosuximide	10–15; or 250 mg bid	20–30; or 1.5 g/day	1–2
Felbamate	15; or 1200 mg/day	30–45; or 3600 mg/day	3–4

(Continued)

Table 12.13   Dosing of Common Anti-epileptic Drugs¶ *(Continued)*

Drug	Initial Daily Dose (mg/kg/day)	Maintenance Daily Dose§ (mg/kg/day)	Number Doses/Day
Gabapentin	5–15; or 300 mg tid	20–100; 2400 mg/day	3
Lacosamide	1; or 50 mg/day	10; or 400 mg/day	2
Lamotrigine*	0.15–0.5	2–10	1–2
Levetiracetam	5–20; 500 mg bid	20–60; or 1500 mg bid	2
Oxcarbazepine	5–10; or 600 mg/day	30–50; 1800 mg/day	2–3
Phenobarbital	3–6	3–6; or 300 mg/day	2
Phenytoin	5	4–10; or 300 mg/day	2
Rufinamide	10; or 400–800 mg/day	45; or 3200 mg/day	2
Topiramate	0.5–1; or 25 mg/day	2–10; or 1600 mg/day	2
Valproic acid	10	30–60	2–3
Vigabatrin (Sabril®)¥	50	100 (< 150 for infantile spasms)	2
Zonisamide	1–2; or 100 mg/day	4–12; max 600 mg/day	2

¶ Each drug has age-specific FDA indications and dosing. See www.FDA.gov/drugs. Pediatric neurologists frequently use medicines in non-FDA doses and indications
* Decrease dosing if co-treating with valproate. Increase dosing if co-treating with enzyme-inducers (carbamazepine, phenobarbital, phenytoin, primidone). See www.FDA.gov/drugs
¥ Can cause vision loss. Requires special consent and frequent ophthalmology exams. Call SHARE program @ 1-888-45-SHARE to enroll a patient
§ Max dose at discretion of treating neurologist: Age, efficacy, and multi-drug therapy all effect decision on maximum acceptable dose

STATUS EPILEPTICUS

DEFINITION:

- Unremitting seizures that are frequent, separated by a period of significantly impaired consciousness, or patients that are medically unstable

EMERGENT CARE:

- ABCs
- Identify underlying cause
- Obtain IV access, lateral decubitus position
- Supply O_2
- Check glucose (if < 70 mg/dL, give 2 mL/kg D_{10}W), electrolytes, arterial blood gas

TREATMENT OF STATUS EPILEPTICUS:

(1) Lorazepam[1]: 0.05–0.1 mg/kg/dose IV or IM, repeat in 5 minutes, *or*
   a. Diazepam: 0.1–0.3 mg/kg IV q 5–10 min (max dose 5 mg [if < 5 yo], 10 mg [if 5–12 yo], 30 mg [if > 12 years old, however, start with smaller dose such as 10 mg]), *or*
   b. Midazolam: 0.1 mg/kg IM or 0.2 mg/kg buccal
(2) Fosphenytoin: 15–20 mg/kg IV (rate 3 mg/kg/min = 5–7 minutes)
(3) Refractory status epilepticus (high-dose sedative therapy may require endotracheal intubation, mechanical ventilation, and blood pressure support)[2,3]

a. Levetiracetam 25–50 mg/kg IV[4,5]
b. Midazolam infusion: 0.15 mg/kg IV × 1, then 1 mcg/kg/min (titrated q 5 min to effect, generally < 30 mcg/kg/min)
c. Pentobarbital: Bolus 5 mg/kg IV × 1, then 1 mg/kg/hr (titrated to max 3 mg/kg/hr)
d. Phenobarbital: 10–20 mg/kg IV load, then 5–10 mg/kg q 15–30 min
e. Propofol: Bolus 1–2 mg/kg IV, then 2 mg/kg/hr (titrated to 15 mg/kg/hr as needed)
f. Valproic acid: Bolus 10–20 mg/kg IV. If seizures abate, continue bid therapy. If seizures continue, consider 5 mg/kg/hr

LABS:

- Complete blood count with differential, complete metabolic panel, urine toxicology, urinalysis, blood and urine cultures, anticonvulsant levels
- For infants: Metabolic workup to include urine organic acids, plasma amino acids and ammonia, pH, blood lactate and pyruvate, CSF amino acids

Abbreviation: CSF: cerebrospinal fluid

IMAGING:

Consider CT head w/o contrast in emergent situation

References:

(1) *Cochrane Rev.* 2008 Jul 16;(3):CD001905.
(2) Abend, et al. *Pediatr Neurol.* 2008;38(6).
(3) Appleton R, et al. *Arch Dis Child.* 2000;83(5):415–419.
(4) Kirmani BF, et al. *Pediatr Neurol.* 2009 Jul;41(1):37–39.
(5) Goraya JS, et al. *Pediatr Neurol.* 2008 Mar;38(3):177–1780.

STROKE

EPIDEMIOLOGY

- Rare (estimated incidence ~2–13/100,000 children per year)
- Types: Arterial ischemic stroke (AIS), venous thrombotic event (VTE), hemorrhage

PRESENTATION

- Acute onset of focal neurologic deficit (hemiparesis most common; can be visual, speech, hearing, balance deficits)
- Differential diagnoses (20% with acute onset, persistent focal neurologic deficit will not have a stroke) include migraine, seizure, postictal paralysis, psychogenic cause, musculoskeletal cause, delirium, tumor, drug toxicity, cerebellitis, AVM, abscess, ADEM

IMAGING (TO BE PERFORMED IN ALL CASES OF PERSISTENT ACUTE NEUROLOGIC DEFICITS)

- CT: Shows bleeding (hemorrhagic stroke) and larger, more established, ischemic strokes
- MRI with diffusion-weighted imaging (DWI): Demonstrates early ischemic stroke
- Magnetic resonance angiography (MRA) of head and neck, if indicated
- Consider axial T1 MRI neck to evaluate for carotid dissection, if indicated

RISK FACTORS

- Most children with AIS have a combination of > 1 thrombophilia risk factor
- Presence of either anticardiolipin antibodies or Factor V Leiden increases AIS risk by 5-fold

Table 12.14   Underlying Illnesses Predisposing to Stroke

Vascular	Moyamoya, arterio-venous malformation (AVM), dissection, fibromuscular dysplasia, Takayasu's arteritis, vasculitis (systemic lupus erythematosus, Kawasaki disease, post-radiation, infection [meningitis]), PHACE syndrome (*P*osterior fossa, *H*emangioma, *A*rterial lesions, *C*ardiac, and *E*ye anomalies)
Hematologic	Inherited: Activated protein C resistance (Factor V Leiden mutation), prothrombin gene mutation G20210A, sickle cell disease Acquired: Anti-phospholipid syndrome, protein C or S deficiency, antithrombin III deficiency
Cardiac	Cardiac surgery/catheterization Valvular disease with vegetation Congenital heart disease (cyanotic, PFO, endocarditis, myocarditis) Arrhythmia
Drugs	Estrogens (OCP), asparaginase chemotherapy, illicit drugs (cocaine)
Other	Hyperhomocysteinemia/homocystinuria (MTHFR variant) Fabry's disease (galactosidase deficiency) MELAS: Mitochondrial encephalopathy, lactic acidosis, and stroke-like episodes Organic acidopathies (methylmalonic, isovaleric, propionic acidemias, glutaric aciduria II) Pregnancy Obesity Trauma Indwelling central venous catheter Immobilization (postoperative, long travel)

MTHFR: Methylenetetrahydrofolate reductase, OCP: Oral contraceptive, PFO: Patent foramen ovale

LABS (CONSULT HEMATOLOGIST)

- Consider complete blood count, d-dimer, fibrinogen, PT, PTT (prolonged with lupus anticoagulant), protein C and S, antithrombin III and homocysteine assays, prothrombin (factor II) and factor V Leiden gene mutation analysis, anticardiolipin and β2 glycoprotein I antibodies (IgG and IgM), lupus anticoagulant (including dilute Russell viper venom time), antinuclear antibodies
- If MELAS suspected: Serum and CSF lactate, mitochondrial genetic testing

Table 12.15   Treatment of Pediatric Patients Based on Type of Stroke

Acute Ischemic Stroke (AIS)	Acute treatment (for up to 1 week after AIS)	• IV UFH***: Bolus 75–100 units/kg IV × 1; maintenance rate ~ 20 units/kg/hr IV (if > 1 year old) or 28 units/kg/hr IV (if < 1 year old), *or* • LMWH*ᵋ: enoxaparin 1 mg/kg SQ q 12 hours (if > 2 mos old) or 1.5 mg/kg SQ q 12 hours (if < 2 months old)

	Chronic treatment	• Evidence of dissection or embolism:
		  ○ LMWH*ᵋ: enoxaparin 0.5 mg/kg SQ q 12 hours (if > 2 months old) or 0.75 mg/kg SQ q 12 hours (if < 2 months old), *or*
		  ○ Warfarin: start 0.1–0.2 mg/kg PO daily × 2 days. Goal INR (2.0–3.0). Usual dose 0.05–0.34 mg/kg PO daily
		 • No evidence of dissection or embolism:
		  ○ Aspirin: 1–5 mg/kg/day × 2 years

(Continued)

Table 12.15 Treatment of Pediatric Patients Based on Type of Stroke *(Continued)*

CSVT (without hemorrhage)	Acute treatment	• IV UFH*: Start 75–100 units/kg IV × 1; maintenance rate ~ 20 units/kg/hr IV, (if > 1 year old) or 28 units/kg/hr IV (if < 1 year old), *or* • LMWH*ᵋ: enoxaparin 1 mg/kg SQ q 12 hours
	Chronic (treat for 6–12 weeks)ᵅ	• LMWH*ᵋ: enoxaparin 0.5 mg/kg SQ q 12 hours, *or* • Warfarin: start 0.1–0.2 mg/kg PO daily × 2 days. Goal INR (2.0–3.0). Usual dose 0.05–0.34 mg/kg PO daily
CSVT (with hemorrhage)	Radiologic monitoring of thrombosis at 5–7 days Anti-coagulation if thrombus propagation noted at 5–7 days	
Sickle Cell Disease	Acute: IV hydration and exchange transfusion (goal sickle Hb level < 30%) Chronic: Transfusion regimen to limit future risk of stroke	
Moyamoya Disease	Revascularization: Indirect vs direct revascularization controversial Anti-coagulants rarely indicated due to risk of hemorrhage	
Migraine	Discontinue estrogen-containing contraceptives Avoid triptans (may cause vasospasm)	
Hemorrhagic	If deficient, replace platelets, clotting factors (goal 100% activity), and/or vitamin K: 1 mg IM × 1 if > 2 kg, 0.5 mg IM × 1 if < 2 kg	
Fabry's Disease	Alpha-galactosidase enzyme replacement	

*Discontinue if platelets < 100 k

*Goal aPTT to correspond with anti-FXa level 0.35–0.7 U/mL

ᵋGoal anti-FXa level for *acute* therapy: 0.5–1 U/mL 4 hours after injection; goal anti-FXa level for *chronic* therapy: 0.1–0.3 U/mL checked every 3–4 weeks on stable dose

ᵅIf persistent CSVT noted on imaging studies after 12 weeks, continue therapy for another 12 weeks

AIS: arterial ischemic stroke; aPTT: activated partial thromboplastin time; anti-FXa: anti Factor Xa assay; CVL: central venous line; CVST: cerebral sinovenous thrombosis; Hb: hemoglobin; INR: international normalized ratio; IV: intravenous; LMWH: low molecular weight heparin; PT: prothrombin time; UFH: unfractionated heparin; UVC: umbilical venous catheter; VKA: vitamin K antagonist (warfarin)

Data from: Roach ES et al. Stroke. 2008;39(9):2644; Monagle P et al. Chest. 2008;133(6 Supple):887S.

RECURRENCE RISK:

- Clinical/radiological recurrence occurs in 6–14% children with AIS
- Silent recurrence and TIA may likely be even more common

Abbreviations: Abs: Antibodies; ADEM: Acute disseminated encephalomyelitis; AIS: Arterial ischemic stroke; AVM: Arterio-venous malformation; CSF: cerebrospinal fluid; PT: Prothrombin time; PTT: Partial thromboplastin time; TIA: Transient ischemic attack; VTE: venous thrombotic event

References: Lynch JK, et al. *Pediatrics*. 2002;109:116–123; Shellhaas RA, et al. *Pediatrics*. 2006;118(2):704–709; Kenet G, et al. *Stroke*. 2000 Jun;31(6):1283–1288; MELAS, Pavlakis, SG et al. *Ann Neurol*. 1984;16(4):481; Roach ES, et al. *Stroke*. 2008;39(9):2644; Monagle P, et al. *Chest*. 2008;133(6 Supple):887S; Muwakkit SA, et al. *Pediatr Neurol*. 2011 Sep;45(3):155–158; Strater R, et al. *Lancet*. 2002;360:1540–154; Ganesan V, et al. *Circulation*. 2006;114:2170–2177.

ALTERED MENTAL STATUS

Table 12.16   Physical Exam Clues to Cause of Altered Mental Status

Mental Status Exam	See section on Glasgow Coma Scale; assign GCS score
Respiratory	Apnea, hyperventilation, hypoventilation, Cheynes-Stokes respiration
Cardiovascular	↑ or ↓ BP, ↑ or ↓ HR? Cushing's triad: ↑ BP, ↓ HR, irregular respiration = ↑ ICP; perfusion?
General	Fever? Signs of infection? Odor or breath? Skin color, rash, bruising; abdominal guarding; hemotympanum; papilledema; nuchal rigidity
Neurologic Exam	Look for focal neurologic findings; Head size/shape, fontanelle; Posturing: decorticate (arms flexed/adducted, legs extended) = cortical or spinal lesion; decerebrate posturing (arms extended/ internally rotated, legs extended) = brain stem lesion Pupils: pinpoint (opioid intoxication, pontine lesion); unilateral dilation (herniation, seizure, CN III lesion); fatigability in response (infant botulism)
Wood's Lamp	Ethylene glycol will illuminate

Table 12.17   Differential Diagnosis of Altered Mental Status

Infection	Meningitis, encephalitis (influenza, enteroviral, post-infectious, others), abscess, subdural empyema, sepsis, HIV, toxoplasmosis, cryptococcus
Increased ICP	Subarachnoid hemorrhage, CVA, AVM, epidural bleed, hydrocephalus, tumor
Systemic Conditions	Hypertensive encephalopathy; connective tissue diseases (SLE); multiple sclerosis, hyperpyrexia, heat stroke, intussusception, hepatic encephalopathy, hypoxia, arrhythmia/syncope/cardiac cause, Wilson's disease, anemia
Endocrine/Metabolic	Hypoglycemia, DKA, hypo-/hypernatremia, uremia, Reye's syndrome, Addisonian crisis
Neoplasms	Acute lymphoblastic leukemia, medulloblastoma, neuroblastoma, craniopharyngioma, glioblastoma, etc.
Trauma	Concussion, subdural/epidural hematoma, drowning, asphyxia
Intoxication/Ingestions	Sedative-hypnotics, narcotics, alcohol, ethylene glycol, salicylates, acetaminophen, carbon monoxide, lead, marijuana, antihistamines
Seizures	Or postictal state
Psychiatric Conditions	Mania, psychosis, medication not taken properly, neuroleptic malignant syndrome, fictitious

Table 12.18   Initial Workup/Interventions in Patient with Altered Mental Status

ABCs always first priority; intubate for GCS < 8
Metabolic panel, glucose, LFTs, ammonia, BUN/Cr CBC with differential, CRP, ESR Urine/blood toxicology, lead Consider ABG, urine/blood/CSF cultures, LP, CT/MRI, TSH, EEG, CXR, ECG
Oxygen: Supply via facemask/nonrebreather **Glucose:** $D_{10}W$ (0.10 g/mL) 2–4 mL/kg IV/IO for neonates $D_{25}W$ [0.25 g/mL] 1–2 mL/kg IV/IO for older children **Naloxone:** < 5 yrs (up to 20 kg): 0.1 mg/kg, ≥ 5 yrs (or > 20 kg): 2 mg, *while awaiting initial workup*
If suspected metabolic disorder: Lactate, pyruvate, serum amino acids, urine organic acids, urine porphyrins, ketone bodies, plasma-free fatty acids, carnitine, creatinine kinase

Data from: *Pediatr Infect Dis J*. 2008;27:390–395; *Am J Emerg Med*. 2002;20:11.

ENCEPHALITIS

Table 12.19   Causes of Encephalitis

Direct Viral Infection of CNS	HSV, VZV, CMV, coxsackie, echovirus, adenovirus, equine encephalitis viruses, West Nile, Japanese encephalitis, St. Louis encephalitis, California encephalitis, mumps, measles, rabies, HIV, influenza, human metapneumovirus
Direct Bacterial Infection	*Listeria monocytogenes, Francisella tularensis, Rickettsia, Mycoplasma, Chlamydia*
Direct Fungal Infection	*Cryptococcus, Blastomyces, Histoplasma, Paracoccidioides*
Direct Parasitic Infection	Naegleria, balamuthia, toxocara
Noninfectious Causes	Immune-mediated: Acute disseminated encephalomyelitis (ADEM), acute hemorrhagic leukoencephalitis, mycoplasma, acute cerebellar ataxia; systemic lupus erythematosus, paraneoplastic syndromes

Table 12.20   Presentation of Encephalitis

Altered mental status (confusion, delirium) Seizures Abnormal neurologic exam (reflexes, eye movements, nystagmus, dysarthria, dysphagia, facial palsies)	Movement disorders Somnolence Decreased feeding (infant) Weak suck (infant) SIADH, adrenal or thyroid abnormalities, autonomic dysfunction (if hypothalamus involved)	Irritability ↓ Head control (infant) Fever Meningeal signs Weakness Altered behavior (agitation, apathy, disinhibited)

Data from: *Pediatrics in Review* Vol. 33 No. 3 March 1, 2012 pp. 122–133.

MOVEMENT DISORDERS

- History and exam crucial to diagnosis
- Toxicology screen for all with acute onset
- Consider imaging (MRI, CT head) and neurology consult

Table 12.21   Ataxia

Uncoordinated voluntary movement, despite normal strength • Disorder of cerebellum. Assess duration. Consider MRI, CT head, EMG, EEG • Exam: Abnormal finger-nose, thumb-digit opposition, wide-based gait		
Acute	• Ingestion • Hydrocephalus • Encephalitis	• Acute post-infectious (particularly varicella) • Guillain-Barré (Miller-Fisher variant) • Stroke • Brain tumor
Chronic	• Friedreich ataxia	• Ataxia telangiectasia • Cerebellar dysgenesis

Data from: *Br J Sports Med.* 2009;43:i76–i84.

Table 12.22 Vertigo

Sensation of movement (spinning) in relation to surrounding
- Disorder of inner ear (labyrinths, hair cells) or brain stem
- Nystagmus should be present; identify otitis media, neurocutaneous signs
- Consider otolaryngology consult and MRI/CT head for recurrent/chronic symptoms

	History	Duration	Hearing	Treatment
Acute Vertigo				
Benign paroxysmal	Occurs with rapid head movement	10–20 seconds	Normal	Head/neck positioning
Labyrinthitis	No trauma or headache	Days	Often impaired	Meclizine
Perilymphatic fistulae	Due to ↑ pressure "pop" at onset	Variable	Fluctuating	Surgical
Labyrinth concussion	Recent trauma	Days	Often impaired	Watch vs surgical
Recurrent Vertigo				
Migraine	Headache	Variable	Normal	See migraine
Ménière's disease	Relapsing	Mins/hrs	↓ Low frequency	

Data from: *Neurologic Clinics.* 23(3) Aug 2005.

Table 12.23 Chorea

Involuntary muscle contractions → twitching and writhing, which often "flow" down extremities, causing flinging "ballistic" movement. Suppressed in sleep

Sydenham's chorea (facial grimacing)	• Associated carditis, arthritis and ↑ ASO titer (rheumatic fever) • May respond to valproic acid, haloperidol, prednisone • Lasts weeks to months; 20% recurrence within 2 years
Other causes	• Wilson's disease, Huntington disease, systemic lupus erythematosus • Drugs: metoclopramide, phenothiazines, haloperidol

Table 12.24 Dystonia

Involuntary, sustained contraction = slow, twisting of trunk, extremities
Occasionally involves eyelid (blepharospasm) or speech muscles (dysphonia)
• Phenothiazines: May respond to diphenhydramine. Remove inciting medication
• Cerebral palsy: Baclofen, benzodiazepines, botulinum injection
• Familial dystonia: Onset 6–12 years, may be levodopa-responsive

ASO: anti-streptolysin O antibody, CT: computed tomography, EEG: electroencephalogram, EMG: electro-myogram, MRI: magnetic resonance imaging

WEAKNESS

Table 12.25   Evaluation of Weakness

Definitions	*Asthenia:* fatigue/exhaustion in the absence of muscle weakness (sleep disorders; depression; chronic heart, lung, and kidney disease; anemia; hypothyroidism; medication; pregnancy) *Hypotonia:* ↓ resistance of muscles to passive stretching *Weakness:* ↓ muscle strength (weak infants are always hypotonic, hypotonic infants may not be weak)
History	Pregnancy history, birth history, detailed PMH, family history, history of consanguinuity Review developmental milestones (any history of regression?) Categorize as acute, chronic, or progressive
General Exam Look for signs of:	Atrophy (longstanding upper or lower motor neuron disease associated with muscle atrophy and possible shortening of extremity) Pseudohypertrophy (muscular dystrophy) Tenderness on muscle palpation (inflammatory process) Fasciculation (caused by denervation/anterior horn cell) Irritability of muscle with percussion (inflammatory process) Myotonia with percussion (problem with muscle membrane) Pain with tapping along spine (entrapped nerve roots)
Assessing Tone	Gentle passive movement of extremities; ↓ tone with acute upper motor neuron problem; tone will ↑ over time (*subacute*)
Signs of proximal muscle *weakness* (more likely to be myopathy)	• Abdominal breathing, accessory muscle use • Head lag, inability to flex neck when supine • Hold child suspended under axillae: "slips through the hands" • Evaluate force of foot withdrawal when stimulated • Gowers maneuver (rise from seated position on floor) • Shoulder elevation, neck flexion and extension
Signs of distal weakness	Weakness in flexion of arms, elevation of legs, foot flexion (more likely to be neuropathy)
Signs of cord lesion	Weakness of BILATERAL lower extremities (may be asymmetric), altered rectal tone, altered perineal sensation
Signs of hypotonia	General posture; position on vertical and horizontal suspension, scissoring or spasticity indicate ↑ tone
Muscle unit, neuromuscular junction, or motor nerve causes (peripheral causes of weakness)	Symmetric or asymmetric ptosis, facial weakness, weak extraocular movements; in neuromuscular junction problems, reflexes are normal. Absent reflexes usually associated with anterior horn cell, neuropathies, and muscle disease. Neuropathy may be associated with sensory changes as well. Small, bell-shaped chest; high-arched palate; tongue fasciculation may be present; may see ↓ muscle tone; toe walking, waddling or hyperlordotic gait
Upper motor neuron lesion (Central cause of weakness)	External rotation legs; arm and wrist are flexed; pronation and drift when standing with arms extended/palms up. Normal to ↑ DTRs on affected side, +/− clonus. Difficult rapid alternating movements. Chest size normal; no tongue fasciculation; toe walking, hemiparetic or spastic gait; +/− unilateral face weakness

Table 12.26   Differential Diagnosis of Weakness

Cerebral Cortex	Vasculitis, cerebral vascular accident, infection (meningitis, encephalitis, abscess), tumor, multiple sclerosis, seizure, migraine*, alternating hemiplegia of childhood
Spinal Cord	Tumor (pain, loss of bowel/bladder function, sensory abnormalities can help to identify level), transverse myelitis (sudden onset), infection, trauma
Anterior Horn Cell	Spinal muscular atrophy*: Infant, DTRs absent, fasciculations Poliomyelitis: Asymmetric, no DTRs, pain, rapid onset, history of diarrhea
Nerves	Guillain-Barré (rapidly progressive, ascending or descending, absent DTRs, may have mild sensory symptoms), peripheral nerve toxins, acute intermittent porphyria
Neuromuscular Junction	Myasthenia gravis* (bulbar symptoms, ptosis, ↑ with exercise/fatigability, DTRs normal, difficulty with breathing, autonomic symptoms), botulism (usually < 1 yr, bulbar symptoms, DTRs nl, fatigability of pupil response), organophosphate or carbamate poisoning
Muscle	Muscular dystrophy* (proximal weakness, pseudohypertrophy, ↓ DTRs), myotonic dystrophy* (temporal balding, intellectual impairment, cataracts, heart sx); myositis (acute onset, tender muscles, myoglobinuria); metabolic: (nontender, normal or ↓ DTRs), rhabdomyolysis, trichinellosis (parasite from raw pork), familial periodic paralysis*, thyroid-related myopathy, dermatomyositis, polymyositis, glycogen storage dieases, lipid storage diseases, mitochondrial disorders
Other	Sepsis, systemic illness, dehydration, renal disease, liver disease, prolonged immobility, hypokalemia, hypophosphatemia, hypocalcemia, hyponatremia, hypernatremia, medication (sulfonamides, corticosteroids, penicillin, isoniazid, nitrofurantoin, zidovudine, Mag sulfate, chemotherapy), psychiatric

*May have positive family history
Data from: http://pedclerk.bsd.uchicago.edu/page/evaluation-child-muscle-weakness. Accessed 1/21/13.

Table 12.27   Workup of Weakness

Perform appropriate studies based on clinical history and exam findings	
Labs	Comprehensive metabolic panel, CK, urine myoglobin, TSH/Free T4; evaluation for infection if suspected
MRI Brain/Spine	Appropriate if spinal cord disease is suspected (emergent); consider as alternative to CT for diagnoses involving the CNS
CT	Indicated to evaluate suspected CNS cause of weakness
Lumbar puncture	Indicated if CNS infection suspected; may be useful in evaluating neuropathies and in spinal cord disease
Nerve Conduction Study	May be indicated when suspecting neuropathies and neuromuscular junction processes
EMG	May be helpful in evaluation of muscle disease
Muscle Biopsy	Gold standard for diagnosis of muscle disease processes

Data from: *Am Fam Physician.* 2005 Apr 1;71(7):1327–1336; *Paediatr Child Health.* 2005;10(7).

CHAPTER 13 ■ NUTRITION

BREASTFEEDING

- American Academy of Pediatrics (AAP) recommends exclusive breastfeeding for the first 6 months of life, and ongoing up to 1 year (longer if desired)
- No pacifier until breastfeeding is well established
- Baby should receive 8–12 feeds/24 hours in the first few weeks of life
- Breastfed infants should get 400 IU vitamin D daily starting within first 2 months of life until child drinking at least 500 mL/day vitamin D supplemented formula or milk
- Breastfed infants should get 0.5–1 mg vitamin K IM after first feed (< 6 hours old)
- Breastmilk storage: Freshly expressed milk can be stored 4–6 hours at room temperature, 24 hours in cooler with ice, 5 days in refrigerator, or 3 months in freezer (2 weeks if freezer is inside refrigerator, 6 months if deep freezer)

Table 13.1   Contents of Breast Milk

Contents of human milk are variable. Primary protein: whey; fats: variable, high in omega-3s and cholesterol; carbohydrate: lactose, oligosaccharides; calories ~ 20/ounce; can add human milk fortifiers to make 24 calories/ounce for preemies

Data from: *Pediatrics.* 2005; 115(2):496–506 and *Pediatrics.* 2008;122(5):1142–1152.

Table 13.2   Benefits of Breastfeeding

Benefits for Baby	Benefits for Mom and Society
Decreased risk of allergies and asthma	↓ Postpartum bleeding
Decreased risk for many infections including diarrhea, meningitis, otitis	↓ Risk breast and ovarian cancer; possible ↓ osteoporosis
↓ SIDS and postneonatal mortality	↓ Time to prepregnancy weight
↓ Risk of type I and II diabetes	↑ Child spacing
↓ Risk certain cancers (leukemia)	↓ Health care costs
↓ Risk of obesity/hypercholesterolemia	↓ Public health costs/special programs
↑ Performance: cognitive development	↓ Environmental burden

Data from: *Pediatrics.* 2005; 115(2):496–506 and *Pediatrics.* 2008;122(5):1142–1152.

Table 13.3   Contraindications to Breastfeeding

Baby with galactosemia	Mother on chemotherapy
Mother with HTLV or HIV infection	Mother taking street/illicit drugs
Mother with untreated tuberculosis	Mother with herpes infection of breast
Mother exposed to radioactive medications/materials	Mother on certain other drugs

HIV: Human immunodeficiency virus, HTLV: Human T-lymphotropic virus, SIDS: Sudden infant death syndrome
Data from: *Pediatrics.* 2005; 115(2):496–506 and *Pediatrics.* 2008;122(5):1142–1152.

Table 13.4   Situations During Which Breastfeeding Is Usually Safe

Hepatitis B surface antigen positive or Hepatitis C positive	Tobacco smoking (try to quit)
Hyperbilirubinemia	Occasional alcohol ingestion*
Cytomegalovirus-positive mother (past conversion), term baby	Certain medications (see below)

*Wait minimum 2 hours after alcohol consumed to breastfeed

Data from: *Pediatrics*. 2005; 115(2):496–506 and *Pediatrics*. 2008;122(5):1142–1152.

Table 13.5   Selected Medications That Are Contraindicated During Breastfeeding

Bromocriptine, ergotamine, phenindione, street drugs (cocaine, phencyclidine, heroin, etc.), chemotherapeutic drugs, radioisotopes, lithium

Data from: *Pediatrics*. 2005; 115(2):496–506 and *Pediatrics*. 2008;122(5):1142–1152.

Table 13.6   Selected Medications That Are Secreted in Breast Milk That May Be Harmful to Infant or Reports of Effects on Infants

Anxiolytics (*diazepam, lorazepam*, etc), antidepressants (*fluoxetine, fluvoxamine*), aspirin, caffeine, chloramphenicol, clemastine, estradiol, haloperidol, mesalamine, metoclopramide, metronidazole, nitrofurantoin, phenobarbital, phenytoin, primidone, pseudoephedrine, sulfasalazine, tinidazole

Data from: *Pediatrics*. 2005; 115(2):496–506 and *Pediatrics*. 2008;122(5):1142–1152.

Table 13.7   Selected Medications That Are Generally Considered Safe While Breastfeeding

Acetaminophen, acyclovir, atenolol, captopril, cefazolin, ceftriaxone, clindamycin, codeine, digoxin, enalapril, folic acid, ibuprofen, isoniazid, medroxyprogesterone, methadone, naproxen, nifedipine, prednisone, rifampin, senna, spironolactone, tetracycline, trimethoprim/sulfamethoxazole, valproic acid, warfarin, levonorgestrel, scopolamine

*For detailed database of medications and breastfeeding, please see http://www.toxnet.nlm.nih.gov/cgi-bin/sis/htmlgen?LACT

Data from: *Pediatrics*. 2005; 115(2):496–506 and *Pediatrics*. 2008;122(5):1142–1152.

Table 13.8   Infant Feeding Guidelines

Age	Frequency	Amount
0–4 weeks	• Every 1–3 hours (timed from the beginning of the feed) • 8–12 feeds/24 hours • Wake after 4 hours to feed	• Breastfeed 20–45+ minutes/feed • 1–3 ounces per feed if using bottle
4–8 weeks	• Every 2–4 hours	• Breastfeed 20–45+ minutes/feed • 2–4 ounces per feed • 18–32 ounces/day
2–6 months	• Every 2–4 hours in day • Every 6–8 hours overnight (may be 10 hours overnight @ 6 months)	• Breastfeed 20–45+ minutes/feed • 4–6 ounces per feed • 24–32 ounces/day
> 6 months	• 4–5 feeds/day, decreases as increase solid foods	• Breastfeed 20–45+ minutes/feed • 6–8 ounces/feed (32 ounces/day)

Data from: *Nutrition Practice Care Guidelines for Preterm Infants in the Community*, 2006; http://public.health.oregon.gov/HealthyPeopleFamilies/wic/Documents/preterm.pdf.

FAILURE TO THRIVE (FTT)

DEFINITION:

No definitive definition exists; consider one of the following:

- Significant weight loss crossing 2 percentile lines on standard growth curves (WHO charts for children < 2 years old, CDC charts for children ≥ 2 years old [see section on growth charts and http://cdc.gov/growthcharts])
- Most FTT occurs in children age < 2 years old
- Insufficient weight or height gain (< 3–5% for age)
- Weight/height or weight/length < 85% mean for age

INDICATIONS FOR HOSPITALIZATION

- Severe FTT (< 85% ideal body weight)
- Absence of weight gain despite intensive outpatient interventions
- Concerning social situation

HISTORY AND PHYSICAL EXAM

- Differentiate FTT from familial short stature, constitutional growth delay, small-for-gestational-age infants, and premature infants "catching-up"
- Diet history:
  - Breastfed versus formula
  - Formula preparation and storage
  - Volume consumed (frequency/duration of feeds)
  - Maternal diet if child breastfed
  - Solid food intake, other liquids (juice, rice water, teas)
- Social history often reveals significant impediments to adequate feeding such as chaotic environment, parenting difficulties, or financial stressors
- Review outpatient 72-hour food diary to assess sufficiency of diet
- Plot current and previous growth parameters on appropriate growth chart
- Physical exam (PE): Look for dysmorphic features that may suggest underlying genetic abnormality. Assess heart (CHF from undiagnosed heart disease can cause FTT)
- Practitioner skilled in lactation consultation should observe breastfeeding
- Neurologic exam: Especially suck/swallow coordination, latch, and tone

Table 13.9   Inadequate Caloric Intake

Psychosocial Problems	Anatomic/Neurologic Problems
• Improperly prepared formula • Inappropriate diet (juice, rice water) • Poverty leading to food shortage • Food phobia following choking • Inadequate breast milk production • Neglect/abuse	• Cleft palate, micrognathia, macroglossia • Poor suck/swallow coordination from: Hypotonia, hypothalamic tumor ("diencephalic syndrome"), neuromuscular weakness (botulism, myasthenia gravis, muscular dystrophy) • Obstructive sleep apnea syndrome

Data from: *Am Fam Phys.* 2003 Sep 1; 68(5):879–884.

Table 13.10   Improper Calorie Utilization

Malabsorption	Metabolism Defects
• Cow's milk protein allergy • Celiac disease • Inflammatory bowel disease • Pancreatic insufficiency • Bacterial overgrowth	• Inborn error of metabolism • Growth hormone deficiency • Glycogen storage disorders

Data from: *Am Fam Phys.* 2003 Sep 1; 68(5):879–884.

Table 13.11   Increased Caloric Needs

• Hyperthyroidism • Congestive heart failure • Prematurity • Malignancy • Chronic liver disease	• Chronic infection: HIV, tuberculosis • Renal disease: Renal tubular acidosis, chronic renal failure, Fanconi syndrome • Chronic lung disease: Bronchopulmonary dysplasia, asthma, cystic fibrosis

Data from: *Am Fam Phys.* 2003 Sep 1; 68(5):879–884.

EVALUATION

- If diagnosis not evident from history and PE, consider laboratory evaluation:
  - ○ Complete blood count with differential, electrolytes, blood urea nitrogen, creatinine, urinalysis with microscopy, albumin, lead level, thyroid stimulating hormone, IgA anti-tissue transglutaminase or anti-endomysial antibodies (evaluate for celiac disease)
  - ○ If concerned for malabsorption: Stool for reducing substances, alpha-1 antitrypsin, fecal calprotectin, qualitative analysis for fat globules

TREATMENT

- Caloric supplementation based on severity of FTT and underlying diagnosis:
  - ○ Infants: "Non-organic" FTT infants need ~ 150% recommended daily calories for "catch-up" growth
    - – If unable to take sufficient volume, mix formula > 20 kcal/oz or add fortifier to pumped breast milk
    - – See tables in Nutrition section for instructions on concentrating formula
  - ○ Toddlers and older children: Consider high-calorie foods such as butter, whole milk, cheese, peanut butter, "instant" breakfast drinks, *PediaSure*®
- Once adequate intake assured, schedule weekly weight checks for several weeks, then monthly as weight velocity increases
- Consider Social Services consult and Child Protective Services referral if significant social aspects underlying FTT

Abbreviations: BUN: Blood urea nitrogen; CHF: Congestive heart failure; FTT: Failure to thrive; TSH: Thyroid stimulating hormone

Reference: *Am Fam Phys.* 2003;68(5):879–884.

GENERAL NUTRITION GUIDELINES

Table 13.12   Calorie Requirements

Age	Calories/day (average)	Kcal/kg/day
0–6 months	650	90–120 kcal/kg/day
6–12 months	850	
1–3 years	1200–1300	75–90 kcal/kg/day
3–7 years	1600–1800	
7–11 years	1800–2000	60–75 kcal/kg/day
11–14 years	Female 2100, male 2500	
15–18 years	Female 2100, male 3000	

Data from: 1999–2002 Dietary Reference Intakes, Institutes of Medicine 2005 Dietary Guidelines.

Table 13.13 Protein Requirements

Age	Grams/day	Grams/kg/day
1–3 years	13	1.1
4–8 years	19	0.95
9–13 years	34	
14–18 years	Female 46, male 52	0.85

Data from: Dietary Reference Intakes: Institute of Medicine 2005 Dietary Guidelines.

Table 13.14 Fat Requirements

Saturated Fat	1–3 years	4–8 years	9–13 years	13–18 years
Total fat (grams/day)	30–50	40–60	60–85	55–95
% of total daily calories	30–35%	25–35%		
Saturated fat	< 10% of calories in kids > 2 years old			

Data from: Dietary Reference Intakes: Institute of Medicine 2005 Dietary Guidelines.

Table 13.15 Daily Vitamin/Fiber Requirements

	1–3 years	4–8 years	9–13 years	13–18 years
Calcium (mg)	500	800	1300	1300
Iron (mg)	7	10	8	Female 15, male 11
Vitamin C (mg)	15	25	45	Female 65, male 75
Vitamin A (mg)	1000	1300	2000	Female 2300, male 3000
Fiber (grams)	~15	~20	~25	Female 20, male 30

Data from: Dietary Reference Intakes: Institute of Medicine 2005 Dietary Guidelines.

INFANT FORMULA REFERENCE

Table 13.16 Infant Formulas

Formula Brand Name	Distinguishing Factors	Indications
Cow's Milk Based		
With Iron Enfamil®, Similac®	• 20 calories/ounce • Protein: whey • Carbohydrate: lactose • Fat: safflower, soy, coconut, palm, sunflower oils. 300 mOsm/kg	• Standard formula • Normal term infants or infants with no specific nutritional needs
Hypercaloric Enfamil 24® or Similac 24®	• 24 calories/ounce • Other components the same as above except ↑ osmolality (360–380 mOsm/kg) and ↑ K, Ca, Phos, Cl concentration	• Used for infants with fluid restrictions and/or ↑ calorie requirements

(Continued)

Table 13.16   Infant Formulas (*Continued*)

Formula Brand Name	Distinguishing Factors	Indications
Cow's Milk Based		
Preterm	• Protein: milk/whey concentrate • Fat: MCT, soy, coconut oil	• ↑ protein concentration and calories for preemies
NeoSure®	• 22 calories/ounce • Carbohydrate: lactose, maltodextrin	
Enfamil Premature®	• 24 calories/ounce • Carbohydrate: corn syrup/ lactose	
Lactose Free	• *Enfamil LactoFree LIPIL, Isomil DF, and Similac Lactose-Free Advance*	• Lactose intolerance
Reflux *Enfamil AR LIPIL®*	• 20 calories/ounce • Protein: nonfat milk • Carbohydrate: lactose/maltodextrin • Fat: palm, soy, coconut, sunflower oil	• Kids with reflux • Thickens in stomach (rice starch added)
Altered Electrolytes *Similac® 60/40*	• 20 calories/ounce • Protein: whey, casein • Carbohydrate: lactose • Fat: soy, coconut, corn oil • 280 mOsm/kg	• For kids with cardiac or renal disease • Lower calcium, phos, iron
Soy Based		
With Iron *Isomil, Prosobee®, Good Start®, Supreme Soy®*	• 20 calories/ounce • Protein: soy/L-methionine (partially hydrolyzed in Good Start®) • Carbohydrate: corn syrup/sucrose (*Isomil*) • Fat: safflower, soy, coconut, palm, sunflower oils • 200 mOsm/kg	• Lactose intolerance • Cow's milk formula intolerance • Galactosemia
Prosobee® 24	• 24 calories/ounce • Same as above except 240 mOsm/kg	Same as above but ↑ calorie needs
Whey Hydrolysate (partial hydrolysate)		
Good Start®, **Good Start Protect Plus®**	• 20 calories/ounce • Carbohydrate: lactose, maltodextrin • Protein: partially hydrolyzed whey • Fats: palm, soybean, safflower, and coconut oils • Protect Plus: added *BIFIDUS BL*	*May* help prevent allergies in high-risk infants
Enfamil Gentlease Lipil®	• 20 calories/ounce • Carbohydrate: corn syrup • Protein: partially hydrolyzed whey • Fats: palm, soybean, safflower, and coconut oils • Indications: fussiness/gas	*Unique features: Partially hydrolysed proteins, decreased lactose, added DHA, ARA, choline*

(Continued)

Table 13.16   Infant Formulas (*Continued*)

Formula Brand Name	Distinguishing Factors	Indications
Casein Hydrolysates		
Shared characteristics of all three:	• 20 calories/ounce • Protein: casein hydrolysate, L-cysteine, L-tyrosine, L-tryptophan	*May* be helpful during acute GI illnesses (diarrhea)
1. Pregestimil®	• Fat: MCT (55%), corn, and sunflower oils • 320 mOsm/kg	Malabsorption (also comes in 24 calories/ounce)
2. Alimentum®	• Fat: MCT (33%), safflower, and soy oils • 370 mOsm/kg	Problems with formulas with intact protein, malabsorption
3. Nutramigen®	• Fat: palm, soy, coconut, and sunflower oils • 320 mOsm/kg	*May* help ↓ allergies in high-risk infants
Amino Acid *Neocate*®, *Elecare*®, *Nutramigen AA*®	• 20 calories/ounce • Protein: simple amino acids • Fat: vegetable oils (MCT in Elecare) • Carbohydrate: corn syrup solids	Child with sensitivity to multiple proteins
High MCT *Portagen*®	• 20 calories/ounce • Protein: caseinate • Fat 85% MCT, corn oils • Carbohydrate: corn syrup/sucrose	↓ lipase/bile salts, fat malabsorption, chylothorax

MCT: medium chain triglycerides

Table 13.17   Enteral Formulas for Older Kids (all have 30 calories/ounce except where noted)

Formula Name	Protein	Fat	Carbohydrate
PediaSure®	Whey/casein	Safflower, soy, MCT	Sucrose, maltodextrin
Kindercal®	Casein	Sunflower, corn, MCT, canola	
Ensure®	Casein/soy	Corn oil	
Boost®	Milk protein	Sunflower, canola, corn	Sucrose/corn
Peptamen Jr.®	Whey hydrolysate	MCT, soy, canola	Corn starch, maltodextrin
Jevity® *(1, 1.2, 1.5 cal/mL)*	Casein/soy	MCT, canola, vegetable oils	Corn syrup/maltodextrin
Neocate Jr +/– prebiotics	Amino acid	Canola, coconut, safflower oils	Corn syrup

MCT: medium chain triglycerides

Table 13.18   Formulas with Special Characteristics for Older Kids and Adolescents

Ensure Plus®, *Deliver*®, and *Two-Cal*®	• ↑ calorie formulas: *Ensure Plus*® = 1.5 calories/mL • *Deliver*® and *Two-cal*® = 2 calories/mL (60 calories/ounces)
Tolerex®, *Vivonex Plus*®, *Neocate Jr.*®	• Amino acid formula • Spoon-feedable food: Neocate Nutra® (not sole source of nutrition)
Peptamen Jr.®	• Hydrolyzed whey formula
Portagen® (long term: need supplements)	• ↑ concentration of MCT (86%); used in patients with ↓ lipase/bile salts, fat malabsorption, chylothorax

MCT: medium chain triglycerides
Adapted from Nutrition Practice Care Guidelines for Preterm Infants in the Community, 2006; http://www.oregon.gov/DHS/ph/wic/docs/preterm.pdf.

FEEDING PRETERM INFANTS

- Preterm infants should gain 20–40 g/day (1–1.5 oz)
- Most preterm or small for gestational age (SGA) infants will have catch-up growth in first 3–8 months; head circumference first, then weight, then length

Table 13.19   Specialized Infant Formulas

Formula Type	Brand Names	Use
Preterm Formulas (24 calories/ounce)	*Enfamil Premature Lipil®, Similac Special Care®*	• Infants weighing less than 2 kg (4 lb 6 oz) and taking less than 500 mL/day • ↑ protein, vitamins A, D, B_6
Transitional Formulas (22 calories/ounce)	*Enfamil EnfaCare Lipil®, Similac NeoSure Advance®*	• ↑ protein, calcium, phosphorus, vitamins, and other minerals
Specialized Formulas	*Pregestimil®, Alimentum®, Nutramigen®, Neocate®, Elecare®, Nutramigen AA®*	• Should be used for formula intolerance • Designed for term infants
Soy Formula	*Isomil®, ProSobee®*	• Not recommended for infants < 1800 g (less weight gain, growth, and albumin levels)

- It is generally recommended that preterm infants stay on transitional formula until 9 months corrected age, but some infants may benefit from transitional formula until 12 months corrected age. Consider on individual basis
- Solids may be started at 6 months corrected age, and cow's milk may be started at 12 months corrected age
- Preterm baby should gain 15 g/kg body weight per day

Table 13.20   Indications of Inadequate Weight Gain of Premature Infants/Children

Corrected Age	Weight Gain
Term to 3 months	< 20 gm/day (< 5 oz/wk)
3–6 months	< 15 gm/day (< 3.5 oz/wk)
6–9 months	< 10 gm/day (< 2 oz/wk)
9–12 months	< 6 gm/day (< 1.5 oz/wk)
1–2 years	< 1 kg/6 months (< 2 pounds/6 months)

CHAPTER 14 ■ ONCOLOGY

BONE MARROW TRANSPLANT COMPLICATIONS

GRAFT VERSUS HOST DISEASE (GVHD)
- Donor T-cells become active against recipient major and minor histocompatibility complex (MHC) antigens
- Acute GVHD: Occurs < 3 months post-transplant; most commonly 2–5 weeks post-transplant
  - Symptoms (each affected organ staged I–IV based on severity)
    - Rash (erythematous, maculopapular), vomiting, diarrhea, anorexia, liver disease (elevated bilirubin, transaminases, alkaline phosphatase)
  - Acute GVHD prophylaxis with immunosuppressives (tacrolimus, glucocorticoids, methotrexate, cyclosporine) may delay engraftment and increase risk of post-transplantation infection
  - Treatment: Glucocorticoids
    - Steroid-resistant GVHD may respond to mycophenolate mofetil, anti-thymocyte globulin, other therapies
- Chronic GVHD: Occurs > 3 months post-transplant; caused by autoantibody production and progressive fibrosis
  - Clinical features include systemic fibrosis of skin, arthritis, joint contractures, bronchiolitis obliterans, cholestasis secondary to bile duct destruction
  - Treatment: glucocorticoids
    - Steroid-refractory chronic GVHD may respond to tacrolimus, cyclosporine, IL-1 receptor antagonists, mycophenolate mofetil
  - May require prolonged (1–3 year) immunosuppression to prevent recurrence
  - Increased risk of secondary cancers (post-transplant lymphoproliferative disorder [PTLD])

VENO-OCCLUSIVE DISEASE (VOD)
- Hepatic sinusoidal damage → fibrin deposition → venule occlusion
- Clinical findings: ascites (weight gain, ↑ abdominal circumference), hepatomegaly, jaundice, right upper quadrant pain
- Lab abnormalities: ↑ D-dimer, ↑ total and direct bilirubin levels, ↓ platelets
- Treatment: No proven efficacious therapies. Options include:
  - Alteplase (tPA), defibrotide, antithrombin III
  - Judicious fluid and electrolyte management, opiates for right-upper quadrant pain, total parenteral nutrition

INFECTIOUS COMPLICATIONS OF STEM CELL TRANSPLANTATION
- *Pneumocystis jiroveci* (*carinii*) pneumonia
  - Preferred prophylaxis:
    - TMP/SMX: 5 mg/kg TMP + 25 mg/kg SMX/day divided bid 3 consecutive days each week
  - Alternative prophylaxis:
    - Dapsone: 2 mg/kg/day PO (max dose 100 mg/day), *or*
    - Dapsone: 4 mg/kg PO once weekly (200 mg/dose), *or*
    - Pentamidine: 300 mg inhaled monthly by Respirgard II nebulizer

FEBRILE NEUTROPENIA

The below guidelines represent a single pathway for diagnosis, initiation, and escalation of therapy, and de-escalation/discontinuation of therapy. Each institution will have variations on what follows:

CRITERIA FOR DIAGNOSING FEBRILE NEUTROPENIA (INSTITUTION-DEPENDENT)
- Temperature > 38.0°C × 1 *or* > 37.8°C × 2 at least 4 hours apart, *and*
- Absolute neutrophil count < 500/mm^3, *or* ANC > 500/mm^3 with *expected* drop
  - ANC = White blood cells × (% neutrophils + % bands)

EVALUATION OF FEBRILE NEUTROPENIC PATIENT
- Culture all lumens of central venous catheters (CVC)
  - Consider peripheral-blood culture concurrent with CVC culture
- If possible, obtain mid-stream, clean-catch urine specimen for analysis and culture
- Obtain chest radiograph only if patient has symptoms of chest infection
- Consider abdominal imaging for moderate–severe abdominal pain or hematochezia

Table 14.1   Common Pathogens in Febrile Neutropenia*

Type	Common Organisms
Gram +	Coagulase-negative staphylococci, *Staphylococcus aureus*, viridans strep
Gram −	*Escherichia coli*, *Pseudomonas* spp, *Klebsiella* spp, *Enterobacter* spp
Fungi	*Candida* spp, *Aspergillus* spp. More common with prolonged fever or prior antibiotics. Shift toward molds with fungal prophylaxis
Viruses	Herpes simplex (HSV), varicella-zoster (VZV), respiratory viruses

* Vary by institution, chemotherapy regimen, and host factors

Table 14.2   Criteria and Treatment Choices for *Monotherapy* of Febrile Neutropenia

Meets low-risk criteria	ANC ≥ 100/mm^3, expected neutropenia ≤ 7 days, conventional solid tumor therapy, maintenance or consolidation of ALL
Absence of comorbidities	Hypotension, DIC, respiratory distress, pneumonia, hypoxia, AMS, severe mucositis, any AML therapy, induction for ALL
First-line therapy*	Cefepime: 50 mg/kg/dose IV q 8 hours (max 2 g/dose), *or* Ceftazidime: 50 mg/kg/dose IV q 8 hours (max 2 g/dose)
Alternative antibiotic choices*	Imipenem + cilastin: 1–3 months old: 25 mg/kg/dose IV q 6 hours, *or* ≥ 3 months old: 15–25 mg/kg/dose IV q 6 hours (max 1 g/dose), *or* Meropenem: 1–3 months old: 20–30 mg/kg/dose IV q 6 hours, *or* ≥ 3 months old: 20 mg/kg/dose IV q 6 hours (max 1 g/dose)

*Adjust dosing interval for renal insufficiency
ALL: Acute lymphoblastic leukemia; AML: Acute myeloid leukemia; AMS: Altered mental status; ANC: Absolute neutrophil count; DIC: Disseminated intravascular coagulation

Table 14.3   Criteria for and Treatment Choices for *Dual Therapy* of Febrile Neutropenia

Meets high-risk criteria	ANC < 100/mm^3, expected neutropenia > 7 days, induction for ALL, high-dose solid tumor therapy, any therapy for AML
Presence of a comorbidity	Hypotension, DIC, respiratory distress, pneumonia, hypoxia, AMS, severe mucositis, any AML therapy, induction for ALL

(Continued)

Conventional therapy as above, plus, consider adding*	Tobramycin: 2.5 mg/kg/dose IV q 8 hours *or* extended-interval dosing: 4.5–7.5 mg/kg/dose IV q 24 hours Gentamicin: Infants/children: 2–2.5 mg/kg/dose IV q 8 hours (max initial dose: 120 mg), *or* extended-interval dosing: 4.5–7.5 mg/kg/dose IV q 24 hours

*Adjust dosing interval for renal insufficiency

ALL: Acute lymphoblastic leukemia; AML: Acute myeloid leukemia; AMS: Altered mental status; ANC: Absolute neutrophil count; DIC: Disseminated intravascular coagulation

INDICATIONS FOR VANCOMYCIN IN FEBRILE NEUTROPENIA

- Hypotension or cardiovascular compromise
- Suspected catheter-related infection
- Colonization with: MRSA or penicillin/cephalosporin-resistant pneumococci
- Blood culture growing gram + cocci
- Also consider for severe mucositis or recent quinolone prophylaxis

ONGOING MANAGEMENT OF FEBRILE NEUTROPENIA

- ≥ 24–72 hours after initiation of treatment
  - ○ Modification of treatment regimen
    - − Do not modify solely based on ongoing fever
    - − Discontinue "double-coverage" for gram-negatives if patient stable and no pathogen identified
    - − If child becomes clinically unstable, ensure coverage of gram +, gram-negative, and anaerobic pathogens
  - ○ Discontinuation of therapy
    - − Afebrile × 24 hours, *plus*
    - − Negative cultures × > 48 hours, *plus*
    - − Evidence of marrow recovery
      - • Consider discharge of low-risk patients ≥ 72 hours into therapy without evidence of marrow recovery if careful follow-up assured
- If still febrile ≥ 96 hours after initiation of treatment
  - ○ Consider initiation of therapy for invasive fungal disease in high-risk patients
    - − AML, relapsed ALL, post-hematopoietic stem cell transplant, *or*
    - − Expected neutropenia (ANC < 100 mm^3) for > 10 days, *or*
    - − Presence of significant mucositis, steroid exposure, elevated CRP

Table 14.4   Empiric Antifungal Treatment in Patients High-Risk for Invasive Fungal Disease

Drug	Dosing
Caspofungin (≥ 3 months old)	Day 1: 70 mg/m^2/dose Subsequent days: 50 mg/m^2/dose
Amphotericin B liposomal*	3–5 mg/kg/dose IV once daily

*For patients who exhibit infusion-related reactions, consider premedication with:
    Acetaminophen: 15 mg/kg/dose PO/IV (max: 1000 mg/dose), *and*
    Diphenhydramine: 1 mg/kg/dose (max: 50 mg/dose)
*For infusion-related chills/rigors, treat with meperidine: 0.5 mg/kg/dose slow IV infusion (max: 25 mg/dose)

Abbreviations: ALL: Acute lymphoblastic leukemia; AML: Acute myeloid leukemia; AMS: Altered mental status; ANC: Absolute neutrophil count; CRP: C-reactive protein; TMP: Trimethoprim; SMX: Sulfamethoxazole; DIC: Disseminated intravascular coagulation

Data from: *J Clin Oncol.* 2012;30(35):4427–4438.

HYPERLEUKOCYTOSIS

- Hyperviscosity from elevated circulating WBC count leads to microvascular stasis and hypoperfusion of tissues (shock)
- Arbitrarily defined as > 50,000–100,000 cells/mm^3
- All organ systems may be involved, but most common systems leading to clinical symptoms are neurologic (altered mental status → seizures → coma) and pulmonary (hypoxemia, pulmonary hypertension)
- Management
  - Intravenous hydration: 20 mL/kg normal saline bolus; repeat as necessary
    - Subsequent IV fluids to run at: 3600 mL/m^2/day
  - Supplemental oxygen as indicated
  - Induction chemotherapy (assuming leukemia-related hyperleukocytosis)
    - Prophylaxis for tumor lysis syndrome should be given
  - Plasmapheresis if available
  - Evaluate for coagulation abnormalities (disseminated intravascular coagulation [DIC], thrombocytopenia)
    - Specific therapy for DIC if suggested by lab evaluation
    - Platelet transfusion if platelet counts < 20,000–30,000/mm^3
  - Avoid transfusing PRBCs unless hemoglobin < 8.5 g/dL, as can contribute to increased plasma viscosity

Abbreviations: DIC: Disseminated intravascular coagulation; PRBC: Packed red blood cells; WBC, White blood cells

MEDIASTINAL MASS

PRESENTING SIGNS AND SYMPTOMS OF MEDIASTINAL MASSES

- Often diagnosed on plain radiography for symptoms due to extrinsic compression or involvement of normal structures such as cough, shortness of breath, hoarseness (recurrent laryngeal nerve), wheezing, Horner's syndrome (involvement of sympathetic ganglion)

Table 14.5   Differential Diagnosis of Mediastinal Mass by Compartment

Anterior (anterior to the pericardium)	Middle (bordered anteriorly and posteriorly by the pericardium)	Posterior (from the posterior pericardial reflection to the vertebral bodies)
Teratoma	Lymphoma (T-cell, Hodgkin's)	Neuroblastoma
Lymphoma	Enlarged lymph nodes	Bronchogenic cyst
Thymoma	Bronchogenic cyst	Ewing sarcoma
Lipoma	Bronchogenic tumor	Paraspinal abscess
Thyroid tumor		Lymphoma

Data from: *Pediatr Anes* 2007 (17)1090–1098.

MANAGEMENT OF MEDIASTINAL MASS

- Assess and stabilize patient
  - Supine position may exacerbate respiratory distress
  - Avoid sedation and procedures that may compromise airway
  - Have advanced airway and cardiovascular support on hand
- Initial post-chest radiography management
  - Complete blood count with differential (CBCd)
    - If CBCd diagnostic (leukemia), treat appropriately
    - If CBCd non-diagnostic, further evaluation

- Subsequent evaluation if CBCd non-diagnostic
  - Evaluate to determine if high risk for anesthesia
    - Clinical signs/symptoms:
      - Orthopnea, facial/upper body edema (superior vena cava [SVC] syndrome)
    - Radiography findings:
      - Pleural effusion, tracheal or bronchial compression
    - Echocardiogram findings:
      - Cardiac dysfunction, great vessel compression, pericardial effusion
    - Pulmonary function test findings:
      - Lung volume loss, flow-loop obstruction
  - Local anesthesia for biopsy may be necessary
- Pleural effusion
  - Consider needle thoracentesis instead of thoracostomy tube, which can lead to reactive pulmonary edema and re-accumulation of fluid
- Emergency chemotherapy and/or radiation to reduce tumor bulk may be lifesaving

Reference: *Pediatr Anes.* 2007;17:1090–1098.

PNEUMOCYSTIS JIROVECI (CARINII) PNEUMONIA (PCP) PROPHYLAXIS

- Preferred prophylaxis:
  - Trimethoprim/sulfamethoxazole (TMP/SMX): 5 mg/kg TMP + 25 mg/kg SMX/day divided bid 3 consecutive days each week
- Alternative prophylaxis:
  - Dapsone: 2 mg/kg daily PO (max dose 100 mg/day), *or*
  - Dapsone: 4 mg/kg PO once weekly (200 mg/dose), *or*
  - Pentamidine: Inhaled monthly treatment by Respirgard II nebulizer
    - < 5 years old: 150 mg/treatment
    - ≥ 5 years old: 300 mg/treatment

SPINAL CORD COMPRESSION

- Can present acutely (numbness, tingling, refusal/inability to ambulate, back pain, incontinence) or with chronic symptoms (pain, constipation, difficulty with ambulation)
- Damage to neurons from both direct compression and vasogenic edema
- Most commonly due to neuroblastoma and Ewing's sarcoma
- Treatment:
  - High-dose corticosteroids
    - Dexamethasone 1–2 mg/kg IV × 1, then
    - Dexamethasone 0.25–0.5 mg/kg IV q 6 hours (max 16 mg/day)
  - Chemotherapy or surgical tumor debulking as dictated by oncologist

CHEMOTHERAPY

Table 14.6   Common Side Effects of Chemotherapeutic Agents Used in Pediatrics

Medication	Most Common Side Effects
L-Asparaginase	Pancreatitis, ↑ blood glucose, platelet dysfunction, coagulopathy, encephalopathy
Bleomycin (Blenoxane)	Nausea/vomiting, pneumonitis/pulmonary fibrosis, stomatitis, Raynaud phenomenon, skin rash
Carboplatin and cisplatin (Platinol)	Nausea/vomiting, allergic reaction/anaphylactic shock, kidney failure, myelosuppression, ototoxicity, tetany, neurologic symptoms
Carmustine (nitrosourea)	Nausea/vomiting, myelosuppression (after weeks); pulmonary fibrosis, stomatitis
Cyclophosphamide (Cytoxan)	Hemorrhagic cystitis (prevent with Mesna and aggressive hydration), nausea/vomiting, allergic reaction/anaphylaxis, myelosuppression, pulmonary fibrosis, SIADH, bladder cancer
Cytarabine (cytosine arabinoside; Ara-C)	Nausea/vomiting, myelosuppression, conjunctivitis, mucositis, neurologic symptoms
Dactinomycin	Nausea/vomiting, extravasation injury, myelosuppression, mucositis
Doxorubicin (Adriamycin), daunorubicin (Cerubidine), idarubicin (Idamycin)	Nausea/vomiting, cardiomyopathy (↓ risk with dexrazoxane [*Zinecard*]), red-colored urine, extravasation injury, myelosuppression, conjunctivitis, dermatitis
Etoposide (VePesid)	Nausea/vomiting, myelosuppression, ↑ risk of secondary leukemia
Ifosfamide (Ifex)	Hemorrhagic cystitis (prevent with Mesna), nausea/vomiting, allergic reaction/anaphylaxis, myelosuppression, pulmonary fibrosis, SIADH, ↑ risk bladder cancer, neurologic symptoms, myocardial cell toxicity
6-Mercaptopurine (Purinethol, 6-MP)	Myelosuppression, hepatitis, mucositis; ↑ toxicity when used with allopurinol
Methotrexate	Myelosuppression, mucositis, rash, hepatitis osteopenia (long term), nephrotoxicity, neurologic symptoms; monitor levels if high dose or in kids with ↓ kidney function, leucovorin rescue when indicated
Pegaspargase (Pegaspar, 6-MP)	Similar to L-asparaginase
Prednisone and Dexamethasone (Decadron)	Cushing syndrome, diabetes, hypertension, osteoporosis, avascular necrosis femoral head, ↑ risk of infection, gastric ulcer, behavioral changes, ophthalmologic complications
Topotecan	Myelosuppression
Tretinoin (all *trans*-retinoic acid) (Versanoid)	Pseudotumor cerebri, dry mouth, hair loss
Vinblastine (Velban)	↓ WBC, extravasation injury
Vincristine (Oncovin)	Peripheral neuropathy, constipation, jaw pain, seizures, abdominal pain/ileus, SIADH

SIADH: syndrome of inappropriate ADH secretion

Table 14.7 Chemotherapeutic Agents Used on Common Pediatric Malignancies

ALL	Vincristine, L-asparaginase, prednisone, methotrexate, daunorubicin (high risk), 6-mercaptopurine, cytarabine, cyclophosphamide, etoposide
AML	Cytarabine, doxorubicin, L-asparaginase
Promyelocytic Leukemia	Tretinoin
Hodgkin Lymphoma	MTX, cytarabine, cyclophosphamide, doxorubicin, bleomycin, vincristine, vinblastine, prednisone, carmustine
Non-Hodgkin Lymphoma	Methotrexate, cytarabine, cyclophosphamide, ifosfamide, doxorubicin, bleomycin, vincristine, vinblastine, prednisone, carmustine, etoposide
Osteosarcoma	MTX, doxorubicin, carboplatin and cisplatin
Medulloblastoma	MTX
Ewing Sarcoma	Cyclophosphamide, dactinomycin, vincristine
Soft Tissue Sarcoma	Cyclophosphamide, ifosfamide
Wilms Tumor	Ifosfamide, dactinomycin, vincristine
Neuroblastoma	Doxorubicin, vincristine, carboplatin, tretinoin
Rhabdomyosarcoma	Dactinomycin, vincristine
Germ Cell Tumors	Bleomycin, carboplatin, etoposide
CNS Tumors	Carmustine, carboplatin

ALL: Acute lymphoblastic leukemia; AML: Acute myeloblastic leukemia; MTX: methotrexate

Data from: *Nelson Textbook of Pediatrics, 19th ed.*, Philadelphia: Elsevier, 2011: Chapter 488.

COMMON PEDIATRIC CANCERS

Table 14.8 Common Childhood Cancers

Cancer Type	Risk Factors/Presentation	Treatment/Other
Acute Lymphoblastic Leukemia (ALL)	↑ risk in neurofibromatosis type 1, Down syndrome, Fanconi anemia, Bloom syndrome, ataxia telangiectasia Presents with symptoms of anemia, ↓ platelets, ↓ WBC; hepatosplenomegaly. > 20% lymphoblasts on marrow biopsy diagnostic	Standard risk: 1–10 years old + leukocyte count $< 50 \times 10^9$/L; High risk: does not meet standard risk criteria Chemo given in 3 phases: induction, consolidation, and maintenance CNS prophylaxis with intrathecal MTX

(Continued)

Table 14.8   Common Childhood Cancers *(Continued)*

Cancer Type	Risk Factors/Presentation	Treatment/Other
Wilms Tumor (most common between 1–5 years old)	95% are unilateral; 10% associated with WAGR (Wilms tumor, aniridia, genitourinary anomalies, mental retardation) syndrome, Beckwith-Wiedemann syndrome, Denys-Drash syndrome, hemihypertrophy. Commonly presents as palpable abdominal mass **Staging:** I: Unilateral, NO capsule extension/ node involvement II: Unilateral, + capsule extension/adherent to adjacent structures, NO nodes affected III: Unilateral + affected node preop tumor rupture, intraoperative tumor spill, incomplete resection, or tumor biopsy only IV: Metastasis to lung, liver, bone, brain, or distant node V: Bilateral tumors	Preoperative chemo may be considered especially if: • Tumor in a solitary kidney • Bilateral Wilms tumor • Tumor in horseshoe kidney • Intravascular extension above the hepatic vena cava • Respiratory distress from metastases Surgical treatment goals: Obtain specimen to confirm diagnosis, look for evidence of metastases, complete resection of tumor, kidney, ureter, nodes Radiation therapy considered for stage III and IV
Neuroblastoma	Stage 1: localized, unilateral, neg nodes, completely excised Stage 2A: localized, unilateral negative nodes, not completely excised Stage 2B: localized, unilateral, positive ipsilateral nodes Stage 3: unresectable, unilateral and infiltrating across the midline, +/– regional node involvement Stage 4: + metastasis to distant nodes, marrow, liver or other organ Stage 4S: localized + metastasis to skin, liver, and marrow but NO cortical bone involvement in infants < 1 year May present with abdominal mass, ↑ BP, neurologic symptoms, Horner syndrome, SVC syndrome, opsoclonus-myoclonus syndrome, periorbital ecchymoses	• Improved prognosis in infants < 1 year old. Survival in neonatal disease is almost 100% • ↑ Vanillylmandelic acid (VMA) and homovanillic acid (HVA) in urine • CT scan is preferred diagnostic study; MRI also useful • Bone marrow biopsy routinely done; core needle biopsy of tumor may be done if not resectable or if candidate for induction chemo • Low Risk: Surgical resection alone with excellent survival rates • Intermediate Risk: Surgery + chemo (cyclophosphamide, doxorubicin, cisplatin, and etoposide) + radiation • High risk: induction chemo for mets (Topotecan +/– cyclophosphamide), then surgery + radiotherapy for local control Etoposide, carboplatin, and melphalan + total body irradiation + BMT may ↑ survival
Ewing's Sarcoma	Usually presents as pain or mass. MRI then imaging guided biopsy for diagnosis. Genetic testing should also be done Once confirmed, CT scan of the chest (look for pulmonary metastases), bone scintigraphy (bony metastases), bone marrow aspirate + biopsy FDG-PET, whole body MRI, and spiral CT also used	Children's Oncology Group studies in North America recognizes 3 groups: localized tumor; lung metastases only; primary tumor + multiple or other metastases. Most common chemo includes vincristine, doxorubicin, cyclophosphamide alternating with ifosfamide and etoposide every 2 weeks
Osteosarcoma	↑ risk if hereditary retinoblastoma, Li-Fraument syndrome, or history of prior radiation Presents with bone pain, tenderness, soft tissue swelling at site Plain X-ray may shows lesion ("Codman triangle," detachment of periosteum from bone); usually at diaphysis	Typically: 10 weeks of chemotherapy (cycles of cisplatin and doxorubicin alternating with cycles of high-dose methotrexate) then surgery

References:
Data from: *Surg Clin North Am.* 2012;92(3):745–767; *Emerg Med Clin North Am.* 2009;27(3):525–544; *Lancet Oncol.* 2010;11(2):184–192.

TUMOR LYSIS SYNDROME

DEFINITION:
Massive lysis of cells results in release of intracellular contents into blood. Increased serum levels of uric acid (metabolite of purine nucleic acids xanthine and hypoxanthine), phosphorus, and potassium

MAJOR CONCERNS:
Direct effects of electrolyte abnormalities and acute kidney injury. Renal tubular precipitants (due to ↑ calcium: phosphorous product > 60 mg/dL^2 and hyperuricosuria) can lead to overall renal dysfunction

RISK FACTORS FOR TUMOR LYSIS SYNDROME
- Large tumor burden
- High tumor proliferation rate
- Sensitivity to cytotoxic therapy (can occur prior to therapy)
- Most commonly associated with Burkitt's lymphoma and ALL

CAIRO-BISHOP CRITERIA FOR TUMOR LYSIS SYNDROME
- Laboratory TLS (see Table 14.9) + 1 or more of the following:
  ○ Increase serum creatinine ≥ 1.5 × normal
  ○ Cardiac arrhythmia (or sudden death)
  ○ Seizure

Table 14.9   Cairo-Bishop Lab Criteria for TLS*

Element	Value	Change from Baseline
Uric Acid	≥ 8 mg/dL	25% increase
Potassium	≥ 6 mEq/L	25% increase
Phosphorus	≥ 6.5 mg/dL	25% increase
Calcium	< 7 mg/dL	25% decrease

*Abnormality in ≥ 2 of the listed elements, and occurs within 3 days before or 7 days after chemotherapy

- Clinical complication grading system: Grades creatinine, arrhythmia, and seizures on a scale of 0–5
  ○ 0: No clinical symptoms
  ○ 1–4: Increasing severity of renal failure, arrhythmias, and seizures
  ○ 5: Death

MANAGEMENT OF HYPERURICEMIA
- Hydration: Intravenous fluids
  ○ If volume depleted or hyponatremic, give normal saline 20 mL/kg boluses until repleted, then:
  ○ D_5 0.2 NS (without K+ or calcium) to run at:
    – 2–4 × maintenance rate, or
    – 2–3 L/m^2 per day of intravenous (IV) fluid
    – In children weighing ≤ 10 kg: 200 mL/kg/day
  ○ Goal urine output
    – 80–100 mL/m^2 per hour
    – In children weighing ≤ 10 kg: 4–6 mL/kg/hour
- Hypouricemic Medications
  ○ Allopurinol (xanthine oxidase inhibitor)

- Prevents conversion of xanthine to uric acid
- 200–300 mg/m^2/day IV in single or divided doses (max 600 mg/day)
- 50% reduction in dose for renal failure
- Small risk for xanthine precipitation/stone formation
○ Recombinant uric oxidase (*Rasburicase: Elitek*™)
- Converts insoluble uric acid to soluble allantoin, resulting in rapid decline in uric acid within 4 hours. Generally well tolerated.
- Dose 0.1–0.2 mg/kg/day for 1–5 days (see Table 14.11)
- FDA Black Box Warning: Anaphylaxis, hemolysis, hemoglobinuria, methemoglobinemia

Table 14.10   Cancer-Specific Risk Stratification for Tumor Lysis Syndrome

Cancer	High Risk	Intermediate Risk	Low Risk
NHL	Burkitt's, B-cell ALL, lymphoblastic	Diffuse large cell B-cell lymphoma	Indolent
ALL	WBC > 100,000/mm^3	WBC 50,000–100,000/mm^3	WBC < 50,000/mm^3
AML	WBC > 50,000/mm^3	WBC 10,000–50,000/mm^3	WBC < 10,000/mm^3
Solid Tumor		Rapid proliferation or rapid expected chemo response	

ALL: Acute lymphoblastic leukemia; AML: Acute myeloid leukemia; NHL: Non-Hodgkin's lymphoma; WBC: White blood cells

Table 14.11   Rasburicase Dosing Based on Tumor Risk Profile and Uric Acid Level

Risk Profile	Uric Acid	Daily Dose × 1–5 Days*
High	> 7.5 mg/dL	0.2 mg/kg
Intermediate	< 7.5 mg/dL	0.15 mg/kg
Low	< 7.5 mg/dL	0.1 mg/kg

*Number of days of rasburicase depends on clinical response to therapy

- Alkalinization: For patients with metabolic acidosis only. Controversial
  ○ D$_5$ 0.2 normal saline (NS) + 25–50 mEq NaHCO$_3$/L
  ○ Goal urine pH: 7.0–7.5
  ○ ↑ solubility of uric acid (as urate) and xanthine with ↑ urine pH
  ○ Possibly ↑ calcium-phosphorous precipitation, especially if urine pH > 7.5
  ○ Decreases ionized calcium, potentially exacerbating clinical hypocalcemia

MANAGEMENT OF HYPERKALEMIA, HYPERPHOSPHATEMIA, AND HYPOCALCEMIA
See sections on potassium, phosphorous, and calcium disturbances

References: *Br J Haematol.* 2004;127(1):3–11; *J Clin Oncol.* 2008;26(16):2767–2778; *Leukemia.* 2005;19(1): 34–38; *Haematol.* 2008;93(12):1877–1885.

ORBITAL AND PRESEPTAL CELLULITIS

ORBITAL CELLULITIS

- Refers to infection of the spaces behind the orbital septum
  - Involves periorbital fat and rectus muscles, but not usually the globe itself
- Frequently secondary to sinusitis (ethmoid [86–98%] > maxillary [60–89%])
- Occasionally orbital cellulitis is due to direct trauma that breaches the septum
- Associated with pain with eye movement, proptosis, diplopia, decreased visual acuity and pupillary abnormalities, and photophobia
- Most common organisms include *S. aureus*, streptococci, and *H. influenzae*

PRESEPTAL (PERI-ORBITAL) CELLULITIS

- Infection of the tissues *anterior* to the orbital septum
- Presents with significant eyelid swelling, redness, and pain
  - No ophthalmoplegia, photophobia, proptosis, diplopia present
- May arise from local trauma (insect bites, scratches), conjunctivitis, dacryocystitis, viral upper respiratory infection, or sinusitis
- Most common organisms include *S. aureus* and streptococci
  - Occasionally *H. influenzae* and anaerobes

EVALUATION

- Fever and leukocytosis common in both orbital and preseptal cellulitis
- CT scan of orbits helps differentiate the entities
  - Orbital cellulitis: Proptosis, retro-orbital stranding, edema of the rectus muscles, subperiosteal abscess
  - Preseptal cellulitis: Edema of the eyelids, absence of other findings

MANAGEMENT

- Empiric antibiotic therapy as noted below
- Consider surgical management for retro-orbital abscess (particularly if > 1 cm in size), significant proptosis, worsening clinical symptoms (pain, visual acuity, photophobia), or no response to therapy in 48 hours
- Simultaneous sinus surgery may be useful/necessary; consult otolaryngology

Table 15.1   Empiric Intravenous Therapy of Orbital or Severe Preseptal Cellulitis

Vancomycin: 60–80 mg/kg/day div q 6 hours (goal trough 15–20 mcg/mL)
and
Ceftriaxone: 50–100 mg/kg/day div q 12–24 hours (max 4 g/day), *or*
Cefotaxime: 150–200 mg/kg/day div q 8 hours (max 12 g/day), *or*
Ampicillin-sulbactam: 300 mg amp component/kg/day div q 6 hours (max 8 g amp/day), *or*
Piperacillin-tazobactam: 240 mg pip component/kg/day div q 6 hours (max 16 g pip/day)

If intracranial extension of infection, cover anaerobes with:
Metronidazole: 30 mg/kg/day IV/PO div q 6 hours (max 2 g/day)

TRANSITION TO OUTPATIENT/ORAL ANTIBIOTICS

- After significant improvement in clinical symptoms, exam, and inflammatory markers (see Table 15.2 for antibiotic options)
- Duration of antibiotic therapy 2–4 weeks
- Longer courses recommended for severe disease and significant ethmoid sinusitis

Table 15.2   Outpatient Oral Treatment of Preseptal Cellulitis

Outpatient therapy if mild disease and child > 1 year old; otherwise treat inpatient with intravenous antibiotics as noted above

Clindamycin*: 30–40 mg/kg/day div q 8 hours (max 1.8 g/day) monotherapy *or*

TMP-SMX: 8–12 mg/kg/day div q 8–12 hours, *and*
One of the following
Amoxicillin: 80–100 mg/kg/day div q 8–12 hours (max 1.75 g/day), *or*
Amoxicillin-clavulanate: 45 mg/kg/day div q 12 hours (max 1.75 g/day), *or*
Cefdinir: 14 mg/kg/day div q 12 hours (max 600 mg/day)

*Clindamycin monotherapy only if fully immunized vs. *H. influenzae*

References: *Int J Pediatr Otorhinolaryngol.* 2008;72:377; *Am J Ophthalmol.* 2007;144:497; *Br J Ophthalmol.* 2008;92:1337; *Pediatrics.* 2011;127:e566; *Pediatr Infect Dis J.* 2006;25:695–699; *Otolaryngol Head Neck Surg.* 2009;140(6): 907–911; *Otolaryngol Head Neck Surg.* 2011;145(5):823–827.

HYPHEMA
- Definition: Blood in anterior chamber of the eye (between cornea and lens)
- Etiology
  - Blunt trauma to eye (by far most common)
  - Rarely: tumor (retinoblastoma), neovascularization (diabetes), vascular anomalies, post-surgical
- Symptoms: Pain, photophobia, vision disturbance/loss, nausea, vomiting, lethargy
- Exam: Blood layered in anterior chamber, decreased visual acuity
- Management: Goal is to reduce rebleeding and ocular hypertension
  - Indication for hospitalization
    - > 1/3 anterior chamber involved
    - Inadequate supervision at home to keep child on bed rest
    - Sickle cell trait or disease (HbSS)
    - Coagulopathy (increased risk of rebleed)
  - Emergent ophthalmologic evaluation (avoid ophthalmic medications until recommended by ophthalmologist)
  - Recumbent position, head of bead elevated 30–45 degrees to allow layering of blood inferiorly via gravity
  - Limit all physical activity for ~5 days
  - Protect eye from further trauma or rubbing (eye shield, no pressure on eye)
  - Treat/prevent emesis (increases intraocular pressure)
  - Manage pain with acetaminophen or opiates
    - Avoid NSAIDs as can theoretically increase bleeding
  - Topical cycloplegics and steroids controversial
  - Aminocaproic acid (*Amicar*™) 50 mg/kg/dose PO q 4 hours (max 30 g/day) *may* limit clot lysis and prevent secondary bleeding
    - Topical aminocaproic acid effective, not available in U.S.
  - Oral glucocorticoids equally effective as aminocaproic acid
    - Prednisone 0.6–1 mg/kg/day
  - Topical antiglaucoma therapy
    - Brimonidine tartrate (*Alphagan*™) 1 gtt tid, *or*
    - Timolol maleate (*Timoptic-XE*™) 0.25% or 0.5% sol: 1 gtt daily, *or*
    - Dorzolamide (*Trusopt*™) 2% sol: 1 gtt tid

- ○ Systemic anti-glaucoma therapy
  - – Acetazolomide: 20 mg/kg/day PO div q 6–8 hours
  - – Methazolomide: 10 mg/kg/day PO div q 6 hours preferred for HbSS patients
- Potential Indications for Surgery
  - ○ Persistence of > 50% hyphema for > 7 days
  - ○ Intraocular pressure > 60 mmHg for > 2 days or > 50 mmHg for > 4 days, despite aggressive medical therapy
  - ○ Total hyphema and intraocular pressure > 25 mmHg for > 5 days
  - ○ Microscopic corneal blood staining
- Outcomes:
  - ○ Glaucoma, secondary bleed, corneal staining, synechiae, optic atrophy
  - ○ Decreased visual acuity in 10–15%
  - ○ Worse outcomes noted in sickle cell trait/disease

CHAPTER 16 ■ PULMONOLOGY

ASTHMA

Definition: Airway reactivity resulting in chronic inflammation and episodes of bronchospasm that are at least partially reversible

Table 16.1   Clinical Characteristics of Asthma

Epidemiology	Affects 1 in 12 children, ↑ incidence in minority and urban children
Symptoms	Intermittent or chronic wheeze, dyspnea, exercise intolerance, cough (including nighttime cough and prolonged coughs)
Triggers	Smoke, exercise, viral infection, animals, grasses, weather change
Signs	Hyperexpanded chest, expiratory wheeze, prolonged expiratory phase, nasal flaring, use of accessory muscles, boggy nasal mucosa, eczema
Severity	In ascending order of severity based on chest exam: Expiratory wheeze < biphasic wheeze < silent (minimal air movement) Paradoxical breathing, cyanosis, respiratory rate > 60/min, significant accessory muscle use associated with more severe disease
Differential diagnosis	Congestive heart failure, cystic fibrosis, foreign body, GERD, bronchiolitis, airway malacia, vascular ring, abnormal bronchus

Table 16.2   Peak Expiratory Flow (PEF)

Ht	43	45	47	49	51	53	55	57	59	61	63	65
PEF	147	173	200	227	254	280	307	334	360	387	413	440

Based on height (ht) in inches, flow in lpm (best of 3 attempts)

INPATIENT MANAGEMENT OF ASTHMA EXACERBATION

Table 16.3   Short-Acting Inhaled Beta₂-Agonists for Acute Asthma Exacerbation

Drug	Dose	Comment
Albuterol nebulized (0.63, 1.25, 2.5 mg/3 mL, or 5 mg/mL)	0.15 mg/kg/dose (min 2.5 mg/dose, max 5 mg/dose) every 20 minutes × 3, *then* 0.15–0.3 mg/kg/dose (2.5–10 mg/dose) every 1–4 hours, *or* 0.5 mg/kg (10–15 mg) continuously over an hour	Dilute to 3 mL Deliver with 6–8 liters per minute gas May mix with ipratropium Use large volume nebulizer
Albuterol MDI (90 mcg/puff)	2–8 puffs every 20 minutes × 3, *then*, every 1–4 hours as needed	Use age-appropriate spacer
Levalbuterol (0.63 mg, 1.25 mg/3 mL, or 1.25 mg/0.5 mL)	0.075 mg/kg (min 1.25 mg, max 2.5 mg) every 20 minutes × 3, *then* 0.075–0.15 mg/kg (1.25–5 mg) every 1–4 hours as needed.	Comparable efficacy to albuterol No data on continuous nebulization
Levalbuterol (45 mcg/puff)	4–8 puffs every 20 minutes × 3, *then*, every 1–4 hours as needed	Use age-appropriate spacer

Table 16.4   Combination Short-Acting Inhaled Beta₂-Agonists + Anticholinergics

Drug	Dose	Comment
Ipratropium (0.5 mg) + **Albuterol** (2.5 mg)/3 mL (*DuoNeb®*)	1.5–3 mL nebulized every 20 minutes × 3	Anticholinergic therapy not shown to be beneficial beyond first 3 hours of therapy
Ipratropium (18 mcg) + **Albuterol** (90 mcg)/puff (*Combivent®*)	4–8 puffs every 20 minutes with age-appropriate spacer, up to 3 hours into therapy	

Table 16.5   Inhaled Anticholinergics for Acute Asthma Exacerbation

Drug	Dose	Comment
Ipratropium (0.25 mg/mL)	0.25–0.5 mg nebulized every 20 minutes × 3 doses, then as needed	**Not first-line therapy** Anticholinergic therapy not shown to be beneficial beyond first 3 hours of therapy
Ipratropium (18 mcg/puff)	4–8 puffs every 20 minutes with age-appropriate spacer, up to 3 hours into therapy	

Table 16.6   Systemic Beta-Agonists for Acute Asthma Exacerbation

Drug	Dose	Comment
Epinephrine (1:1000 = 1 mg/mL)	0.01 mg/kg SQ (max 0.3–0.5 mg) every 20 minutes × 3 doses	Likely no significant benefit over aerosolized therapy
Terbutaline (1 mg/mL)	0.01 mg/kg SQ (max 0.25 mg) every 20 minutes × 3 doses, *then* every 2–6 hours as needed	

Table 16.7   Systemic Corticosteroids for Acute Asthma Exacerbation

Drug	Dose	Comment
Prednisolone (5 mg/5 mL, 15 mg/5 mL), *or* **Methylprednisolone** (Solu-Medrol), *or* **Prednisone** (2.5-, 5-, 10-, 20-mg tabs; 5 mg/5 mL soln)	1–2 mg/kg/day (max 60–80 mg/day) PO/IV either daily or divided bid	No advantage to higher dosing No advantage to intravenous over oral route if GI tract functioning
Outpatient "Burst": 1–2 mg/kg/day (max 60 mg/day) PO daily or divided bid × 3–10 days total (inpatient + outpatient), depending on severity of exacerbation. Unlikely to need to taper with ≤ 10-day "burst," unless requires > 2–3 bursts/year		

Table 16.8   Adjunctive Therapies

Drug	Dose	Comment
Magnesium sulfate	25–75 mg/kg IV (max 2 g/dose)	Studies show mixed benefit Consider for severe exacerbations not responding to high-dose inhaled albuterol

THERAPIES NOT RECOMMENDED

- Mucolytics, chest percussive therapy, cough suppressant, and incentive spirometry all may trigger worsening bronchospasm
- Methylxanthine (theophylline, aminophylline) side effects (tachycardia, arrhythmias, seizures) limit their usefulness. Not generally recommended
  - May be useful in exacerbations refractory to beta-agonists
- Antibiotics not indicated unless purulent sputum or bacterial sinusitis present

CYSTIC FIBROSIS

Inherited disorder with defective cystic fibrosis transmembrane conductance regulator (CFTR) leads to inspissation of secretions in lungs, pancreas, and other organs. Defective mucociliary clearance in the lungs leads to a cycle of mucous obstruction, inflammation, and chronic infection

PULMONARY INFECTIONS

- Avoid close contact (cohorting) between hospitalized patients with CF
- Infants and younger children: *Staph aureus* and *H. influenzae*
- Older children, adolescents, and adults: *Pseudomonas aeruginosa*
  - Chronic mucoid *P. aeruginosa* infection leads to decreased lung function
- *Burkholderia cepacia* (associated with more advanced disease and worse lung function), *Stenotrophomonas maltophilia*, *Achromobacter xylosoxidans* are becoming more prevalent

INTRAVENOUS ANTIBIOTICS

Choose appropriate regimen based on child's previous culture and sensitivities, degree of illness of child, as well as local antibiotic resistance patterns

(1) Aminoglycosides[1,2]
  - Antibacterial effect proportional to peak tissue concentrations
  - ↑ volume of distribution and renal clearance: Require higher dosing
  - Measure trough 18 hours post-dose. Goal < 0.5–1 mcg/mL
  - Check creatinine with all levels. Adjust dose if creatinine rising
    1. Tobramycin 10 mg/kg IV once daily, *or*
    2. Gentamicin 10 mg/kg IV once daily, *or*
    3. Amikacin 30 mg/kg IV once daily
(2) Cephalosporins
  - Bactericidal effect related to maintaining tissue concentration above minimum inhibitory concentration (MIC) throughout dosing interval
    1. Cefepime 50 mg/kg IV q 8 hours (max 2 g/dose), *or*
    2. Ceftazidime 50 mg/kg IV q 8 hours (max 2 g/dose)
(3) Carbepenems
  - Meropenem 40 mg/kg IV q 8 hours (max 2 g/dose), *or*
  - Imepenem/Cilastin 25 mg/kg IV q 6 hours (max 1 g/dose)
(4) Beta-Lactam + Beta-Lactamase Inhibitor
  - Piperacillin-tazobactam: 100 mg piperacillin component/kg IV q 8 hours (max 4 g piperacillin/dose), *or*
  - Ticarcillin-clavulanate: 50 mg ticarcillin component/kg IV q 6 hours (max 3 mg ticarcillin/dose)
(5) Quinolones
  - Ciprofloxacin 10 mg/kg IV q 8 hours (max 400 mg/dose), *or*
  - Ciprofloxacin 20 mg/kg PO bid (max 1000 mg/dose)
(6) Colistimethate sodium (*Colistin*)
  - Do not use concurrently with aminoglycosides due to renal toxicity
  - 2.5–5 mg/kg/day IV divided q 8 hours (max 100 mg/day)
(7) Macrolide prophylaxis (> 6 years old with pseudomonas infection)[3,4]
  - Azithromycin 250 mg 3×/week (15–39 kg child), *or*
  - Azithromycin 500 mg 3×/week (≥ 40 kg child)
(8) *Burkholderia cepecia* complex and *Stenotrophomonas maltophilia*
  - Unclear if pathogens or colonizers. If choose to treat, consider:
  - Trimethoprim-sulfamethoxazole (TMP-SMX): Consider 50% increase dose due to rapid clearance[13]
  - Alternates: Meropenem, minocycline, tigecycline (Steno), levofloxacin (Steno), cefepime (Burk), colisitin/polymixin B (Steno)

APPETITE STIMULATION[5]
- 1–12 years old: megestrol acetate 7 mg/kg PO daily
- > 12 years old: megestrol acetate 400 mg PO daily, or Megace ES® 625 mg PO daily

AIRWAY CLEARANCE
- High-frequency chest wall oscillation ("vest therapy," *Theravest*®)[6]
  - Consider Minnesota protocol: 6 cycles, each 5 minutes long

Table 16.9   Minnesota Protocol for High-Frequency Chest Wall Oscillation

Cycle (each 5 minutes long)	1	2	3	4	5	6
Frequency (Hz)	8	9	10	18	19	20
Pressure setting*	10	10	10	6	6	6

*May decrease if child not tolerating well

Data from: *Chest*. 2007; 132(4): 1227–1232.

- Beta-agonist therapy (albuterol 0.5–5 mg) nebulized bid–qid with vest therapy
- Dornase alfa (*Plumozyme*®)[7]: 2.5 mg inhaled bid for patients > 6 years old
- Hypertonic saline 3–7%, 4 mL inhaled bid for patients > 6 years old
  - Can be associated with bronchospasm; consider coupling with beta-agonist
- Chronic inhaled corticosteroids not recommended unless diagnosed with asthma or allergic bronchopulmonary aspergillosis (ABPA)

NUTRITIONAL THERAPY
- Height is an independent risk factor for pulmonary function
- High-calorie, high-protein diet (120–200% RDA for age)
  - Conflicting evidence as to whether supplemental high-calorie "shakes" improve outcomes. Generally recommended if patient desires
- Pancreatic enzyme replacement therapy
  - Birth–2 years: 2000 U lipase/120 mL formula *or* nursing session[14]
    - Can increase to 5000 U lipase/feed
  - > 2 years old: 500–2500 U lipase/kg/meal[15]
  - Max: 2500 U lipase/kg/feed, and 10,000 U lipase/kg/day to limit risk of fibrosing colonopathy
  - Overnight tube feeds: Give 1–2 capsules of standard enzymes at initiation and discontinuation of feeds. May need to be titrated based on signs of fat malabsorption
- Sodium chloride (NaCl) supplementation
  - Birth–6 months: ⅛ teaspoon/day[14]
  - 6 months–2 years: ¼ teaspoon/day[14]
  - > 2 years: Unrestricted NaCl in diet
- Vitamin D: check vitamin D status yearly (preferably at end of winter). Goal 25-OH vitamin D > 30 ng/mL (75 nmol/L). Routine initial dosing as follows[9]:
  - Birth–12 months: 400–500 IU daily (max 2000 IU daily)
  - > 12 months–10 years: 800–1000 IU daily (max 4000 IU daily)
  - > 10–18 years old: 800–2000 IU daily (max 10,000 IU daily)
- Oral magnesium therapy 300 mg PO daily shown in single study to increase respiratory muscle function[10]

INVESTIGATIONAL THERAPIES

- Ibuprofen 10 mg/kg/dose bid for patients > 6 years old and forced expiratory volume in 1 second (FEV_1) > 60%[7]
  - Need to monitor levels ensure therapeutic and nontoxic
- Inhaled mannitol 400 mg bid may improve FEV_1 if used chronically[8]

CYSTIC FIBROSIS RELATED DIABETES (CFRD)

- Prevalence: 2% children, 19% adolescents, 40–50% adults[11]
- Insulin sensitivity decreases significantly during acute exacerbations
- Oral glucose tolerance test (OGTT): 1.75 g CHO/kg (max 75 g). Check fasting blood glucose (FBG) and 2 hours post CHO load (2hPG)[12]
  - Normal: FBG < 126 mg/dL, 2hPG < 140 mg/dL
  - Impaired glucose tolerance: FBG < 126 mg/dL, 2hPG 140–199 mg/dL
  - CFRD without fasting hyperglycemia: FBG < 126 mg/dL, 2hPG > 200 mg/dL
  - CFRD + fasting hyperglycemia: FBG > 126 mg/dL, 2hPG > 200 mg/dL
- Management (Initial doses given. Titration based on subsequent BG results)
  - Basal: 0.25 units/kg/day sq glargine (generally given at night)
  - Meal: 0.5–1 unit rapid-acting insulin/15 g CHO
    - Check 2 h post-prandial glucose and adjust based on results
  - Pre-meal correction: 1 unit/rapid-acting insulin/50 mg/dL > 150 mg/dL
  - If on continuous overnight feeds: Consider single dose isophane (NPH)/regular insulin (70:30 insulin) to cover overnight feeds
- Dietary Goals in CFRD[12]
  - Total calories: 120% recommended
  - Fat: 40% total energy intake
  - Carbohydrates: 40–50% total energy intake
  - Protein: 200% of recommended daily intake for age
  - Salt: increased requirement—unrestricted intake

Abbreviations: CF: Cystic fibrosis; CFRD: cystic fibrosis related diabetes; CHO: carbohydrates; FBG: fasting blood glucose; NPH: isophane insulin; TMP: trimethoprim

References:

(1) *Am J Respir Crit Care Med.* 2009; 180: 802–808.

(2) *Cochrane Database Syst Rev.* 2010:CD002009.

(3) *JAMA.* 2003; 290: 1749–1756.

(4) *Eur Respir J.* 2007; 30: 487–495.

(5) *J Pediatr.* 2002; 140: 439–444.

(6) *Chest.* 2007; 132(4): 1227–1232.

(7) *Am J Respir Crit Care Med.* 2007; 176(10): 957–969.

(8) *Am J Respir Crit Care Med.* 2012; 185: 645–652.

(9) *J Clin Endocrinol Metab.* 2012; 97(4).

(10) *Am J Clin Nutr.* 2012; 96: 50–56.

(11) *Diabetes Care.* 2009 Sep; 32(9): 1626–1632.

(12) *Pediatric Diabetes.* 2009; 10 (Suppl.12): 43–50.

(13) *J Pediatr.* 1984; 104(2): 303.

(14) *J Pediatr.* 2009; 155: S73–93.

(15) *J Am Diet Assoc.* 2008; 108: 832–839.

FOREIGN BODY: AIRWAY

Table 16.10   Foreign Bodies (FB)—General Considerations

Symptoms of ingestion	• Often asymptomatic • Possible symptoms include gagging, choking, vomiting, dysphagia, drooling, tachypnea, ongoing emesis
Evaluation	• Plain radiographs of neck, chest, abdomen as indicated • If symptomatic despite normal X-rays, consider computed tomography, barium esophagram, esophagoscopy (EGD)
Common sites of obstruction	• Thoracic inlet • Gastroesophageal junction • Pylorus (if FB > 2 cm wide) • Duodenum (if FB > 5 cm long) • Ileocecal valve

Table 16.11   Foreign Body (FB) Aspiration

Peak 1–3 years old, > 50% unwitnessed, ~50% diagnosed ≥ 24 hours after event	
Symptoms	Choking, gagging, wheezing, chronic cough, recurrent pneumonia
Exam	• Most often normal • Can have ↓ breath sounds, stridor, drooling, cough
Evaluation	• Obtain AP, lateral, and inspiratory/expiratory films • Lateral decubitus films (in lieu of inspiratory/expiratory films) may show air trapping and failure to compress lung on side with FB when dependent. > 50% X-rays normal despite presence of FB
Treatment	• Acute airway obstruction: Heimlich maneuver or back blows as appropriate • Rigid bronchoscopy: Consider in symptomatic patients or if high clinical suspicion, even if X-rays negative

FOREIGN BODY: GI SYSTEM

Table 16.12   Management of Gastrointestinal Foreign Bodies

Object	X-rays	Esophageal Management	Beyond Esophagus
Coin	AP: circular disk Lateral: linear	Urgent removal: EGD or bougie dilator via esophagus	Weekly X-rays Average 4–21 days to pass
Battery	AP: 2 densities Lateral: Step-off of cathode	Urgent removal: Mucosal burn occurs < 4 hours, can lead to fistula, perforation, scarring	Watch and wait. If in stomach ≥ 3 days, consider removal
Sharp object	May be negative	Urgent removal	Watch and wait Follow with X-rays

*Instruct patients to return immediately for fever, emesis, pain, or melena

PERTUSSIS

Vaccine-preventable disease characterized by multiphase illness resulting in prolonged cough. Particularly high morbidity/mortality in infants age < 4 months old

THREE CLINICAL STAGES

- *Catarrhal stage*: Lasts 1–2 weeks, rhinorrhea, cough gradually worsens
- *Paroxysmal stage*: Severe coughing, often in bursts (paroxysms) without intervening inspiration. May have posttussive "whoop" (often absent in infants). Often well-appearing between paroxysms. Average 15 paroxysms/24 hours, ↑ at night
- *Convalescent stage*: Cough wanes over 2–3 weeks. May last > 6 weeks
- Consider pertussis in patients of any age with: Paroxysmal cough + inspiratory whoop (present in two-thirds of adolescents and adults), cough persisting > 2 weeks, posttussive emesis, apnea and/or bradycardia in an infant, apparent life-threatening event (ALTE)

DEFINITIONS

- *Clinical case*: Cough × 2 weeks with ≥ one of the following:
  - Paroxysm of coughing, inspiratory whoop, or posttussive emesis
- *Confirmed case*:
  - Any cough illness with positive culture for B pertussis, *or*
  - Patient meeting "clinical case" definition with positive B pertussis polymerase chain reaction assay (PCR), or
  - Patient meeting "clinical case" definition with a direct epidemiologic link to a case confirmed by PCR or culture
- *Probable case*:
  - Patient meeting "clinical case" definition without confirmatory lab testing (culture or PCR) or epidemiologic link to confirmed case

Table 16.13   Confirmatory Tests for Pertussis
Check with local lab for collection techniques

Culture	Specificity: 100%, Sensitivity: 30–60% early on, but as low as 1–3% by third week of paroxysmal stage. 7- to 14-day turn-around-time. Best yield in catarrhal and early paroxysmal phases. ↓ sensitivity if immunized, late in disease course, or received antibiotics
PCR Testing	Turnaround time 1–3 days, higher sensitivity than culture. Lab-specific false positive rates may be high. CDC still recommends culture confirmation. May remain positive later in disease (and after treatment), as does not require live organism
DFA Testing	Useful for rapid screening where PCR not available, but not used for *confirmation*. Variable specificity, low sensitivity (high false negative rate)
Serologic Testing	Tests IgG and IgA antibodies to pertussis toxin. Useful late in paroxysmal stage or after antibiotics. Collect at least 2 weeks after onset of symptoms, and again in convalescent phase

DFA: Direct fluorescence antibody

TREATMENT AND POSTEXPOSURE PROPHYLAXIS

Early therapy (during catarrhal stage, before onset of paroxysms) shortens duration of symptoms and communicability. Patients are infectious from onset of catarrhal stage through third week of paroxysmal stage or until 5 days after antibiotic therapy begins

CHEMOPROPHYLAXIS

Should be given, regardless of age or immunization status, to:
- All household and "close contacts" as defined as any one of the following:
  - Face-to-face contact within 3 feet of symptomatic patient, *or*
  - Direct contact with respiratory, oral, or nasal secretions from symptomatic patient (sneeze in the face, shared drink/utensils, medical examination of mouth, nose, or throat), *or*
  - Shared confined space with symptomatic patient for an hour or longer

- Patients at high risk of developing severe symptoms include:
  - Infants age < 1 year
  - Immune deficient
  - Chronic lung disease, cystic fibrosis, respiratory insufficiency

Table 16.14   Treatment and Chemoprophylaxis of Pertussis

Drug	Dosage			
	< 1 month old	1–5 months old	≥ 6 months old	Adolescents and Adults
Azithromycin	10 mg/kg/day × 5 days	10 mg/kg/day × 5 days	10 mg/kg on day 1, then 5 mg/kg on days 2–5	500 mg on day 1, then 250 mg on days 2–5
Erythromycin	Not preferred	40–50 mg/kg/day in four divided doses × 14 days	40–50 mg/kg/day in four divided doses × 14 days	500 mg four times per day × 14 days
Clarithromycin	Not recommended	15 mg/kg/day in two divided doses × 7 days	15 mg/kg/day in two divided doses × 7 days	500 mg twice daily × 7 days
Trimethoprim-sulfamethoxazole (TMP-SMX)	Contraindicated for infants < 2 months of age For infants 2–5 months of age: 8 mg/kg/day of TMP and SMX 40 mg/kg/day in two divided doses for 14 days		8 mg/kg/day of TMP and SMX 40 mg/kg/day in two divided doses for 14 days	TMP 320 mg/day and SMX 1600 mg/day in two divided doses × 14 days

Data from: *AAP Redbook* 2009:504–519.

IMMUNIZATION FOR PERTUSSIS

- If less than 7 years of age and under-immunized, initiate catch-up according to current Centers for Disease Control and Prevention–Advisory Committee on Immunization Practices (CDC–ACIP) standards with DTaP
- If ≥ 7 years of age, then consider booster dose with Tdap (FDA approval: Adacel® ≥ 11 yrs old, Boostrix® ≥ 10 yrs old) per provisional CDC–ACIP and state public health department guidelines

COMPLICATIONS OF PERTUSSIS

- Infants < 1 year of age: 57% hospitalization rate, 23% pneumonia rate, 1–2% seizure rate, > 50% have apnea, 1–2% mortality (most deaths in infants < 4 months of age).
- Malignant pertussis: Severe leukocytosis (> 100,000/mm³) can lead to hyperviscosity and underperfusion, seizures, progressive respiratory failure and hypoxia, and pulmonary hypertension. Transfer to intensive care. Consider exchange transfusion, nitric oxide, high-frequency oscillation

References: *MMWR*. 2005;54(RR-14):1–16; *MMWR*. 2006;55(RR-17):1–37; *AAP Red Book*. 2009:504–519; *JAMA*. 2003;290(22):2968–2975; *Pediatr Crit Care Med*. 2011 Mar;12(2):e107–9.

PLEURAL EFFUSION

Pleural effusion: Fluid in the pleural space

Parapneumonic: Fluid in the pleural space associated with lung infection

Table 16.15   Characteristics and Common Causes of Pleural Effusion

Type	Characteristic	Common Causes
Transudate	pH: ~7.4, LDH < 1000 U/mL, WBC < 1000/mm³, glucose = serum, protein < 3 g/dL	Congestive heart failure Cirrhosis Nephrotic syndrome Hypoalbuminemia
Exudate	pH: ≤ 7.4, LDH ≥ 1000 U/mL, WBC ≥ 1000/mm³, glucose ≤ serum, protein ≥ 3 g/dL	Infection Oncologic/neoplastic Hemothorax Intra-abdominal abscess

PATHOPHYSIOLOGY OF PARAPNEUMONIC EFFUSION

- Inflammation and infection of lung parenchyma spreads to the pleura → sterile accumulation of proteins → WBCs and fluid in the pleural space → bacterial invasion → purulence. Over time the body's defenses cordon off the infection, resulting in empyema
- Pathogens that lead to parapneumonic effusion: *Strep pneumonia* and *Staph aureus* most common pathogens. Less commonly viridans strep, group A strep, and *Actinomyces*

Table 16.16   Radiographic Evaluation: Chest X-ray (With Decubitus Films)

< 1 cm effusion, *or* < 25% hemithorax	• Thoracentesis, thoracostomy tube, and VATS not routinely indicated
> 1 cm effusion, *but* < 50% hemithorax	• Perform diagnostic/therapeutic thoracentesis • Consider thoracostomy + fibrinolysis, *or* VATS for ○ Labs suggestive of empyema ○ Presence of respiratory distress or loculations • Persistent fever or poor response to antibiotics
> 50% hemithorax	Perform thoracostomy + fibrinolysis, *or* VATS

If further information needed, consider ultrasound or computed tomography (CT)

VATS: Video-assisted thoracoscopic surgery

Data from: *Clin Infect Dis.* 2011;53(7):e25.

ANTIBIOTIC THERAPY

- Per section on pneumonia

THORACENTESIS

- LDH, pH, glucose not necessary, but, if not abnormal, raise suspicion of mycobacterial or oncologic source. Consider cytology if not classic for infection
- Typical bacterial effusion has pH < 7.2, glucose < 40 mg/dL, LDH > 1000 U/mL, WBC > 50,000 cells/mL
- 10–50,000 WBC/mL can be seen in early infections or tuberculosis (monos)

THORACOSTOMY TUBE + FIBRINOLYTIC THERAPY (UROKINASE, STREPTOKINASE)

- Place thoracostomy tube and allow fluid to drain
  - ○ Instill urokinase (10,000 units/10 mL if < 1 year old, 40,000 units/40 mL if ≥ 1 year old) and clamp tube × 4 hours. Repeat q 12 hours × 3 days. If temp > 38.0°C or ultrasound evidence of significant residual fluid at 4 days after therapy initiation, proceed to VATS
- Remove thoracostomy tube when no air-leak and drainage < 1 mL/kg/day

VIDEO-ASSISTED THORACOSCOPIC SURGERY (VATS)

- Previously shown to decrease length of stay and thoracostomy tube need

References: *Thorax.* 2005; 60:suppl 1; *Am J Respir Crit Care Med.* 2006;174(2):221; *Pediatrics. 2005; 115:1652; Clin Infect Dis.* 2011;53(7):e25; *J Pediatr Surg.* 2009;44(1):289.

PNEUMONIA

DIAGNOSIS

- Suspect in children with tachypnea, fever, decreased localized breath sounds, decreased SpO_2 (< 92%). Infants may have lethargy, poor feeding, irritability. Lower lobe disease associated with abdominal pain
- Elevated WBC (> 20,000/mm³), CRP suggestive, but not entirely specific for bacterial etiology
- Lobar process on chest radiograph suggestive of pneumococcal disease
- Rapid viral tests of nasopharyngeal aspirates for influenza, adenovirus, RSV, and parainfluenza are valuable in differentiating viral from bacterial illness

INDICATIONS FOR HOSPITAL ADMISSION

- Infants < 3–6 months of age, pneumatocele, empyema, effusion, underlying chronic illness, immunodeficiency, respiratory distress (respiratory rate > 60/min, SpO_2 < 92%), dehydration, persistent vomiting

CRITERIA FOR INTENSIVE CARE UNIT ADMISSION

- Indicated for SpO_2 < 92% on $FiO_2 \geq 50\%$, altered mental status, patient requiring CPAP or BiPAP, concern for impending respiratory failure

INPATIENT ANTIBIOTIC MANAGEMENT

- Anti-pneumococcal antibiotics (If MIC ≤ 2.0 ug/mL)
  - Ampicillin 150–200 mg/kg/day divided 4–6 hours (preferred agent)
  - Ceftriaxone 50–100 mg/kg/day divided q 12–24 hours, *or*
  - Cefotaxime 150 mg/kg/day divided q 8 hours
  - Alternatives: Clindamycin 40 mg/kg/day divided q 8 hours, *or*
    - Vancomycin 60 mg/kg/day divided q 6 hours
- If concern for methicillin-sensitive *Staphylococcus aureus*
  - Cefazolin 150 mg/kg/day divided q 8 hours
- If concern for Methicillin-resistant *Staphylococcus aureus*
  - Vancomycin 60 mg/kg/day divided q 6 hours, *or*
  - Clindamycin 40 mg/kg/day divided q 6 hours, *or*
  - Linezolid 30 mg/kg/day divided q 8 hours if < 12 years old, *or*
  - Linezolid 20 mg/kg/day divided q 12 hours if ≥ 12 years old
- If concern for *Mycoplasma pneumonia*
  - Azithromycin 10 mg/kg PO/IV day 1, then 5 mg/kg/day daily × 4 days, *or*
  - Doxycycline 4 mg/kg/day PO divided bid if > 8 years old
- Aspiration: Oral/nasopharyngeal secretions enter lung. Cover oral anaerobes
  - Chemical pneumonitis and bacterial aspiration difficult to distinguish
  - Unclear if oral water/food restriction beneficial in preventing events
  - Clindamycin 40 mg/kg/day divided q 6 hours, *plus*
  - Ceftriaxone 50 mg/kg/day daily or divided q 12 hours, *or*
  - Piperacillin-tazobactam (> 9 months old to < 40 kg) 300 mg piperacillin component/kg/day divided q 8 hours as monotherapy
    - > 40 kg, severe infection: 4.5 g piperacillin component IV q 6 hours

Table 16.17 Transition to Outpatient Antibiotics for Pneumonia

Age	Management Options
1–6 months	• Amoxicillin 80–100 mg/kg day divided bid × 7–10 days, *or* • Erythromycin 40 mg/kg/day div qid if suspect pertussis or *Chlamydia pneumoniae*
6 months to 4 years	• Amoxicillin 80–100 mg/kg/day divided bid–qid, *or* • Azithromycin 10 mg/kg day 1 (max 500 mg), then 5 mg/kg day 2–5 (max 250 mg/day)
≥ 4 years	• Azithromycin 10 mg/kg day 1, then 5 mg/kg day 2–5 • If > 8 years old, consider doxycycline 4 mg/kg/day div bid

Data from: *Cochrane Database Sys Rev.* 2012 Sep 12;9:CD005303; *Clin Infect Dis.* 2011; :e1-5216.

References: *Cochrane Database Sys Rev.* 2012 Sep 12;9:CD005303; *Clin Infect Dis.* 2011; :e1–e52.

PULMONARY EDEMA

- **Definition:** Increased fluid in pulmonary interstitium due to decreased oncotic pressure (hypoalbuminemia), increased pulmonary capillary pressures (CHF) or increased capillary permeability (sepsis, pneumonia, etc.)
- **Symptoms:** Cough, increased work of breathing (grunting, nasal flaring, use of accessory muscles/retractions)
- **Signs:** Crackles on inspiration, tachypnea, hypoxia
- **Treatment:**
  - ○ Positive end-expiratory pressure (PEEP): Initiate continuous positive airway pressure (CPAP) at 4–6 mmHg
  - ○ Consider Bilevel positive airway pressure (BiPAP) or endotracheal intubation for severe cases
  - ○ Diuretics: Furosemide 1 mg/kg IV/PO

Reference: *Crit Care Med.* 2005;33:2651–2658.

HEMOPTYSIS

Definition: Coughing up blood that originated in bronchopulmonary tree as a result of pulmonary or bronchial bleeding

Table 16.18   Causes of Hemoptysis in Children

Lower respiratory tract infection	Trauma (accidental or non-accidental, including suffocation)	Bleeding disorder or ↑ risk for bleeding due to chemotherapy
Foreign body aspiration	GI tract or nasal source	Immunocompromised child
Pulmonary tuberculosis	Congenital heart disease	Goodpasture's syndrome
Pulmonary AVM	Pulmonary embolism	Idiopathic pulmonary hemosiderosis
Pulmonary hypertension	Pulmonary tumors	Bronchiectasis
Systemic lupus erythematosus	Cystic fibrosis	

AVM: arteriovenous malformation

Table 16.19   Evaluation of the Child with Hemoptysis

- Stabilize patient
- CXR: AP and lateral for signs of localized hemorrhage or clues to diagnosis
- Chest CT with contrast; can identify cavitary lesions or pulmonary AVM
- Bronchoscopy is definitive diagnostic tool. Bronchoalveolar lavage (BAL) to look for hemosiderin-laden macrophages. Hemosiderin-laden macrophages most likely to be seen if BAL done between 3–14 days after bleed. Lung biopsy is rarely necessary
- If etiology not clear from bronchoscopy and BAL, consider echocardiography. May also consider workup for connective tissue disease or pulmonary-renal syndromes. If BAL negative and patient has no further evidence of hemoptysis, may observe and follow

Data from: American Academy of Family Physicians. Hemoptysis: diagnosis and management. 2005. http://www.aafp.org/afp/2005/1001/p1253.html; *Ped Pulmonol.* 2004;37(6):476–484.

RESPIRATORY DISTRESS

Table 16.20   Physical Exam Findings in Respiratory Distress

Retractions	Tripod positioning	Decreased LOC
Stridor	Head bobbing	Decreased air movement
Nasal flaring	Cyanosis	Decreased chest excursion
Grunting	Tachypnea	Agitation
Cough	Crackles	Unable to speak in full sentences
Decreased oral intake	Tachycardia	
Wheezing	Lethargy	
Low O_2 saturation		

Table 16.21   Normal Respiratory Rates

Age	Normal Respiratory Rate
Newborn	35–70 breaths/min
1–12 months	30–55 breaths/min
1–2 years	25–45 breaths/min
2–4 years	20–35 breaths/min
4–12 years	20–30 breaths/min
> 12 years	12–18 breaths/min

Table 16.22   Pathophysiology of Respiratory Failure

Failure of nervous system, musculature, chest wall, conducting airways	Leads to →	Hypercapnia
Failure of alveolar units, gas exchange	Leads to →	Primarily hypoxia

Table 16.23   Types of Respiratory Failure

Type I (failure of oxygenation) Most common	Alveolar hypoventilation; ↑ CO_2 also present
	V/Q mismatch; most common cause of hypoxemia; caused by asthma, pulmonary edema, ARDS
	Shunt; some venous blood returning to systemic circulation without passing through alveolar unit; may be intracardiac or intrapulmonary; 100% FiO_2 will NOT ↑ oxygenation
	Low FiO_2 (i.e., high altitude, inhalation), impairment of diffusion
Type II (CO₂ retention)	Hypoventilation, ↑ dead space (caused by hypovolemia, ↓ cardiac output, PE, ↑ airway pressure), ↑ CO_2

Table 16.24   Signs of Respiratory Failure

- Severely increased work of breathing (seesaw respirations)
- Decreased or absent air movement (asthmatics may stop wheezing)
- Increasing CO_2 ($PaCO_2$ > 60 mmHg)
- Cyanosis on > 40% FiO_2 or hypoxemia despite oxygen therapy (PaO_2 < 60 mmHg with FiO_2 > 0.6)
- pH < 7.3
- Irregular breathing pattern (tachypnea, bradypnea, or apnea)
- Altered mental status, decreased response to pain
- Diaphoresis
- Bradycardia
- Vital capacity < 15 mL/kg

Table 16.25   Causes of Respiratory Distress

Upper airway obstruction (stridor or stertor)	Croup, retropharyngeal or parapharyngeal abscess, epiglottitis, foreign body, congenital anomaly (vascular ring, TEF, polyp, papilloma, palate anomaly, laryngomalacia, tracheomalacia, subglottic stenosis), nasal congestion, hypotonia/tongue obstruction, thyromegaly, mediastinal mass, hemangioma, vocal cord paralysis, psychogenic, chemical or thermal injury, bacterial tracheitis
Lower airway obstruction (wheezing, hyperinflation, prolonged expiration)	Asthma, viral bronchiolitis, foreign body aspiration (focal signs), anaphylaxis/allergic reaction, GERD, laryngeal cleft, vascular ring, tumor, ciliary dyskinesia, cystic fibrosis, alpha-1 antitrypsin deficiency, immunodeficiency, bronchomalacia, CHF, vocal cord dysfunction, lobar emphysema (congenital or acquired), bronchopulmonary dysplasia (BPD), idiopathic pulmonary hemosiderosis, bronchiolitis obliterans
Alveolar/interstitial (lower airway)	Pneumonia, pulmonary edema, pneumonitis, atypical pneumonia (*Mycoplasma*, *Chlamydia*), interstitial pneumonitis, pulmonary edema, GERD, transient tachypnea of newborn, meconium aspiration, near drowning, foreign body aspiration, atelectasis, embolism, hemorrhage, high-altitude pulmonary edema, thermal/chemical exposures, pulmonary fibrosis (including drug-induced), PCP pneumonia
Other thoracic	Pneumothorax, tension pneumothorax, pneumomediastinum, empyema, hemothorax, chylothorax, diaphragmatic hernia, congenital malformations (CCAM: polyhydramnios, cysts on CXR that compress normal lung), allergic bronchopulmonary aspergillosis (ABPA; low-grade fever, productive cough; seen in cystic fibrosis)
Altered mental or neurologic status (neuromuscular weakness or absent airway reflexes)	Head injury, meningitis/encephalitis, seizures, toxic ingestion, abnormal neuromuscular control (muscular dystrophy, spinal muscular atrophy [Werdnig-Hoffman], spinal cord injury), brain tumor, other neurologic insult
Hematologic/altered oxygen delivery	Severe anemia, carbon monoxide poisoning, methemoglobinemia, polycythemia
Systemic/other	Febrile illness, sepsis, shock, cardiac causes (congenital heart disease, CHF, myocarditis, pericarditis), metabolic derangements (acidosis [including diabetes], hypothermia, salicylates, liver/kidney disease), abdominal pain (including appendicitis and other causes of acute abdomen)

Table 16.26   Management of Respiratory Distress

Airway Stabilization	• If airway obstruction from foreign body: Heimlich > 1 year old, back/chest blows < 1 year old • Suction nose/mouth • Position head with head tilt/jaw thrust if appropriate • Oral airway or nasopharyngeal airway if appropriate • Endotracheal intubation if indicated (see below) • Needle crichothyrotomy (emergent artificial airway to sustain life if upper airway obstruction cannot otherwise be relieved and tracheostomy not immediately available) • Tracheostomy (in OR) if upper airway obstruction not relieved by intubation
Noninvasive Ventilation (Requires patient compliance, GCS > 13, and upper airway must be open/intact; intact gag; appropriate for trial in hypoxemic respiratory failure, airway obstruction, asthma, bronchiolitis, pneumonia, BPD exacerbation, CF)	**Oxygen administration options:** • Bag Valve Mask Ventilation • High-Flow Nasal Cannula: Up to 8 L/min in infants • Face Mask: Non-rebreather or Venturi-style allows control of FiO$_2$. FiO$_2$ at 100% for acute treatment (not long term) and humidity close to 100% • Heliox (80:20): Use for reactive airways disease, RSV bronchiolitis, post-extubation, BPD, post radiation. Risk of hypothermia and hypoxemia • Nitric Oxide: Pulmonary vasodilator, useful in pulmonary hypertension, PPHN. Monitor methemolglobin • CPAP: Ideal for neonate/infant • Settings: Pressure 4–10 cm H$_2$O; FiO$_2$ to maintain PaO$_2$ 50–70 mmHg • BiPAP: Cycles between higher inspiratory pressures and lower expiratory pressures. Can adjust inspiration time • Combitude™: Double lumen airway that is blindly inserted through the mouth • Laryngeal Mask Airway (LMA): May be useful if unable to intubate. Does not prevent aspiration

BPD: Bronchopulmonary dysplasia; CF: Cystic fibrosis; GCS: Glasgow coma scale; RSV: Respiratory syncytial virus

Table 16.27   Indications for Intubation in Children

- Failed noninvasive ventilation (hypoxemia: $PaO_2 < 60$ mmHg with $FiO_2 > 0.6$; $PaCO_2 > 60$ mmHg)
- Lower airway/parenchymal disorders causing hypoxemia and/or hypercarbia
- Upper airway obstruction (impending or real)
- Hemodynamically unstable patient (actual or anticipated)
- CNS dysfunction (lack of protective reflexes, decreased LOC, neuromuscular weakness)
- Therapeutic hyperventilation (pulmonary hypertension, metabolic acidosis)
- Management of pulmonary secretions
- Emergency drug administration

CNS: Central nervous system; LOC: Level of consciousness

Table 16.28   Individual Disease Processes That Cause Respiratory Distress

Croup	Steeple sign on CXR (see section on croup)
Retropharyngeal Abscess (Group A strep, *S. aureus*, mixed gram +/–, or anaerobes)	Usually child < 4 years old; high fever, drooling, dyspnea. Lateral neck X-ray (in extension, during inspiration) shows marked thickening of the prevertbral space (wider than width of one vertebral body); consider CT scan of neck with IV contrast, ENT consultation, IV antibiotics (and possibly drainage)
Parapharyngeal Abscess (Group A strep, *S. aureus*, mixed gram positive/gram negatives, or anaerobes)	Present similar to retropharyngeal abscess, but may also have torticollis and tender neck swelling. CT is diagnostic. IV antibiotics and surgical drainage
Epiglottitis (Group A strep, *S. aureus*, *Haemophilus influenzae* type B, also consider *Candida albicans* if white patches)	Rapidly progressive stridor, fever, dysphagia, drooling, toxicity, dyspnea. Child sits with neck extended. First step is to stabilize airway, in OR if possible, then culture and start antibiotics. X-ray (after stabilized) shows "thumb print sign," epiglottic enlargement. Steroid use may be considered
Foreign Body Aspiration	+/– history of choking. Object may lodge in trachea or mainstem bronchus (usually right side). Radio-opaque objects can be identified on plain films of chest/neck. Inspiratory/expiratory films or left lateral decub films may show air trapping. Bronchoscopy to confirm and treat
Vocal Cord Dysfunction	True vocal cords paradoxically close during inspiration, associated with dyspnea. Often psychogenic
Vocal Cord Paralysis	Often presents in neonatal period; weak, hoarse cry, stridor, feeding problems. Bilateral: may be associated with hydrocephalus, Arnold-Chiari malformation, other nervous system anomalies. Unilateral: may be associated with congenital heart defects
Laryngomalacia	Stridor in newborn, increase when feeding, crying, or supine. Usually resolves by 18 months of age. Endoscopy is required to rule out other causes
Pulmonary Edema	Cardiogenic and noncardiogenic (ARDS); fluid accumulates in alveoli and interstitium; CXR shows peribronchial and perivascular cuffing early, and diffuse patchy densities late. Cardiomegaly when associated with CHF. Cardiogenic edema is treated with inotropic support, afterload reduction and diuretics (see also CHF)
Interstitial Pneumonitis/Interstitial Lung Disease	Restrictive pattern. Diffuse infiltrates on CXR. Seen with neuroendocrine cell hyperplasia in infancy (NEHI) and pulmonary interstitial glycogenesis (PIG), desquamative interstitial pneumonitis (DIP)
Bronchiolitis Obliterans	Presents with unresolving cough and wheeze after short respiratory illness (often adenovirus; leads to chronic nonprogressive course). May occur after Stevens-Johnson syndrome (progressive and often requires lung transplant) adenovirus, or post- transplant patients. CT: Mosaic perfusion, vascular attenuation, central bronchiectasis; PFTs: fixed obstructive lung disease
Idiopathic Pulmonary Hemosiderosis	Cough, respiratory distress, hemoptysis, and drop in hematocrit. Consider autoimmune workup and testing for von Willebrand disease

(Continued)

Table 16.28 Individual Disease Processes That Cause Respiratory Distress *(Continued)*

Bronchopulmonary Dysplasia (BPD)	Seen in premature infants who are treated with positive pressure ventilation and oxygen. Associated with increased airway resistance, reactivity, and obstruction and decreased lung compliance. May see pulmonary hypertension; CXR: decreased lung volumes, patchy atelectasis/hyperinflation, pulmonary edema, and pulmonary interstitial emphysema. Children with BPD are often treated with furosemide (or other diuretic), bronchodilators (beta agonist or ipratropium bromide), theophylline, caffeine, corticosteroids (dexamethasone after 1 month old). Follow RSV prophylaxis guidelines
Carbon Monoxide Poisoning	May present with shortness of breath, headache, dizziness, nausea. Measure blood carboxyhemoglobin concentration (venous sample adequate) or noninvasive CO-oximetry monitors. May be falsely elevated in infants < 3 months old
Tension Pneumothorax	Dyspnea, unilateral breath sounds, tracheal shift, ↑ neck veins, cardiorespiratory collapse 18- to 22-gauge needle in second ICS midclavicular line and/or chest tube fourth and fifth ICS midaxillary line
Pneumothorax (non-tension)	If large/significant, requires chest tube and possible surgical intervention

See individual sections on asthma, bronchiolitis, anaphylaxis, GERD, cystic fibrosis, pneumonia, stridor, heart disease, and apnea

ARDS: Acute respiratory distress syndrome; BPD: Bronchopulmonary dysplasia; CF: Cystic fibrosis; CHF: Congestive heart failure; CXR: Chest X-ray; ENT: Ear, nose, and throat (specialty); GCS: Glasgow coma scale; ICS: Intercostal space; PFT: Pulmonary function test; RSV: Respiratory syncytial virus

Data from: *Curr Opin Pediatr.* 2008 Jun;20(3):272–278; *Paediatr Respir Rev.* 2010 Dec;11(4):233–9. Epub 2010 Aug 19.

Table 16.29 Studies to Consider in Workup of Respiratory Distress

CBC with differential Serum electrolytes CRP/ESR Viral swabs (RSV, influenza, paraflu) Sweat chloride (CF)		
Arterial or venous blood gas IgE (ABPA, allergic processes) Blood carboxyhemoglobin		
Fungal serology *Mycoplasma pneumoniae* serology Urine for glucose and ketones		
Consider imaging: CXR: AP/lateral, lateral decubitus, and/or inspiratory/expiratory Lateral neck films: extended, inspiratory Barium swallow pH probe CT scan	**If suspect immunodficiency:** Quantitative immunoglobulins, IgG subclasses, tetanus, diphtheria, polyvalent pneumococcal vaccine, and *Haemophilus influenzae* type B antibodies, complement (C3, C4, CH50), and lymphocyte subsets (via flow cytometry)	
	If interstitial disease: Genetic testing for *SFTPB* and *ABCA3*	**If suspect cardiac cause:** Lactate ECG Echocardiogram

Useful equations when dealing with respiratory distress/failure:

Arterial oxygen content (CaO_2) equation: (normal $= 17$–24 mL/dL)
    Reflects overall oxygen carrying capacity of arterial blood
    $CaO_2 = (Hgb \times 1.34 \times SaO_2) + (0.0031 \times PaO_2)$
Mixed venous oxygen content (CvO_2) equation: (normal $= 12$–17 mL/dL)
    Reflects oxygen content of venous blood returning to the heart
    $CvO_2 = (Hgb \times 1.34 \times SvO_2) + (0.0031 \times PvO_2)$
Alveolar gas equation:
    $P_AO_2 = (FiO_2 [P_{atm} - P_{H20}]) - (Pa_{CO2} / RQ)$
    $P_{atm} = 760$ mmHg, $P_{H20} = 47$ mmHg, RQ usually $= 0.8$
Alveolar-arterial oxygen gradient (A-a gradient; $P_AO_2 - PaO_2$):
    $([P_{atm} - P_{H20}] FiO_2) - (Pa_{CO2}/0.8) - PaO_2$
    $P_{atm} = 760$ mmHg, $P_{H20} = 47$ mmHg; PaO_2 obtained from ABG
    Normal on room air $= 15$–20 (age [years]/4 + 4)
    Ventilation/perfusion (V/Q) mismatch $= 50$–300
    Shunting $= > 300$
Bohr equation (physiologic dead space): $Vd/Vt = PaCO_2 - PeCO_2/PaCO_2$
Capillary oxygen content: $CcO_2 = (Hgb \times 1.34) + (0.0031 \times PaO_2)$
Mean Airway Pressure $= ([rate][IT][PIP] + [60 - (rate)(IT)(PEEP)])/60$

MANAGEMENT OF INTUBATED PATIENT

Table 16.30   Endotracheal Intubation*

Endotracheal tube:	Procedure
Infant Size: 3.0: Newborn	Insure suction available
3.5: 3–8 months	Preoxygenate with 100% FiO_2
4.0: 9–24 months	Monitoring in place
Size $= (Age/4) + 4$	Vascular access in place
Cuffed tube: add half a size	Sedative/hypnotic, and neuromuscular blockade
For children over 14 years, use 7.0 for females and 8.0	Cricoid pressure
for males.	Laryngoscopy and intubation (watch tube pass through
Laryngoscope Blade:	vocal cords)
Size 1: ≤ 1 year	Confirm: breath sounds, $ETCO_2$, colorimetric CO_2 detector,
Size 2: 2–11 years	chest movement, CXR
Size 3: ≥ 12 years	Secure tube

*See also critical care chapter

Table 16.31   Rapid-Sequence Intubation

1. Preoxygenation (positive-pressure ventilation with BVM)
2. Adjunctive agents ➤ Atropine 0.01 mg/kg (1 mg max [helps prevent bradycardia]) ➤ Lidocaine 1.5 mg/kg (if suspect increased ICP)
3. Are you able to ventilate patient if intubation fails? If not, do not proceed
4. Cricoid pressure
5. Paralyzing agent options: ➤ Rocuronium 0.6–1 mg/kg (fewer side effects, lasts 25–60 minutes) ➤ Succinylcholine 1–2 mg/kg (shorter duration 3–12 minutes) ➤ Vecuronium 0.1–0.2 mg/kg (onset within 90 seconds, lasts 2 hours)
6. Sedation options (conditions in which drug is particularly beneficial): ➤ Thiopental 3–5 mg/kg (status epilepticus, head injury without hypotension) ➤ Etomidate 0.3 mg/kg (head injury with mild hypotension) ➤ Ketamine 1–2 mg/kg (hypotension, status asthmaticus)
7. Consider NG/OG tube
8. Neostigmine + atropine may be needed to reverse rocuronium if some spontaneous recovery already seen

Table 16.32 Ventilator Basics

VOLUME VENTILATION	PRESSURE VENTILATION
• Most commonly used for infants < 8 kg • Volume delivery and inspiratory flow are constant • Inspiratory pressure variable	• Most commonly used for pediatric patients > 8 kg • Inspiratory pressure constant • Volume delivery and inspiratory flow vary
Initial Settings	
Settings • **Rate:** start with rate that is close to child's age reference • **FiO$_2$:** 100% to start, decrease as tolerated (based on SpO$_2$ or ABG results) • **PEEP:** 3–5 mmHg • **TV:** 8–10 mL/kg, or **PIP:** 14–20 mmHg • **Pressure support:** 5–10 • **Mode: A/C** (controls every breath); **SIMV** (control some breaths)	

Table 16.33 Initial HFOV Settings

• Mean airway pressure (MAP): 2–10 cms > MAP of conventional mandatory ventilation • Frequency (Hz) based on body size and disease process: ○ 2–12 kg = 10 Hz; 13–20 kg = 8 Hz; 21–34 kg = 7 Hz; > 35 kg = 6 Hz • Power set at 4.0 • FiO$_2$ at 1.0 (100%)

STRIDOR

Definition: High-pitched sound caused by turbulent airflow through the supraglottis, glottis, subglottis, and/or trachea

Table 16.34 Classification of Stridor

Inspiratory stridor	Noted with inspiration only; usually associated with obstruction at the level of the larynx
Expiratory stridor	Noted with expiration; usually associated with obstruction at tracheobronchial level
Biphasic stridor	Both inspiratory and expiratory; usually suggests glottis or subglottic pathology

- **History:** Associated symptoms (drooling, voice/crying changes, feeding difficulties, fever, cough, cyanosis, respiratory distress, GERD symptoms, weight loss or poor weight gain), positional changes, precipitating events (feeding), birth history (maternal condyloma, intubation)
- **Exam:** Defer detailed exam of toxic child with stridor until airway support is available. Avoid irritating child if moderate to severe stridor. Aside from assessing vitals and respiratory status and comprehensive physical exam, note craniofacial anomalies, cutaneous anomalies (hemangiomas), growth parameters

Table 16.35 Differential Diagnosis of Acute Stridor

Croup (see below)	Retropharyngeal abscess	Epiglottitis
Foreign body aspiration	Bacterial tracheitis (S. aureus	Spasmodic croup
Anaphylaxis	following croup)	Peritonsillar abscess

Table 16.36   Differential Diagnosis of Chronic Stridor

Larygomalacia (75% of cases of stridor in newborn; increase with cry/ feeding; improved in prone position. Usually resolves but intervention necessary if significant obstruction or weight loss) **Vocal cord paralysis** (weak cry, biphasic stridor. Congenital or post cardiac/thoracic surgery; L > R)	**Subglottic stenosis** (inspiratory or biphasic; congenital or acquired after intubation) **Laryngeal web** **Laryngeal cyst or hemangioma** **Papillomas** (vertical transmission of HPV) **Macroglossia** **Micrognathia**	**Tracheal stenosis** (congenital caused by complete tracheal rings; can also be caused by compression by vascular slings or double aortic arch; also consider thoracic mass) **Tracheomalacia** (expiratory stridor) **Gastroesophageal reflux**

Data from: *B-ENT*, 2005, 1, Suppl. 1, 113–125.

- **Workup:** Consider AP/lateral CXR, as well as left lateral decubitus films or inspiratory and expiratory films to demonstrate air trapping/foreign body. Lateral neck films to evaluate epiglottitis
  - ○ Barium esophagram if suspect esophageal abnormalities.
  - ○ Echocardiography for suspected vascular/cardiac anomalies. pH probe if suspect GER
  - ○ MRI or CT used to confirm extrinsic mass detected on endoscopy
  - ○ Direct laryngoscopy and bronchoscopy are best way to make definitive diagnosis
  - ○ Laryngeotracheobronchoscopy indicated for severe stridor, progressive stridor, stridor associated with cyanosis, apnea, dysphagia, FTT, radiographic abnormality
- **Treatment:** Depends on cause of stridor
  - ○ Otolaryngology consultation may be indicated (except in routine cases of croup and anaphylaxis)
  - ○ Admit children with significant respiratory distress, stridor at rest, toxicity, poor feeding or dehydration, unclear etiology of significant stridor

Reference: *B-ENT.* 2005; 1(1):113–125.

LAB EVALUATION IN RHEUMATOLOGIC DISEASES

Table 17.1 Common Lab Evaluation in Pediatric Rheumatologic Diseases

C-reactive protein (CRP)	Helps in diagnosis of infection, monitoring treatment response acutely; also useful in conjunction with ESR to monitor chronic inflammation
ESR	Marker of inflammation, acute phase reactant
CBCd	Cytopenias can be present in rheumatologic disorders, or as a result of treatment
Anti-SSA/Ro and anti-SSB/La antibodies	Associated with Sjogren's syndrome, SLE, and congenital heart block
Anti-U1 small nuclear ribonucleoprotein antibodies	High specificity for mixed connective tissue disease
Cytoplasmic anti-neutrophil antibodies	Wegener's granulomatosis
Hereditary periodic fever syndromes (most have specific genetic tests)	Familial Mediterranean fever: mutations in MEFV gene; Hyperimmunoglobulinemia D syndrome: MK gene for mevalonate kinase
Antinuclear antibodies (ANA), anti-Smith antibodies	Useful in diagnosis, determining prognosis, and facilitating follow-up in children with SLE ANA + children with juvenile idiopathic arthritis (JIA) have much higher risk of anterior uveitis
Anti-double stranded DNA (dsDNA) antibodies	Correlates with lupus nephritis Increased titer usually indicates increased disease activity
Human leukocyte antigen-B27	Ankylosing spondylitis and Reiter's syndrome
Rheumatoid factor	Helpful in identifying/differentiating juvenile idiopathic arthritides
C3, C4	Useful in follow-up of SLE and membranoproliferative glomerulonephritis
Ferritin	Hallmark of primary and secondary hemophagocytic lymphohistiocytosis
ASO titers	To confirm a diagnosis of acute rheumatic fever; anti-hyaluronidase, anti-deoxyribonuclease (DNase) B, and anti-streptokinase (ASO) antibodies are other markers of strep infection
Anti-phospholipid (aPL) antibodies	Associated with repeated spontaneous abortions, thrombocytopenia, thrombosis (venous or arterial)
Complement split products	Correlates with disease activity, reflects especially extra-renal involvement
Lupus nephritis renal panel	Helps identify active kidney inflammation Measures: CC-chemokine ligand 2, neutrophil gelatinase-associated lipocalin (NGAL), hepcidin-20 and hepcidin-25, lipocalin-like prostaglandin D synthetase, α-1-acid-glycoprotein (orosomucoid), ceruloplasmin, and transferrin
Cell-bound, genomic (blood), and urinary biomarkers	Likely to be helpful in coming years

Data from: *Semin Arthritis Rheum.* 2010 Aug;40(1):53–72. Epub 2009 Feb 26.

PEDIATRIC SYSTEMIC LUPUS ERYTHEMATOSUS (pSLE)

- Also known as childhood-onset SLE, juvenile onset SLE (diagnosis made < 16 yrs old, most commonly between 12–14 yrs of age)
- 15–20% of lupus cases have onset in childhood; 20% male
- Glucocorticoids and immunosuppressive therapy necessary for most children and teens with lupus

Table 17.2   Signs/Symptoms of Pediatric Lupus by Organ System

Kidney	Nephritis or nephrotic syndrome
Musculoskeletal	Arthritis; avascular necrosis (AVN) affects large weight-bearing bones. Increased risk if 15–20 years old, aPL positive, other thrombotic risk factors, unclear if associated with steroid treatment
Blood	Hemolytic anemia, thrombocytopenia, leukopenia, or lymphopenia; thrombophlebitis
Neurologic	Psychosis, seizures, cognitive disorders, peripheral neuropathies
Pulmonary	Pulmonary hemorrhage, fibrosis, or infarct
Cardiac	Valvulitis and carditis, pericarditis
Gastrointestinal	Abdominal pain, diarrhea, malabsorption, protein-losing enteropathy

Table 17.3   Diagnosis of Pediatric Systemic Lupus Erythematosus

Requires at least 4 of the following findings:		
Mucocutaneous findings	Non-mucocutaneous findings	Lab findings
Malar rash Naso-oral ulcers Photosensitive rash Discoid rash	Arthritis Carditis or pleuritis Encephalitis (seizure or psychosis) Nephritis (Proteinuria, hematuria)	Hemolytic anemia, thrombocytopenia, leukopenia, or lymphopenia Positive anti-dsDNA, anti-Smith, or antiphospholipid antibody Positive antinuclear antibody (ANA)

Table 17.4   Treatment Options for Pediatric Systemic Lupus Erythematosus*

Medication	Indications	Dose	Comments
Naproxen	Musculoskeletal symptoms	10–20 mg/kg/day Max 500 mg bid	Avoid if renal damage
Ibuprofen	Musculoskeletal symptoms	20–40 mg/kg/day Max 800 mg q 8 hour	Avoid if renal damage

(Continued)

Table 17.4   Treatment Options for Pediatric Systemic Lupus Erythematosus* *(Continued)*

Medication	Indications	Dose	Comments
Prednisone	Rapid relief of moderate–severe acute symptoms OR low dose for maintenance	0.5–2 mg/kg/day Max 60 mg/day	Dose decreased over time or alternate day regimen if possible
Methylprednisolone (PO)	Moderate–severe acute symptoms	0.5–2 mg/kg/day PO Max 60 mg/ day	Use if liver signs
Methylprednisolone (IV)	Acute neuropsychiatric symptoms, heme or kidney disease	10–30 mg/ dose IV Max 1000 mg/dose	May give daily for ≤ 3 days
Azathioprine	Moderate–severe disease	0.5–2.5 mg/kg/day PO Max 200 mg PO/day	CBCd, LFTs at baseline, 1 month, and q 3 months. Can check thiopurine methyltransferase
Cyclophosphamide (PO)	Severe organ involvement	0.5–2 mg/kg/day Max 150 mg PO q day	Renal panel and CBCd on days of infusion and 7–10 days after dose; Can cause leukopenia and impaired gonadal function. PCP prophylaxis recommended
Cyclophosphamide (IV)	Severe organ involvement	500–1000 mg/m² 2500 mg/dose (initially given monthly then less often)	
Mycophenolate mofetil (*CellCept*)	Nephritis	1200 mg/m²/day Max 1000 mg bid	Side effects include abdominal pain, diarrhea, rash. Check CBCd, LFTs at baseline, 1 month, and q 3 months. May check levels to adjust dose
Rituximab (Anti CD-20 monoclonal antibody)	Moderate–severe disease	375 mg/ m²/dose Max 4 doses at weekly intervals	Benefits might be limited to a subgroup patients; monitor B cell panel prior to Rx and 6–8 wk after. Update Iz before Rx if possible. Monitor IgG levels and Rx if necessary
Hydroxychloroquine (Plaquenil)	Reduces flares, skin disease, and autoantibody production	5–7 mg/kg/day Max 400 mg PO q day	Monitor CBC, CK, liver panel baseline, at 1 month, then q 3 months. Skin hyperpigmentation possible
Dapsone	Skin disease	2 mg/kg/day Max 100 mg PO q day	
Immunoglobulins	Heme disease		
Methotrexate	Arthritis	25 mg/week PO	Avoid in kidney disease

(Continued)

Table 17.4   Treatment Options for Pediatric Lupus* *(Continued)*

Medication	Indications	Dose	Comments
Aspirin	aPL positive		
Vitamin D	Support bone health	600 IU to 4000 IU/ day	
Calcium	Support bone health	1000–3000 mg/day (> 9 years old)	

*No medication specifically approved for treatment of pediatric SLE; dosing not well established

Table 17.5   Short-Term Follow-Up Care of Children with SLE

Every 3 months (other testing may be indicated depending on individual)
CBC with differential (CBCd), C3, C4, ESR, renal panel, hepatic panel, anti-dsDNA antibodies Urinalysis, urine protein/creatinine, urine microalbumin

Table 17.6   Yearly Follow-up Care of Children with SLE

Labs: aPL, anti-Ro, anti-La, anti-Sm, anti-RNP (do not need to repeat if positive) TSH, FT4 25-hydroxyvitamin D (goal 50 nmol/L) Serum lipid profile	Ophthalmologic exam (especially if on Plaquenil; more frequent if complications present)	Health-related quality of life evaluation using validated measure Discuss cardiovascular risk factors, weight management, and sun protection

Other:
- Dual-energy X-ray absorptiometry (DXA) of the lumbar spine and body (except head) at diagnosis and every 1–2 years after
- Avoid live-attenuated vaccines (measles, mumps, rubella [MM]; varicella)
- Vaccination against pneumococcus, meningococcus, *Haemophilus influenzae* type B highly recommended
  - Discuss risks/benefits of hep B, human papillomavirus (HPV) vaccines
- Counsel regarding contraception, especially if on mycophenolate, ACE inhibitors, methotrexate, or anticoagulants

Prognosis:
- Disease course often more severe when diagnosed in childhood
- Poor prognostic indicators are renal disease, severe disease flares, infections, and neuropsychiatric symptoms

JUVENILE IDIOPATHIC ARTHRITIS

- Arthritis for at least 6 weeks in children < 16 years old
- Usually have pain in the morning or after long period of rest
- Diagnosis mostly clinical. Labs helpful. MRI is most useful radiologic technique for indicating disease activity. Nuclear imaging, CT, ultrasound, plain films sometimes indicated
- Admit child with systemic flare, unable to ambulate, unclear diagnosis, pericarditis

Table 17.7   ILAR Classification of Juvenile Idiopathic Arthritis

Systemic-onset JIA	Spiking fevers 1–2 times daily, usually predictable pattern/time; may appear toxic Salmon-colored macular rash at trunk/extremities Hepatomegaly, lymphadenopathy, serositis, myalgia sometimes present Lower risk of uveitis but need to be screened yearly Watch for signs of macrophage activating syndrome (MAS) with ↓ ESR, platelets, WBC, fibrinogen, and ↑ LFTs and ferritin. DIC and hemorrhage may be present
Persistent or extended oligoarthritis	< 4 joints affected, usually large weight-bearing joints May see leg length discrepancy, muscle atrophy, or contractures X-ray if only one joint affected (soft-tissue swelling, osteopenia, joint space narrowing) Anterior uveitis common (20%) requiring exam every 3 months × 4 years if ANA positive. If uveitis not present, examine q 6 months until 7 years after diagnosis, then yearly
Rheumatoid factor (RF)-positive polyarthritis	5 or more joints affected in first 6 months of diagnosis, weight-bearing joints and hands. May see rheumatoid nodules and hands. Lower risk of uveitis than oligoarticular but still requires regular screening
RF-negative polyarthritis	Same as RF positive but no nodules
Psoriatic JIA	Skin findings of psoriasis typically present; also look for nail pits and dactylitis. Half of kids have monoarticular arthritis and DIP involvement
Enthesitis-related arthritis	Pediatric spondyloarthropathy. Evening pain; buttock pain that improves with activity. Pain at insertion of tendon/ligament to bone AND arthritis OR either enthesitis or arthritis PLUS 2 of the following: sacroiliitis, HLAB27 positive, onset in boy > 6 years, acute symptomatic anterior uveitis, or family history of ankylosing spondylitis, enthesitis-related arthritis, IBD with sacroiliitis, reactive arthritis, or acute anterior uveitis
Undifferentiated	Does not fulfill criteria of any one category, or meet criteria from more than 1 category

Data from: *Journal of Rheumatology* 2004; 31:2.

Table 17.8   American College of Rheumatology Treatment Recommendations for Juvenile Idiopathic Arthritis

Arthritis in 4 or fewer joints	NSAIDs, intra-articular steroid injections, methotrexate (or sulfasalazine for enthesitis-related arthritis), TNF-alpha inhibitors
Arthritis in 5 or more joints	Low disease activity or moderate activity without poor prognostic indicators* may start with NSAIDs/intra-articular injections All others start with methotrexate or leflunomide If no response after 3–6 months, switch to TNF-alpha inhibitor Abatacept or rituximab if still symptomatic despite above therapies

(Continued)

Table 17.8   American College of Rheumatology Treatment Recommendations for Juvenile Idiopathic Arthritis *(Continued)*

Active sacroiliac arthritis	Trial of NSAIDs and methotrexate but may move more quickly to TNF-alpha inhibitor
Systemic JIA with active systemic features but *without* active arthritis	2-week trial of NSAIDs then systemic glucocorticoids. Patients who are more ill may be started on systemic glucocorticoids as a first step Patients who develop fever while on steroids can be started on anakinra. (IL-1 receptor antagonist) Tocilizumab (*Actemra*; monoclonal Ab vs IL-6 receptor) approved for treatment of children > 2 years old with JIA
Systemic JIA with active arthritis but without active systemic features	NSAIDs, joint injections, then methotrexate if needed; consider anakira, or TNF-alpha inhibitor, or abatacept for active arthritis not responding to above therapies

*Hip or cervical spine involvement, positive RF or anti-cyclic citrullinated peptide antibodies, radiographic signs of joint damage

Data from: *Arthritis Care & Research* Vol. 63, No. 4, April 2011, pp 465–482.

MIXED CONNECTIVE TISSUE DISEASE

Table 17.9   Symptoms/Findings of Mixed Connective Tissue Disease

Arthritis Raynaud's phenomenon Positive anti-RNP antibodies	Scleroderma Rash typical of SLE ANA often high	Rash typical of dermatomyositis Fever RF often positive	Esophageal dysmotility Cardiac, muscle, pulmonary, CNS, kidney inflammation

ANA: Antinuclear antibodies; CNS: Central nervous system; SLE: Systemic lupus erythematosus; RNP: Ribonucleoprotein

Data from: American College of Rheumatology 2011 Recommendations for the Treatment of JIA, www.rheumatology.org, accessed 5/29/13.

DERMATOMYOSITIS

SYMPTOMS
- Symmetric, proximal muscle (hip girdle and leg) weakness +/– pain
- Purple discoloration of upper eyelids (heliotrope)
- Erythematous papulosquamous eruption over dorsal surfaces knuckles (Gottron's papules)
- Dyspnea, dysphagia
- Rash (symmetric, red, atrophic changes at extensor surfaces)
- Malar rash (nasolabial folds not spared)
- May see soft-tissue calcification on X-ray
- Usual onset 4–10 years of age, girls predominate 2:1
- Vasculitis may lead to intestinal perforation

Table 17.10   Tests Commonly Used in Evaluation Dermatomyositis

CK, AST, ALT, aldolase, LDH, serum neopterin, von Willebrand factor (elevated)
MRI can show edema/ inflammation in muscles
Muscle biopsy

TREATMENT

- Glucocorticoids are first line (usually prednisone)
- Azathioprine (*Azasan, Imuran*) or methotrexate (*Trexall, Rheumatrex*, or generic)
- Intravenous immunoglobulin (IVIG)
- Tacrolimus, cyclosporine, cyclophosphamide, rituximab (*Rixutan*), TNF-alpha inhibitors may be used for more severe disease

NEONATAL LUPUS

Neonatal Lupus = disease caused by the passage of maternal antibodies across placenta; affects children < 6 months old

Table 17.11   Symptoms of Neonatal Lupus

Cardiac	Risk for 3rd-degree (complete) heart block 1–5/100 chance if mother is anti-Ro or La antibody + May be detected between weeks 20–30 of pregnancy 20–30% mortality in infancy > 50% require pacemaker
Liver	Hepatomegaly, elevated ALT/AST, conjugated hyperbilirubinemia
CNS	Hydrocephalus, macrocephaly
Skin	66% present at birth, others present at 1–5 months of age Annular red plaques mostly on neck, face, scalp Telangiectasias, petechiae, cutis marmorata
Hematologic	Hemolytic anemia, severe thrombocytopenia, neutropenia Usually present at 2 weeks old and resolve around 2 months of age
Splenic	Splenomegaly

RISK FACTORS

Presence of anti-SSA/Ro, anti-SSB/La, human leukocyte antigen B8 (HLA-B8), and human leukocyte antigen DR3 (HLA-DR3) in mother puts infant at increased risk (mother may not have SLE). Higher risk of heart block if mother has had previous infant with heart block

DIAGNOSIS

Clinical finding plus presence of maternal antibodies

TREATMENT

- Skin, liver, CNS, and hematologic manifestations are often transient and self-resolve
- Heart block often requires pacemaker; maternal glucocorticoids are sometimes used when second-degree heart block noted in utero in effort to decrease progress to third-degree block

PROGNOSIS

Infants with neonatal lupus do not necessarily go on to develop SLE, though there is increased risk to any child of mother with SLE, especially females

CHAPTER 18 ■ TRAUMA

Trauma is the number one cause of childhood death and disability, with approximately 20,000 yearly deaths, 120,000 newly disabled children, and 500,000 hospitalizations from 1.5 million injuries. Most of these injuries are caused by motor vehicle crashes, burns, and falls.

PREHOSPITAL TRAUMA PREPARATION

Upon receiving preliminary information regarding the extent of injuries to the child, notify appropriate specialized personnel (pediatric surgeon, neurosurgery, trauma team, intensivist, anesthesiologist) based on suspicion of any of the following:

- Impaired airway, breathing, or circulation
- Depressed level of consciousness
- Suspected spinal cord injury
- Extensive burns
- Penetrating trauma
- Abdominal trauma

DIFFERENCES BETWEEN ADULT AND PEDIATRIC TRAUMA PATIENTS

- **Surface area**: Children have large surface area: volume ratios, increasing heat loss, resulting in rapid hypothermia
- **Skeleton**: Elastic bones allow for internal injuries without overlying fractures
- **Head/airway relationship**: Large occiput can create flexion obstruction of airway in supine position, necessitating shoulder roll to straighten neck/open airway

PRIMARY SURVEY

Identical to adult patients, including cervical spine immobilization with appropriate size collar (or manual immobilization). Of note, children often become "combative" to emergency personnel when restrained and in an unfamiliar environment. Engaging the conscious child in a conversation using their native language frequently helps minimize anxiety and allows for improved evaluation of the extent of injuries

- **Airway**: Cervical spine tends to flex due to large occiput. Generally, a small shoulder roll will bring the neck to neutral position, relieving any flexion-induced obstruction (while maintaining c-spine precautions). The larynx tends to be anterior in children and the trachea is soft and short. Coupled with large tongue, this often makes intubation more difficult. Consider straight laryngoscope (Miller) blade in infants less than 12 months of age (see rapid-sequence intubation table)
- **Surgical airway**: When a surgical airway is needed, remember that a cricothyroidotomy is contraindicated in children. Instead, a temporary needle cricothyroidotomy followed by a formal tracheostomy should be performed
- **Breathing**: Underlying lung trauma without rib fractures is possible due to elasticity of ribs. Always consider occult lung injury, pneumothorax, or hemothorax, especially in presence of poor ventilation or oxygenation despite proper endotracheal tube placement. In addition, remember that infants are obligate nasal breathers and therefore an OGT should be used in place of an NGT

Table 18.1 Quick Reference for Pediatric Trauma

Age	Preemie	Neonate (0–30 days)	1 mo	4 mos	8 mos	1 yr	2 yrs	3 yrs	4 yrs	5 yrs	6 yrs	8 yrs	10 yrs	12 yrs
Weight	< 3 kg	3.5 kg	4 kg	6 kg	8 kg	10 kg	12 kg	14 kg	16 kg	18 kg	20 kg	25 kg	32 kg	40 kg
HR Range (beats/min)	120–160	100–180	100–180	120–170	110–170	110–170	90–150	80–140	75–135	65–135	60–130	60–120	60–120	60–120
Respiratory Rate (per minute)	40–60	40–60	40–60	30–50	25–45	20–40	20–40	20–30	20–30	20–30	15–25	12–25	12–25	12–25
Systolic Blood Pressure (mmHg)	40–60	65–85	65–90	65–95	70–105	70–110	70–110	80–110	80–110	80–110	90–115	90–115	95–120	95–120
Endotracheal Tube Size	2.5–3.0	3.0	3.0–3.5	3.5	3.5	4.0	4.0 – 4.5	4.5	4.5–5.0	5.0–5.5	5.5	5.5–6.0	6.0–6.5	7.0–7.5
Laryngoscopy Blade	0 Miller	1 Miller	1 Miller	1 Miller	1 Miller	1 Miller	1–2	1–2	1–2	2	2	2–3	2–3	3
Chest Tube (Fr)	8–10	10–12	10–12	10–12	12–16	16–20	16–20	20–24	20–24	24–28	24–28	24–28	28–32	32–42
Femoral Vein Line (Fr)		3	4	4	4	4	4–5	5	5	5	5	5–7	6–7	7

- **Circulation**: Children have impressive physiologic reserve to counteract blood loss and dehydration. Normal vital signs or mild tachycardia may precede hypotensive shock. Once the "crash" occurs, it may be too late. Assume pediatric blood volume is 80–90 mL/kg (8–9% of total body weight)

- **Vascular Access**: Peripheral access is preferred. Alternative access method (intraosseous or central venous line) should be used after 3 unsuccessful attempts at peripheral access, or 90 seconds if child is in shock

All fluids should be warmed to prevent hypothermia. In cases of hypotension, 2 boluses of crystalloid (20 mL/kg) may be given. If the patient continues to have hypotension, give 10 mL/kg of blood as the patient is being prepared for either the operating room or angiography

- **Intraosseous (IO) line**: Provides rapid, secure access to vascular space
  - *All* resuscitation fluids, medication (including "code" meds and vasoactive drips) and blood products can be given via the IO line
  - **Sites:** Proximal tibia on flat, medial surface, 1–2 cm below the tibial tuberosity. Second option is distal anterior femur 2–3 cm above knee
  - **Contraindication:** Previous IO attempt on same bone, or fracture of extremity (or pelvis) proximal to IO site
  - **Risk:** Osteomyelitis, infusion into soft tissue resulting in compartment syndrome

- **Disability**: Assess pupils, movement of extremities, GCS (see Pediatric Coma Score table). Avoid secondary injury from hypotension or hypoxia

- **Exposure**: Expose the patient thoroughly to look for all signs of injury (roll patient, maintaining c-spine precautions if indicated). Then quickly place a warm blanket to prevent hypothermia

- **Prevention**: Large potential to significantly impact death and disability: Bicycle helmets, car seats, safe storage of firearms, smoke detectors, fire-retardant clothing/pajamas, pool safety

SPECIAL CIRCUMSTANCES THAT RELATE TO PEDIATRIC TRAUMA

- **Airway**: Difficulties with intubation may be caused by:
  - Anterior located larynx
  - Large occiput causing flexion of the neck
  - Short, soft trachea

- **Visceral injury without overlying fracture**:
  - Children have soft, pliable bones and may have significant brain or other internal organ injury without an overlying fracture

- **Aspiration**:
  - Children swallow large amounts of air, particularly with crying. NGT (or OGT placement for obligate nose breathers/infants) can prevent over-distension of the stomach and subsequent emesis with aspiration

- **Spinal cord injury without radiographic abnormality (SCIWORA)**:
  - Due to pliable bones
  - Normal C-spine studies

- **Abnormal C-spine studies**:
  - Skeletal growth plates
  - Pseudosubluxation

- **Normal vital signs**:
  - Children have a large physiologic reserve and will have normal blood pressure until just prior to decompensation ("crashing")

○ Tachycardia should be present long before hypotensive shock. Differential diagnosis of tachycardia includes hypovolemia, pain, anxiety, and fever

- **Child Abuse**: Historical or physical exam findings listed below should increase concern for intentionally inflicted injuries

  ○ Repeat visits or delay in accessing care

  ○ Discrepancy in story over repeated histories, or discrepancy in severity of injury not well explained by the history

  ○ Bites, burns

  ○ Peri-oral or genital injuries

  ○ Retinal hemorrhages

  ○ Injuries of varying ages

CHAPTER 19 ■ PEDIATRIC CRITICAL CARE

BASIC AND ADVANCED LIFE SUPPORT ALGORITHMS

Begin CPR if pulse < 60/min + poor perfusion despite good ventilation and oxygenation

↓

Assess × 10 seconds after 2 minutes: Continue CPR for poor perfusion and HR < 60/min

↓

- **Compressions: at least 100/min**
  Depth: 1/3 AP diameter of chest (Infants: 1.5 inches, Children: 2 inches)
  Allow complete recoil after each compression
- **One rescuer:** 30 compressions: 2 breaths
- **Two rescuers:** 15 compressions: 2 breaths
- **Goal Spo₂:** > 94% but < 100%

↓

Check Rhythm
Follow appropriate PALS algorithm below

↓

PALS ALGORITHMS

PULSELESS VFIB/VTACH

- **Defibrillate** (2 J/kg)
- **CPR** × 2 mins (5 cycles)
- **Defibrillate** (4 J/kg) every 2 minutes
  if rhythm remains shockable
- **Epinephrine** q 3–5 minutes
  IV/IO: 0.01 mg/kg (0.1 mL/kg,
  1:10,000 soln), max 1 mg/dose
  ETT: 0.1 mg/kg (0.1 mL/kg, 1:1000 soln)
- **Antiarrhythmics:**
  Amiodarone 5 mg/kg IV/IO (max
  300 mg/dose)
  Magnesium 25–50 mg/kg IV for
  torsades de pointes (max 2 gm/dose)
- **Treat reversible causes:** (see PEA
  below)

BRADYCARDIA (CV UNSTABLE)

- **CPR** if HR < 60 and poor perfusion despite
  adequate oxygenation and ventilation
- **Epinephrine** q 3–5 minutes
  IV/IO: 0.01 mg/kg (0.1 mL/kg, 1:10,000 soln);
  max 1 mg/dose
  ETT: 0.1 mg/kg (0.1 mL/kg, 1:1000 soln)
- **Atropine** for ↑ vagal tone or 1° AV block
  IV/IO: 0.02 mg/kg (min: 0.1 mg/dose,
  max: 1 mg/dose)
  ETT: 0.03 mg/kg/dose
- **Identify and treat reversible causes**
  (see PEA below)
- **Consider vasoactive drips**
  Epinephrine 0.1–1 mcg/kg/min, *or*
  Dopamine 2–20 mcg/kg/min

PEA/ASYSTOLE

- **Continue CPR**
- **Epinephrine** q 3–5 minutes IV/IO: 0.01
  mg/kg (0.1 mL/kg, 1:10,000 soln), max
  1 mg/dose
  ETT: 0.1 mg/kg (0.1 mL/kg,
  1:1000 soln)
- **Identify and treat reversible
  causes:**
  Hypoxemia, tension pneumothorax,
  pericardial tamponade, pulmonary
  embolus, hypothermia,
  hypovolemia, hypo/hyperkalemia,
  acidosis, hypoglycemia, toxins

TACHYCARDIA

Wide QRS (> 0.09 sec)
- **Cardioversion** (if unstable): Initial:
  0.5–1 J/kg, repeat: up to 2 J/kg
- **Medications:**
  Amiodarone 5 mg/kg over 20–60 min,
  or
  Procainamide 15 mg/kg over 30 min,
  or
  Adenosine (for monomorphic QRS
  with regular rhythm). Dose below
Narrow QRS (< 0.09 sec = SVT)
- **Adenosine:** IV rapid push (1–3 sec)
  0.05–0.1 mg/kg (max 12 mg/dose)
  Repeat q 1–2 min PRN
- **Cardioversion** if unstable
- **Antiarrhythmics** post-conversion

Figure 19.1 Pediatric Basic Life Support Algorithm

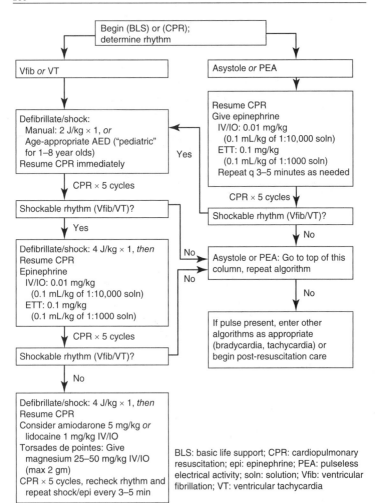

Figure 19.2 Pulseless Arrest Algorithm

Data from: *Pediatric Crit Care Med* 2012;13(1) Suppl.

EMERGENCY DRUG SHEETS

EMERGENCY DRUG SHEET: 3 kg

Table 19.1A   Resuscitation Equipment: 3 kg

Item	Size	Other
Endotracheal tube (ETT) (16 + age (yr) / 4)	3–3.5 Uncuffed	O_2 mask: Newborn
		Oral airway: Infant
Laryngoscope blade	1 Miller	Foley: 5- or 6-Fr
		Self-inflating bag: Infant (250 mL)
ETT depth of insertion (cm) (3× internal diameter of tube)	9–10 cm	Femoral line: 4-Fr
		Chest tube: 10- to 12-Fr

Table 19.1B   Rapid-Sequence Intubation: 3 kg

	Dosing	Dose	Concentration	Volume
Premedication				
Atropine*	0.02 mg/kg[†]	0.1 mg	0.1 mg/mL	1 mL
Lidocaine	1–2 mg/kg	3–6 mg	20 mg/mL	0.15–0.3 mL
Sedation				
Midazolam	0.05–0.1 mg/kg	0.15–0.3 mg	1 mg/mL	0.15–0.3 mL
Etomidate	0.2–0.3 mg/kg	0.6–0.9 mg	2 mg/mL	0.3–0.45 mL
Ketamine#	1–2 mg/kg	3–6 mg	50 mg/mL	0.06–0.12 mL
Paralysis				
Rocuronium	0.6–1.2 mg/kg	1.8–3.6 mg	10 mg/mL	0.18–0.36 mL
Succinylcholine§	1–2 mg/kg	3–6 mg	20 mg/mL	0.15–0.3 mL

Contraindication: *Glaucoma or thyrotoxicosis; #elevated intracranial pressure; §burn or crush injury, glaucoma, neuromuscular disease, or malignant hyperthermia.
[†]Minimum dose 0.1 mg

Table 19.1C   Cardiopulmonary Resuscitation Medications: 3 kg

Drug	Dosing	Dose	Concentration	Volume
Epinephrine 1:10,000	0.01 mg/kg	0.03 mg	0.1 mg/mL	0.3 mL
Epinephrine 1:1000	0.1 mg/kg	0.3 mg	1 mg/mL	0.3 mL
Atropine	0.02 mg/kg	0.1 mg	0.1 mg/mL	1 mL

(Continued)

Table 19.1C   Cardiopulmonary Resuscitation Medications: 3 kg *(Continued)*

Drug	Dosing	Dose	Concentration	Volume
Calcium chloride 10%	20 mg/kg	60 mg	100 mg/mL	0.6 mL
Sodium bicarbonate 4.2%	1 mEq/kg	3 mEq	0.5 mEq/mL	6 mL

Table 19.1D   Defibrillation and Cardioversion: 3 kg

Defibrillation	2 J/kg, then 4 J/kg	6 J, then 10 J
Cardioversion	½ J/kg, then 1 J/kg (max 2 J/kg)	1 J, then 3 J (max 6 J)

Table 19.1E   Other Emergency Medications: 3 kg

Drug	Dosing	Dose	Concentration	Volume
Adenosine	0.1–0.2 mg/kg	0.3–0.6 mg	3 mg/mL	0.1–0.2 mL
Amiodarone	5 mg/kg/dose	15 mg	50 mg/mL	0.3 mL
Benadryl	1.25 mg/kg	4 mg	50 mg/mL	0.08 mL
Glucose ($D_{10}W$)	0.5–1 g/kg	1.5–3 g	0.5 g/mL	6 mL (2 mL/kg)
Flumazenil	0.01 mg/kg	0.03 mg	0.1 mg/mL	0.3 mL
Hydrocortisone	1–5 mg/kg	3–15 mg	50 mg/mL	0.06–0.3 mL
Lidocaine	1 mg/kg	3 mg	20 mg/mL	0.15 mL/dose
Lorazepam	0.05–0.1 mg/kg	0.15–0.3 mg	2 mg/mL	0.08–0.15 mL
Magnesium	25–50 mg/kg/dose	75–150 mg	500 mg/mL	0.15–0.3 mL
Naloxone	0.1 mg/kg	0.3 mg	1 mg/mL	0.3 mL

EMERGENCY DRUG QUICK REFERENCE: 4 kg

Table 19.2A   Resuscitation Equipment: 4 kg

Item	Size	Other
Endotracheal tube (ETT) (16 + age (yr) / 4)	3.5 Uncuffed	O_2 mask: Newborn
		Oral airway: Infant/small
Laryngoscope blade	1 Miller	Foley: 5- or 6-Fr
		Self-inflating bag: Infant (250 mL)
ETT depth of insertion (cm) (3 × internal diameter of tube)	~10 cm	Femoral line: 4-Fr
		Chest tube: 10- to 12-Fr

Table 19.2B   Rapid-Sequence Intubation: 4 kg

	Dosing	Dose	Concentration	Volume
Premedication				
Atropine*	0.02 mg/kg†	0.1 mg	0.1 mg/mL	1 mL
Lidocaine	1–2 mg/kg	4–8 mg	20 mg/mL	0.2–0.4 mL
Sedation				
Midazolam	0.05–0.1 mg/kg	0.2–0.4 mg	1 mg/mL	0.2–0.4 mL
Etomidate	0.2–0.3 mg/kg	0.8–1.2 mg	2 mg/mL	0.4–0.6 mL
Ketamine#	1–2 mg/kg	4–8 mg	50 mg/mL	0.08–0.16 mL
Paralysis				
Rocuronium	0.6–1.2 mg/kg	2.4–4.8 mg	10 mg/mL	0.24–0.48 mL
Succinylcholine§	1–2 mg/kg	4–8 mg	20 mg/mL	0.2–0.4 mL

Contraindications: *Glaucoma, thyrotoxicosis; #elevated intracranial pressure; §burn or crush injury, glaucoma, neuromuscular disease, malignant hyperthermia
†Minimum dose: 0.1 mg

Table 19.2C   Cardiopulmonary Resuscitation Medications: 4 kg

Drug	Dosing	Dose	Concentration	Volume
Epinephrine 1:10,000	0.01 mg/kg	0.04 mg	0.1 mg/mL	0.4 mL
Epinephrine 1:1000	0.1 mg/kg	0.4 mg	1 mg/mL	0.4 mL
Atropine	0.02 mg/kg	0.1 mg	0.1 mg/mL	1 mL
Calcium chloride 10%	20 mg/kg	80 mg	100 mg/mL	0.8 mL
Sodium bicarbonate 4.2%	1 mEq/kg	4 mEq	0.5 mEq/mL	8 mL

Table 19.2D   Defibrillation and Cardioversion: 4 kg

Defibrillation	8 J (2 J/kg), then 20 J (4 J/kg); max 40 J (10 J/kg)
Cardioversion	2 J (½ J/kg), then 4 J (1 J/kg); max 8 J (2 J/kg)

Table 19.2E   Other Emergency Medications: 4 kg

Drug	Dosing	Dose	Concentration	Volume
Adenosine	0.1–0.2 mg/kg	0.4–0.8 mg	3 mg/mL	0.13–0.27 mL
Amiodarone	5 mg/kg/dose	20 mg	50 mg/mL	0.4 mL
Benadryl	1.25 mg/kg	5 mg	50 mg/mL	0.1 mL
Glucose (D$_{150}$W)	0.2 g/kg	0.8 gm	0.1 g/mL	8 mL (2 mL/kg)
Flumazenil	0.01 mg/kg	0.04 mg	0.1 mg/mL	0.4 mL

(Continued)

Table 19.2E   Other Emergency Medications: 4 kg *(Continued)*

Drug	Dosing	Dose	Concentration	Volume
Hydrocortisone	1–5 mg/kg	4–20 mg	50 mg/mL	0.08–0.4 mL
Lidocaine	1 mg/kg	4 mg	20 mg/mL	0.2 mL/dose
Lorazepam	0.05–0.1 mg/kg	0.2–0.4 mg	2 mg/mL	0.1–0.2 mL
Magnesium	25–50 mg/kg/dose	100–200 mg	500 mg/mL	0.2–0.4 mL
Naloxone	0.1 mg/kg	0.4 mg	1 mg/mL	0.4 mL

EMERGENCY DRUG QUICK REFERENCE: 5 kg

Table 19.3A   Resuscitation Equipment: 5 kg

Item	Size	Other
Endotracheal tube (ETT) (16 + age (yr) / 4)	3.5 Uncuffed	O$_2$ mask: Newborn
		Oral airway: Infant/small
Laryngoscope blade	1 Miller	Foley: 5- or 6-Fr
		Self-inflating bag: Infant (250 mL)
ETT depth of insertion (cm) (3 × internal diameter of tube)	~10 cm	Femoral line: 4-Fr
		Chest tube: 10- to 12-Fr

Table 19.3B   Rapid-Sequence Intubation: 5 kg

	Dosing	Dose	Concentration	Volume
Premedication				
Atropine*	0.02 mg/kg†	0.1 mg	0.1 mg/mL	1 mL
Lidocaine	1–2 mg/kg	5–10 mg	20 mg/mL	0.25–0.5 mL
Sedation				
Midazolam	0.05–0.1 mg/kg	0.25–0.5 mg	1 mg/mL	0.25–0.5 mL
Etomidate	0.2–0.3 mg/kg	1–1.5 mg	2 mg/mL	0.5–0.75 mL
Ketamine#	1–2 mg/kg	5–10 mg	50 mg/mL	0.1–0.2 mL
Paralysis				
Rocuronium	0.6–1.2 mg/kg	3–6 mg	10 mg/mL	0.3–0.6 mL
Succinylcholine§	1–2 mg/kg	5–10 mg	20 mg/mL	0.25–0.5 mL

Contraindications: *Glaucoma, thyrotoxicosis; #elevated intracranial pressure; §burn or crush injury, glaucoma, neuromuscular disease, malignant hyperthermia
†Minimum dose: 0.1 mg

Table 19.3C   Cardiopulmonary Resuscitation Medications: 5 kg

Drug	Dosing	Dose	Concentration	Volume
Epinephrine 1:10,000	0.01 mg/kg	0.05 mg	0.1 mg/mL	0.5 mL
Epinephrine 1:1000	0.1 mg/kg	0.5 mg	1 mg/mL	0.5 mL
Atropine	0.02 mg/kg	0.1 mg	0.1 mg/mL	1 mL
Calcium chloride 10%	20 mg/kg	100 mg	100 mg/mL	1 mL
Sodium bicarbonate 4.2%	1 mEq/kg	5 mEq	0.5 mEq/mL	10 mL

Table 19.3D   Defibrillation and Cardioversion: 5 kg

Defibrillation	10 J (2 J/kg), then 20 J (4 J/kg); max 50 J (10 J/kg)
Cardioversion	2 J (½ J/kg), then 5 J (1 J/kg); max 10 J (max 2 J/kg)

Table 19.3E   Other Emergency Medications: 5 kg

Drug	Dosing	Dose	Concentration	Volume
Adenosine	0.1–0.2 mg/kg	0.5–1 mg	3 mg/mL	0.17–0.33 mL
Amiodarone	5 mg/kg/dose	25 mg	50 mg/mL	0.5 mL rapid IV bolus
Benadryl	1.25 mg/kg	6.25 mg	50 mg/mL	0.13 mL
Glucose (D$_{50}$W)	0.5–1 g/kg	2.5–5 g	0.5 g/mL	Dilute 5–10 mL 1:1 with sterile water
Flumazenil	0.01 mg/kg	0.05 mg	0.1 mg/mL	0.5 mL
Hydrocortisone	1–5 mg/kg	5–25 mg	50 mg/mL	0.1–0.5 mL
Lidocaine	1 mg/kg	5 mg	20 mg/mL	0.25 mL/dose
Lorazepam	0.05–0.1 mg/kg	0.25–0.5 mg	2 mg/mL	0.13–0.25 mL
Magnesium	25–50 mg/kg/dose	125–250 mg	500 mg/mL	0.25–0.5 mL
Naloxone	0.1 mg/kg	0.5 mg	1 mg/mL	0.5 mL

EMERGENCY DRUG QUICK REFERENCE: 6 kg

Table 19.4A   Resuscitation Equipment: 6 kg

Item	Size	Other
Endotracheal tube (ETT) (16 + age (yr) / 4)	3.5–4 Uncuffed	O$_2$ mask: Newborn
		Oral airway: Small
Laryngoscope blade	1 Miller	Foley: 6-Fr
		Self-inflating bag: Infant (250 mL)
ETT depth of insertion (cm) (3 × internal diameter of tube)	10–12 cm	Femoral line: 4-Fr
		Chest tube: 10- to 14-Fr

Table 19.4B   Rapid-Sequence Intubation (RSI) (see section on RSI for details): 6 kg

	Dosing	Dose	Concentration	Volume
Premedication				
Atropine*	0.02 mg/kg†	0.1–0.12 mg	0.1 mg/mL	1–1.2 mL
Lidocaine	1–2 mg/kg	6–12 mg	20 mg/mL	0.3–0.6 mL
Sedation				
Midazolam	0.05–0.1 mg/kg	0.3–0.6 mg	1 mg/mL	0.3–0.6 mL
Etomidate	0.2–0.3 mg/kg	1.2–1.8 mg	2 mg/mL	0.6–0.9 mL
Ketamine#	1–2 mg/kg	6–12 mg	50 mg/mL	0.12–0.24 mL

(Continued)

Table 19.4B   Rapid-Sequence Intubation (RSI) (see section on RSI for details): 6 kg *(Continued)*

	Dosing	Dose	Concentration	Volume
Paralysis				
Rocuronium	0.6–1.2 mg/kg	3.6–7.2 mg	10 mg/mL	0.36–0.72 mL
Succinylcholine§	1–2 mg/kg	6–12 mg	20 mg/mL	0.3–0.6 mL

Contraindications: *Glaucoma, thyrotoxicosis; #elevated intracranial pressure; $burn or crush injury, glaucoma, neuromuscular disease, §malignant hyperthermia
†Minimum dose: 0.1 mg

Table 19.4C   Cardiopulmonary Resuscitation Medications: 6 kg

Drug	Dosing	Dose	Concentration	Volume
Epinephrine 1:10,000	0.01 mg/kg	0.06 mg	0.1 mg/mL	0.6 mL
Epinephrine 1:1000	0.1 mg/kg	0.6 mg	1 mg/mL	0.6 mL
Atropine	0.02 mg/kg	0.12 mg	0.1 mg/mL	1.2 mL
Calcium chloride 10%	20 mg/kg	120 mg	100 mg/mL	1.2 mL
Sodium bicarbonate 8.4%	1 mEq/kg	6 mEq	1 mEq/mL	6 mL

Table 19.4D   Defibrillation and Cardioversion: 6 kg

Defibrillation	10 J (2 J/kg), then 20 J (4 J/kg); max 60 J (10 J/kg)
Cardioversion	3 J (½ J/kg), then 6 J (1 J/kg); max 12 J (2 J/kg)

Table 19.4E   Other Emergency Medications: 6 kg

Drug	Dosing	Dose	Concentration	Volume
Adenosine	0.1–0.2 mg/kg	0.6–1.2 mg	3 mg/mL	0.2–0.4 mL rapid IV
Amiodarone	5 mg/kg/dose	30 mg	50 mg/mL	0.6 mL
Benadryl	1.25 mg/kg	7.5 mg	50 mg/mL	0.15 mL
Glucose ($D_{50}W$)	0.5–1 g/kg	3–6 g	0.5 g/mL	Dilute 6–12 mL 1:1 with sterile water
Flumazenil	0.01 mg/kg	0.06 mg	0.1 mg/mL	0.6 mL
Hydrocortisone	1–5 mg/kg	6–30 mg	50 mg/mL	0.12–0.6 mL
Lidocaine	1 mg/kg	6 mg	20 mg/mL	0.3 mL/dose
Lorazepam	0.05–0.1 mg/kg	0.3–0.6 mg	2 mg/mL	0.15–0.3 mL
Magnesium	25–50 mg/kg/dose	150–300 mg	500 mg/mL	0.3–0.6 mL
Naloxone	0.1 mg/kg	0.6 mg	1 mg/mL	0.6 mL

EMERGENCY DRUG QUICK REFERENCE: 7 kg

Table 19.5A   Resuscitation Equipment: 7 kg

Item	Size	Other
Endotracheal tube (ETT) (16 + age (yr) / 4)	3.5–4 Uncuffed	O₂ mask: Small
		Oral airway: Small
Laryngoscope blade	1 Miller	Foley: 6-Fr
		Self-inflating bag: Infant or child
ETT depth of insertion (cm) (3 × internal diameter of tube)	10–12 cm	Femoral line: 4-Fr
		Chest tube: 12- to 14-Fr

Table 19.5B   Rapid-Sequence Intubation (RSI) (see section on RSI for details): 7 kg

	Dosing	Dose	Concentration	Volume
Premedication				
Atropine*	0.02 mg/kg†	0.14 mg	0.1 mg/mL	1.4 mL
Lidocaine	1–2 mg/kg	7–14 mg	20 mg/mL	0.35–0.7 mL
Sedation				
Midazolam	0.05–0.1 mg/kg	0.35–0.7 mg	1 mg/mL	0.35–0.7 mL
Etomidate	0.2–0.3 mg/kg	1.4–2.1 mg	2 mg/mL	0.7–1.5 mL
Ketamine#	1–2 mg/kg	7–14 mg	50 mg/mL	0.14–0.28 mL
Paralysis				
Rocuronium	0.6–1.2 mg/kg	4.2–8.4 mg	10 mg/mL	0.42–0.84 mL
Succinylcholine§	1–2 mg/kg	7–14 mg	20 mg/mL	0.35–0.7 mL

Contraindications: *Glaucoma, thyrotoxicosis; #elevated intracranial pressure; §burn or crush injury, glaucoma, neuromuscular disease, malignant hyperthermia

†Minimum dose: 0.1 mg

Table 19.5C   Cardiopulmonary Resuscitation Medications: 7 kg

Drug	Dosing	Dose	Concentration	Volume
Epinephrine 1:10,000	0.01 mg/kg	0.07 mg	0.1 mg/mL	0.7 mL
Epinephrine 1:1000	0.1 mg/kg	0.7 mg	1 mg/mL	0.7 mL
Atropine	0.02 mg/kg	0.14 mg	0.1 mg/mL	1.4 mL
Calcium chloride 10%	20 mg/kg	140 mg	100 mg/mL	1.4 mL
Sodium bicarbonate 8.4%	1 mEq/kg	7 mEq	1 mEq/mL	7 mL

Table 19.5D   Defibrillation and Cardioversion: 7 kg

Defibrillation	10 J (2 J/kg), then 30 J (4 J/kg); max 70 J (10 J/kg)
Cardioversion	3 J (½ J/kg), then 7 J (1 J/kg); max 14 J (max 2 J/kg)

Table 19.5E   Other Emergency Medications: 7 kg

Drug	Dosing	Dose	Concentration	Volume
Adenosine	0.1–0.2 mg/kg	0.7–1.4 mg	3 mg/mL	0.23–0.47 mL
Amiodarone	5 mg/kg/dose	35 mg	50 mg/mL	0.7 mL
Benadryl	1.25 mg/kg	8.75 mg	50 mg/mL	0.18 mL
Glucose ($D_{50}W$)	0.5–1 g/kg	3.5–7 g	0.5 g/mL	Dilute 7–14 mL 1:1 with sterile water
Flumazenil	0.01 mg/kg	0.07 mg	0.1 mg/mL	0.7 mL
Hydrocortisone	1–5 mg/kg	7–35 mg	50 mg/mL	0.14–0.7 mL
Lidocaine	1 mg/kg	7 mg	20 mg/mL	0.35 mL/dose
Lorazepam	0.05–0.1 mg/kg	0.35–0.7 mg	2 mg/mL	0.18–0.35 mL
Magnesium	25–50 mg/kg/dose	175–350 mg	500 mg/mL	0.35–0.7 mL
Naloxone	0.1 mg/kg	0.7 mg	1 mg/mL	0.7 mL

EMERGENCY DRUG QUICK REFERENCE: 8 kg

Table 19.6A   Resuscitation Equipment: 8 kg

Item	Size	Other
Endotracheal tube (ETT) (16 + age (yr) / 4)	4 Uncuffed	O_2 mask: Child
		Oral airway: Small
Laryngoscope blade	1 Miller	Foley: 6-Fr
		Self-inflating bag: Child
ETT depth of insertion (cm) (3 × internal diameter of tube)	12 cm	Femoral line: 4- or 5-Fr
		Chest tube: 12- to 16-Fr

Table 19.6B   Rapid-Sequence Intubation (RSI) (see section on RSI for details): 8 kg

	Dosing	Dose	Concentration	Volume
Premedication				
Atropine*	0.01–0.02 mg/kg[†]	0.1–0.16 mg	0.1 mg/mL	1–1.6 mL
Lidocaine	1–2 mg/kg	8–16 mg	20 mg/mL	0.4–0.8 mL
Sedation				
Midazolam	0.05–0.1 mg/kg	0.4–0.8 mg	1 mg/mL	0.4–0.8 mL
Etomidate	0.2–0.3 mg/kg	1.6–2.4 mg	2 mg/mL	0.8–1.2 mL
Ketamine#	1–2 mg/kg	8–16 mg	50 mg/mL	0.16–0.32 mL
Paralysis				
Rocuronium	0.6–1.2 mg/kg	4.8–9.6 mg	10 mg/mL	0.48–0.96 mL
Succinylcholine§	1–2 mg/kg	8–16 mg	20 mg/mL	0.4–0.8 mL

Contraindications: *Glaucoma, thyrotoxicosis; #elevated intracranial pressure; §burn or crush injury, glaucoma, neuromuscular disease, malignant hyperthermia
†Minimum dose: 0.1 mg

Table 19.6C   Cardiopulmonary Resuscitation Medications: 8 kg

Drug	Dosing	Dose	Concentration	Volume
Epinephrine 1:10,000	0.01 mg/kg	0.08 mg	0.1 mg/mL	0.8 mL
Epinephrine 1:1000	0.1 mg/kg	0.8 mg	1 mg/mL	0.8 mL
Atropine	0.02 mg/kg	0.16 mg	0.1 mg/mL	1.6 mL
Calcium chloride 10%	20 mg/kg	160 mg	100 mg/mL	1.6 mL
Sodium bicarbonate 8.4%	1 mEq/kg	8 mEq	1 mEq/mL	8 mL

Table 19.6D   Defibrillation and Cardioversion: 8 kg

Defibrillation	20 J (2 J/kg), then 30 J (4 J/kg); max 80 J (10 J/kg)
Cardioversion	4 J (½ J/kg), then 8 J (1 J/kg); max 16 J (2 J/kg)

Table 19.6E   Other Emergency Medications: 8 kg

Drug	Dosing	Dose	Concentration	Volume
Adenosine	0.1–0.2 mg/kg	0.8–1.6 mg	3 mg/mL	0.27–0.53 mL
Amiodarone	5 mg/kg/dose	40 mg	50 mg/mL	0.8 mL
Benadryl	1.25 mg/kg	10 mg	50 mg/mL	0.2 mL
Glucose ($D_{50}W$)	0.5–1 g/kg	4–8 g	0.5 g/mL	Dilute 8–16 mL 1:1 with sterile water
Flumazenil	0.01 mg/kg	0.08 mg	0.1 mg/mL	0.8 mL
Hydrocortisone	1–5 mg/kg	8–40 mg	50 mg/mL	0.16–0.8 mL
Lidocaine	1 mg/kg	8 mg	20 mg/mL	0.4 mL/dose
Lorazepam	0.05–0.1 mg/kg	0.4–0.8 mg	2 mg/mL	0.2–0.4 mL
Magnesium	25–50 mg/kg/dose	200–400 mg	500 mg/mL	0.4–0.8 mL
Naloxone	0.1 mg/kg	0.8 mg	1 mg/mL	0.8 mL

EMERGENCY DRUG QUICK REFERENCE: 9 kg

Table 19.7A   Resuscitation Equipment: 9 kg

Item	Size	Other
Endotracheal tube (ETT) (16 + age (yr) / 4)	4 Uncuffed	O₂ mask: Child
		Oral airway: Small
Laryngoscope blade	1 Miller	Foley: 6-Fr
		Self-inflating bag: Child
ETT depth of insertion (cm) (3 × internal diameter of tube)	12 cm	Femoral line: 4- or 5-Fr
		Chest tube: 12- to 18-Fr

Table 19.7B   Rapid-Sequence Intubation (RSI) (see section on RSI for details): 9 kg

	Dosing	Dose	Concentration	Volume
Premedication				
Atropine*	0.01–0.02 mg/kg[†]	0.1–0.18 mg	0.1 mg/mL	1–1.8 mL
Lidocaine	1–2 mg/kg	9–18 mg	20 mg/mL	0.45–0.9 mL
Sedation				
Midazolam	0.05–0.1 mg/kg	0.45–0.9 mg	1 mg/mL	0.45–0.8 mL
Etomidate	0.2–0.3 mg/kg	1.8–2.6 mg	2 mg/mL	0.9–1.35 mL
Ketamine#	1–2 mg/kg	9–18 mg	50 mg/mL	0.18–0.36 mL
Paralysis				
Rocuronium	0.6–1.2 mg/kg	5.4–10.8 mg	10 mg/mL	0.54–1.08 mL
Succinylcholine§	1–2 mg/kg	9–18 mg	20 mg/mL	0.45–0.9 mL

Contraindications: *Glaucoma, thyrotoxicosis; #elevated intracranial pressure; §burn or crush injury, glaucoma, neuromuscular disease, malignant hyperthermia
[†]Minimum dose: 0.1 mg

Table 19.7C   Cardiopulmonary Resuscitation Medications: 9 kg

Drug	Dosing	Dose	Concentration	Volume
Epinephrine 1:10,000	0.01 mg/kg	0.09 mg	0.1 mg/mL	0.9 mL
Epinephrine 1:1000	0.1 mg/kg	0.9 mg	1 mg/mL	0.9 mL
Atropine	0.02 mg/kg	0.18 mg	0.1 mg/mL	1.8 mL
Calcium chloride 10%	20 mg/kg	180 mg	100 mg/mL	1.8 mL
Sodium bicarbonate 8.4%	1 mEq/kg	9 mEq	1 mEq/mL	9 mL

Table 19.7D   Defibrillation and Cardioversion: 9 kg

Defibrillation	20 J (2 J/kg), then 40 J (4 J/kg); max 90 J (10 J/kg)
Cardioversion	4 J (½ J/kg), then 9 J (1 J/kg); max 18 J (2 J/kg)

Table 19.7E   Other Emergency Medications: 9 kg

Drug	Dosing	Dose	Concentration	Volume
Adenosine	0.1–0.2 mg/kg	0.9–1.8 mg	3 mg/mL	0.3–0.6 mL
Amiodarone	5 mg/kg/dose	45 mg	50 mg/mL	0.9 mL
Benadryl	1.25 mg/kg	11.25 mg	50 mg/mL	0.23 mL
Glucose (D$_{50}$W)	0.5–1 g/kg	4–8 g	0.5 g/mL	Dilute 9–18 mL 1:1 with sterile water
Flumazenil	0.01 mg/kg	0.09 mg	0.1 mg/mL	0.9 mL
Hydrocortisone	1–5 mg/kg	9–45 mg	50 mg/mL	0.18–0.9 mL
Lidocaine	1 mg/kg	9 mg	20 mg/mL	0.45 mL/dose

(Continued)

Table 19.7E   Other Emergency Medications: 9 kg *(Continued)*

Drug	Dosing	Dose	Concentration	Volume
Lorazepam	0.05–0.1 mg/kg	0.45–0.9 mg	2 mg/mL	0.23–0.5 mL
Magnesium	25–50 mg/kg/dose	225–450 mg	500 mg/mL	0.45–0.9 mL
Naloxone	0.1 mg/kg	0.9 mg	1 mg/mL	0.9 mL

EMERGENCY DRUG QUICK REFERENCE: 10 kg

Table 19.8A   Resuscitation Equipment: 10 kg

Item	Size	Other
Endotracheal tube (ETT) (16 + age (yr) / 4)	4–4.5 Uncuffed	O$_2$ mask: Child
		Oral airway: Small
Laryngoscope blade	1–2 Miller	Foley: 6- to 8-Fr
		Self-inflating bag: Child
ETT depth of insertion (cm) (3 × internal diameter of tube)	12–14 cm	Femoral line: 4- or 5-Fr
		Chest tube: 16- to 20-Fr

Table 19.8B   Rapid-Sequence Intubation (RSI) (see section on RSI for details): 10 kg

	Dosing	Dose	Concentration	Volume
Premedication				
Atropine*	0.01–0.02 mg/kg†	0.1–0.2 mg	0.1 mg/mL	1–2 mL
Lidocaine	1–2 mg/kg	10–20 mg	20 mg/mL	0.5–1 mL
Sedation				
Midazolam	0.05–0.1 mg/kg	0.5–1 mg	1 mg/mL	0.5–1 mL
Etomidate	0.2–0.3 mg/kg	1.8–2.6 mg	2 mg/mL	1–1.5 mL
Ketamine#	1–2 mg/kg	10–20 mg	50 mg/mL	0.2–0.4 mL
Paralysis				
Rocuronium	0.6–1.2 mg/kg	6–12 mg	10 mg/mL	0.6–1.2 mL
Succinylcholine§	1–2 mg/kg	10–20 mg	20 mg/mL	0.5–1 mL

Contraindications: *Glaucoma, thyrotoxicosis; #elevated intracranial pressure; §burn or crush injury, glaucoma, neuromuscular disease, malignant hyperthermia

†Minimum dose: 0.1 mg

Table 19.8C   Cardiopulmonary Resuscitation Medications: 10 kg

Drug	Dosing	Dose	Concentration	Volume
Epinephrine 1:10,000	0.01 mg/kg	0.1 mg	0.1 mg/mL	1 mL
Epinephrine 1:1000	0.1 mg/kg	1 mg	1 mg/mL	1 mL
Atropine	0.02 mg/kg	0.2 mg	0.1 mg/mL	2 mL
Calcium chloride 10%	20 mg/kg	200 mg	100 mg/mL	2 mL
Sodium bicarbonate 8.4%	1 mEq/kg	10 mEq	1 mEq/mL	10 mL

Table 19.8D   Defibrillation and Cardioversion: 10 kg

Defibrillation	20 J (2 J/kg), then 40 J (4 J/kg); max 100 J (10 J/kg)
Cardioversion	5 J (½ J/kg), then 10 J (1 J/kg); max 20 J (2 J/kg)

Table 19.8E   Other Emergency Medications: 10 kg

Drug	Dosing	Dose	Concentration	Volume
Adenosine	0.1–0.2 mg/kg	1–2 mg	3 mg/mL	0.33–0.67 mL
Amiodarone	5 mg/kg/dose	50 mg	50 mg/mL	1 mL
Benadryl	1.25 mg/kg	12.5 mg	50 mg/mL	0.25 mL
Glucose ($D_{50}W$)	0.5–1 g/kg	5–10 g	0.5 g/mL	Dilute 10–20 mL 1:1 with sterile water
Flumazenil	0.01 mg/kg	0.1 mg	0.1 mg/mL	1 mL
Hydrocortisone	1–5 mg/kg	10–50 mg	50 mg/mL	0.2–1 mL
Lidocaine	1 mg/kg	10 mg	20 mg/mL	0.5 mL/dose
Lorazepam	0.05–0.1 mg/kg	0.5–1 mg	2 mg/mL	0.25–0.5 mL
Magnesium	25–50 mg/kg/dose	250–500 mg	500 mg/mL	0.5–1 mL
Naloxone	0.1 mg/kg	1 mg	1 mg/mL	1 mL

EMERGENCY DRUG QUICK REFERENCE: 12 kg

Table 19.9A   Resuscitation Equipment: 12 kg

Item	Size	Other
Endotracheal tube (ETT) (16 + age (yr) / 4)	4.0–4.5 Uncuffed	O_2 mask: Child
		Oral airway: Small
Laryngoscope blade	1–2 Miller or Mac	Foley: 6- to 8-Fr
		Self-inflating bag: Child
ETT depth of insertion (cm) (3 × internal diameter of tube)	12–14 cm	Femoral line: 4- or 5-Fr
		Chest tube: 16- to 20-Fr

Table 19.9B   Rapid-Sequence Intubation (RSI (see section on RSI for details): 12 kg

	Dosing	Dose	Concentration	Volume
Premedication				
Atropine*	0.01–0.02 mg/kg[†]	0.12–0.24 mg	0.1 mg/mL	1.2–2.4 mL
Lidocaine	1–2 mg/kg	12–24 mg	20 mg/mL	0.6–1.2 mL
Sedation				
Midazolam	0.05–0.1 mg/kg	0.6–1.2 mg	1 mg/mL	0.6–1.2 mL
Etomidate	0.2–0.3 mg/kg	2.4–3.6 mg	2 mg/mL	1.2–1.8 mL

(Continued)

Table 19.9B Rapid-Sequence Intubation (RSI) (see section on RSI for details): 12 kg *(Continued)*

	Dosing	Dose	Concentration	Volume
Sedation				
Ketamine#	1–2 mg/kg	12–24 mg	50 mg/mL	0.24–0.48 mL
Paralysis				
Rocuronium	0.6–1.2 mg/kg	7.2–14.4 mg	10 mg/mL	0.72–1.44 mL
Succinylcholine§	1–2 mg/kg	12–24 mg	20 mg/mL	0.6–1.2 mL

Contraindications: *Glaucoma, thyrotoxicosis; #elevated intracranial pressure; ‡burn or crush injury, §glaucoma, neuromuscular disease, malignant hyperthermia
†Minimum dose: 0.1 mg

Table 19.9C Cardiopulmonary Resuscitation Medications: 12 kg

Drug	Dosing	Dose	Concentration	Volume
Epinephrine 1:10,000	0.01 mg/kg	0.12 mg	0.1 mg/mL	1.2 mL
Epinephrine 1:1000	0.1 mg/kg	1.2 mg	1 mg/mL	1.2 mL
Atropine	0.02 mg/kg	0.24 mg	0.1 mg/mL	2.4 mL
Calcium chloride 10%	20 mg/kg	240 mg	100 mg/mL	2.4 mL
Sodium bicarbonate 8.4%	1 mEq/kg	12 mEq	1 mEq/mL	12 mL

Table 19.9D Defibrillation and Cardioversion: 12 kg

Defibrillation	20 J (2 J/kg), then 50 J (4 J/kg); max 120 J (10 J/kg)
Cardioversion	6 J (½ J/kg), then 10 J (1 J/kg); max 25 J (2 J/kg)

Table 19.9E Other Emergency Medications: 12 kg

Drug	Dosing	Dose	Concentration	Volume
Adenosine	0.1–0.2 mg/kg	1.2–2.4 mg	3 mg/mL	0.4–0.8 mL
Amiodarone	5 mg/kg/dose	60 mg	50 mg/mL	1.2 mL
Benadryl	1.25 mg/kg	15 mg	50 mg/mL	0.3 mL
Glucose ($D_{50}W$)	0.5–1 g/kg	6–12 g	0.5 g/mL	Dilute 12–24 mL 1:1 with sterile water
Flumazenil	0.01 mg/kg	0.12 mg	0.1 mg/mL	1.2 mL
Hydrocortisone	1–5 mg/kg	12–60 mg	50 mg/mL	0.24–1.2 mL
Lidocaine	1 mg/kg	12 mg	20 mg/mL	0.6 mL/dose
Lorazepam	0.05–0.1 mg/kg	0.6–1.2 mg	2 mg/mL	0.3–0.6 mL
Magnesium	25–50 mg/kg/dose	300–600 mg	500 mg/mL	0.6–1.2 mL
Naloxone	0.1 mg/kg	1.2 mg	1 mg/mL	1.2 mL

EMERGENCY DRUG QUICK REFERENCE: 14 kg

Table 19.10A Resuscitation Equipment: 14 kg

Item	Size	Other
Endotracheal tube (ETT) (16 + age (yr) / 4)	4.5–5 Uncuffed	O_2 mask: Child
		Oral airway: Small/medium
Laryngoscope blade	1–2 Miller or Mac	Foley: 8-Fr
		Self-inflating bag: Child
ETT depth of insertion (cm) (3 × internal diameter of tube)	13–15 cm	Femoral line: 4- or 5-Fr
		Chest tube: 20- to 24-Fr

Table 19.10B Rapid-Sequence Intubation (RSI) (see section on RSI for details): 14 kg

	Dosing	Dose	Concentration	Volume
Premedication				
Atropine*	0.01–0.02 mg/kg†	0.14–0.28 mg	0.1 mg/mL	1.4–2.8 mL
Lidocaine	1–2 mg/kg	14–28 mg	20 mg/mL	0.7–1.4 mL
Sedation				
Midazolam	0.05–0.1 mg/kg	0.7–1.4 mg	1 mg/mL	0.7–1.4 mL
Etomidate	0.2–0.3 mg/kg	2.8–4.2 mg	2 mg/mL	1.4–2.8 mL
Ketamine#	1–2 mg/kg	14–28 mg	50 mg/mL	0.28–0.56 mL
Paralysis				
Rocuronium	0.6–1.2 mg/kg	8.4–16.8 mg	10 mg/mL	0.84–1.68 mL
Succinylcholine§	1–2 mg/kg	14–28 mg	20 mg/mL	0.7–1.4 mL

Contraindications: *Glaucoma, thyrotoxicosis; #elevated intracranial pressure; §burn or crush injury, §glaucoma, neuromuscular disease, malignant hyperthermia
†Minimum dose: 0.1 mg

Table 19.10C Cardiopulmonary Resuscitation Medications: 14 kg

Drug	Dosing	Dose	Concentration	Volume
Epinephrine 1:10,000	0.01 mg/kg	0.14 mg	0.1 mg/mL	1.4 mL
Epinephrine 1:1000	0.1 mg/kg	1.4 mg	1 mg/mL	1.4 mL
Atropine	0.02 mg/kg	0.28 mg	0.1 mg/mL	2.8 mL
Calcium chloride 10%	20 mg/kg	280 mg	100 mg/mL	2.8 mL
Sodium bicarbonate 8.4%	1 mEq/kg	14 mEq	1 mEq/mL	14 mL

Table 19.10D Defibrillation and Cardioversion: 14 kg

Defibrillation	30 J (2 J/kg), then 50 J (4 J/kg); max 140 J (10 J/kg)
Cardioversion	7 J (½ J/kg), then 10 J (1 J/kg); max 30 J (2 J/kg)

Table 19.10E Other Emergency Medications: 14 kg

Drug	Dosing	Dose	Concentration	Volume
Adenosine	0.1–0.2 mg/kg	1.4–2.8 mg	3 mg/mL	0.47–0.93 mL
Amiodarone	5 mg/kg/dose	70 mg	50 mg/mL	1.4 mL
Benadryl	1.25 mg/kg	17.5 mg	50 mg/mL	0.35 mL
Glucose (D$_{50}$W)	0.5–1 g/kg	7–14 g	0.5 g/mL	Dilute 14–28 mL 1:1 with sterile water
Flumazenil	0.01 mg/kg	0.14 mg	0.1 mg/mL	1.4 mL
Hydrocortisone	1–5 mg/kg	14–70 mg	50 mg/mL	0.28–1.4 mL
Lidocaine	1 mg/kg	14 mg	20 mg/mL	0.7 mL/dose
Lorazepam	0.05–0.1 mg/kg	0.7–1.4 mg	2 mg/mL	0.35–0.7 mL
Magnesium	25–50 mg/kg/dose	350–700 mg	500 mg/mL	0.7–1.4 mL
Naloxone	0.1 mg/kg	1.4 mg	1 mg/mL	1.4 mL

EMERGENCY DRUG QUICK REFERENCE: 16 kg

Table 19.11A Resuscitation Equipment: 16 kg

Item	Size	Other
Endotracheal tube (ETT) (16 + age (yr) / 4)	5–5.5 Uncuffed or cuffed	O$_2$ mask: Child
		Oral airway: Medium
Laryngoscope blade	1–2 Miller or Mac	Foley: 8–10 Fr
		Self-inflating bag: Child
ETT depth of insertion (cm) (3 × internal diameter of tube)	15–17 cm	Femoral line: 4–5 Fr
		Chest tube: 20–24 Fr

Table 19.11B Rapid Sequence Intubation (RSI) (see section on RSI for details): 16 kg

	Dosing	Dose	Concentration	Volume
Premedication				
Atropine$^\alpha$	0.01–0.02 mg/kg	0.16–0.32 mg	0.1 mg/mL	1.6–3.2 mL
Lidocaine	1–2 mg/kg	16–32 mg	20 mg/mL	0.8–1.6 mL
Sedation				
Midazolam	0.05–0.1 mg/kg	0.8–1.6 mg	1 mg/mL	0.8–1.6 mL
Etomidate	0.2–0.3 mg/kg	3.2–4.8 mg	2 mg/mL	1.6–2.4 mL
Ketamine$^\beta$	1–2 mg/kg	16–32 mg	50 mg/mL	0.32–0.64 mL
Paralysis				
Rocuronium	0.6–1.2 mg/kg	9.6–19.2 mg	10 mg/mL	0.96–1.92 mL
Succinylcholine§	1–2 mg/kg	16–32 mg	20 mg/mL	0.8–1.6 mL

Contraindications: $^\alpha$Glaucoma or thyrotoxicosis; $^\beta$elevated intracranial pressure; §burn or crush injury, glaucoma, neuromuscular disease or malignant hyperthermia

$^\alpha$Minimum dose: 0.1 mg

Table 19.11C   Cardiopulmonary Resuscitation Medications: 16 kg

Drug	Dosing	Dose	Concentration	Volume
Epinephrine 1:10,000	0.01 mg/kg	0.16 mg	0.1 mg/mL	1.6 mL
Epinephrine 1:1000	0.1 mg/kg	1.6 mg	1 mg/mL	1.6 mL
Atropine	0.02 mg/kg	0.32 mg	0.1 mg/mL	3.2 mL
Calcium chloride 10%	20 mg/kg	320 mg	100 mg/mL	3.2 mL
Sodium bicarbonate 8.4%	1 mEq/kg	16 mEq	1 mEq/mL	16 mL

Table 19.11D   Defibrillation and Cardioversion: 16 kg

Defibrillation	30 J (2 J/kg), then 50 J (4 J/kg); max 160 J (10 J/kg)
Cardioversion	8 J (½ J/kg), then 20 J (1 J/kg); max 30 J (2 J/kg)

Table 19.11E   Other Emergency Medications: 16 kg

Drug	Dosing	Dose	Concentration	Volume
Adenosine	0.1–0.2 mg/kg	1.6–3.2 mg	3 mg/mL	0.53–1.07 mL
Amiodarone	5 mg/kg/dose	80 mg	50 mg/mL	1.6 mL
Benadryl	1.25 mg/kg	20 mg	50 mg/mL	0.4 mL
Glucose (D_{50}W)	0.5–1 gm/kg	8–16 gm	0.5 gm/mL	Dilute 16–32 mL 1:1 with sterile water
Flumazenil	0.01 mg/kg	0.16 mg	0.1 mg/mL	1.6 mL
Hydrocortisone	1–5 mg/kg	16–80 mg	50 mg/mL	0.32–1.6 mL
Lidocaine	1 mg/kg	16 mg	20 mg/mL	0.8 mL/dose
Lorazepam	0.05–0.1 mg/kg	0.8–1.6 mg	2 mg/mL	0.4–0.8 mL
Magnesium	25–50 mg/kg/dose	400–800 mg	500 mg/mL	0.8–1.6 mL
Naloxone	0.1 mg/kg	1.6 mg	1 mg/mL	1.6 mL

EMERGENCY DRUG QUICK REFERENCE: 18 kg

Table 19.12A   Resuscitation Equipment: 18 kg

Item	Size	Other
Endotracheal tube (ETT) (16 + age (yr) / 4)	5–5.5 Uncuffed or cuffed	O_2 mask: Child
		Oral airway: Medium
Laryngoscope blade	2	Foley: 8- to 10-Fr
		Self-inflating bag: Child
ETT depth of insertion (cm) (3 × internal diameter of tube)	15–17 cm	Femoral line: 4- or 5-Fr
		Chest tube: 24- to 28-Fr

Table 19.12B   Rapid-Sequence Intubation (RSI) (see section on RSI for details): 18 kg

	Dosing	Dose	Concentration	Volume
Premedication				
Atropine*	0.01–0.02 mg/kg†	0.18–0.36 mg	0.1 mg/mL	1.8–3.6 mL
Lidocaine	1–2 mg/kg	18–36 mg	20 mg/mL	0.9–1.8 mL
Sedation				
Midazolam	0.05–0.1 mg/kg	0.9–1.8 mg	1 mg/mL	0.9–1.8 mL
Etomidate	0.2–0.3 mg/kg	3.6–5.4 mg	2 mg/mL	1.8–2.7 mL
Ketamine#	1–2 mg/kg	18–36 mg	50 mg/mL	0.36–0.72 mL
Paralysis				
Rocuronium	0.6–1.2 mg/kg	10.8–21.6 mg	10 mg/mL	1.08–2.16 mL
Succinylcholine§	1–2 mg/kg	18–36 mg	20 mg/mL	0.9–1.8 mL

Contraindications: *Glaucoma, thyrotoxicosis; #elevated intracranial pressure; §burn or crush injury, glaucoma, neuromuscular disease, malignant hyperthermia
†Minimum dose: 0.1 mg

Table 19.12C   Cardiopulmonary Resuscitation Medications: 18 kg

Drug	Dosing	Dose	Concentration	Volume
Epinephrine 1:10,000	0.01 mg/kg	0.18 mg	0.1 mg/mL	1.8 mL
Epinephrine 1:1000	0.1 mg/kg	1.8 mg	1 mg/mL	1.8 mL
Atropine	0.02 mg/kg	0.36 mg	0.1 mg/mL	3.6 mL
Calcium chloride 10%	20 mg/kg	360 mg	100 mg/mL	3.6 mL
Sodium bicarbonate 8.4%	1 mEq/kg	18 mEq	1 mEq/mL	18 mL

Table 19.12D   Defibrillation and Cardioversion: 18 kg

Defibrillation	30 J (2 J/kg), then 50 J (4 J/kg); max 180 J (10 J/kg)
Cardioversion	9 J (½ J/kg), then 20 J (1 J/kg); max 36 J

Table 19.12E   Other Emergency Medications: 18 kg

Drug	Dosing	Dose	Concentration	Volume
Adenosine	0.1–0.2 mg/kg	1.8–3.6 mg	3 mg/mL	0.6–1.2 mL
Amiodarone	5 mg/kg/dose	90 mg	50 mg/mL	1.8 mL
Benadryl	1.25 mg/kg	22.5 mg	50 mg/mL	0.45 mL
Glucose (D$_{50}$W)	0.5–1 g/kg	9–18 g	0.5 g/mL	Dilute 18–36 mL 1:1 with sterile water
Flumazenil	0.01 mg/kg	0.18 mg	0.1 mg/mL	1.8 mL
Hydrocortisone	1–5 mg/kg	18–90 mg	50 mg/mL	0.36–1.8 mL

(Continued)

Table 19.12E   Other Emergency Medications: 18 kg *(Continued)*

Drug	Dosing	Dose	Concentration	Volume
Lidocaine	1 mg/kg	18 mg	20 mg/mL	0.9 mL/dose
Lorazepam	0.05–0.1 mg/kg	0.9–1.8 mg	2 mg/mL	0.45–0.9 mL
Magnesium	25–50 mg/kg/dose	450–900 mg	500 mg/mL	0.9–1.8 mL
Naloxone	0.1 mg/kg	1.8 mg	1 mg/mL	1.8 mL

EMERGENCY DRUG QUICK REFERENCE: 20 kg

Table 19.13A   Resuscitation Equipment: 20 kg

Item	Size	Other
Endotracheal tube (ETT) (16 + age (yr) / 4)	5.5 Uncuffed or cuffed	O$_2$ mask: Child
		Oral airway: Medium
Laryngoscope blade	2	Foley: 8- to 10-Fr
		Self-inflating bag: Child
ETT depth of insertion (cm) (3 × internal diameter of tube)	17 cm	Femoral line: 5-Fr
		Chest tube: 24- to 28-Fr

Table 19.13B   Rapid-Sequence Intubation (RSI) (see section on RSI for details): 20 kg

	Dosing	Dose	Concentration	Volume
Premedication				
Atropine*	0.01–0.02 mg/kg†	0.2–0.4 mg	0.1 mg/mL	2–4 mL
Lidocaine	1–2 mg/kg	20–40 mg	20 mg/mL	1–2 mL
Sedation				
Midazolam	0.05–0.1 mg/kg	1–2 mg	1 mg/mL	1–2 mL
Etomidate	0.2–0.3 mg/kg	4–6 mg	2 mg/mL	2–3 mL
Ketamine#	1–2 mg/kg	20–40 mg	50 mg/mL	0.4–0.8 mL
Paralysis				
Rocuronium	0.6–1.2 mg/kg	12–24 mg	10 mg/mL	1.2–2.4 mL
Succinylcholine§	1–2 mg/kg	20–40 mg	20 mg/mL	1–2 mL

Contraindications: *Glaucoma, thyrotoxicosis; #elevated intracranial pressure; §burn or crush injury, glaucoma, neuromuscular disease, malignant hyperthermia
†Minimum dose: 0.1 mg

Table 19.13C   Cardiopulmonary Resuscitation Medications: 20 kg

Drug	Dosing	Dose	Concentration	Volume
Epinephrine 1:10,000	0.01 mg/kg	0.2 mg	0.1 mg/mL	2 mL
Epinephrine 1:1000	0.1 mg/kg	2 mg	1 mg/mL	2 mL

(Continued)

Table 19.13C Cardiopulmonary Resuscitation Medications: 20 kg *(Continued)*

Drug	Dosing	Dose	Concentration	Volume
Atropine	0.02 mg/kg	0.4 mg	0.1 mg/mL	4 mL
Calcium chloride 10%	20 mg/kg	400 mg	100 mg/mL	4 mL
Sodium bicarbonate 8.4%	1 mEq/kg	2 mEq	1 mEq/mL	20 mL

Table 19.13D Defibrillation and Cardioversion: 20 kg

Defibrillation	30 J (2 J/kg), then 50 J (4 J/kg); max 200 J (10 J/kg)
Cardioversion	10 J (½ J/kg), then 20 J (1 J/kg); max 40 J (2 J/kg)

Table 19.13E Other Emergency Medications: 20 kg

Drug	Dosing	Dose	Concentration	Volume
Adenosine	0.1–0.2 mg/kg	2–4 mg	3 mg/mL	0.67–1.33 mL
Amiodarone	5 mg/kg/dose	100 mg	50 mg/mL	2 mL
Benadryl	1.25 mg/kg	25 mg	50 mg/mL	0.5 mL
Glucose ($D_{50}W$)	0.5–1 g/kg	10–20 g	0.5 g/mL	Dilute 20–40 mL 1:1 with sterile water
Flumazenil	0.01 mg/kg	0.2 mg (max)	0.1 mg/mL	2 mL
Hydrocortisone	1–5 mg/kg	20–100 mg	50 mg/mL	0.4–2 mL
Lidocaine	1 mg/kg	20 mg	20 mg/mL	1 mL/dose
Lorazepam	0.05–0.1 mg/kg	1–2 mg	2 mg/mL	0.5–1 mL
Magnesium	25–50 mg/kg/dose	500–1000 mg	500 mg/mL	1–2 mL
Naloxone	0.1 mg/kg	2 mg (max)	1 mg/mL	2 mL

EMERGENCY DRUG QUICK REFERENCE: 25 kg

Table 19.14A Resuscitation Equipment: 25 kg

Item	Size	Other
Endotracheal tube (ETT) (16 + age (yr) / 4)	5.5–6.5	O₂ mask: Child
		Oral airway: Medium
Laryngoscope blade	2	Foley: 8- to 10-Fr
		Self-inflating bag: Child
ETT depth of insertion (cm) (3 × internal diameter of tube)	17–20 cm	Femoral line: 5-Fr
		Chest tube: 24- to 28-Fr

Table 19.14B   Rapid-Sequence Intubation (RSI) (see section on RSI for details): 25 kg

	Dosing	Dose	Concentration	Volume
Premedication				
Atropine*	0.01–0.02 mg/kg[†]	0.25–0.5 mg	0.1 mg/mL	2.5–5 mL
Lidocaine	1–2 mg/kg	25–50 mg	20 mg/mL	1.25–2.5 mL
Sedation				
Midazolam	0.05–0.1 mg/kg	1.25–2.5 mg	1 mg/mL	1.25–2.5 mL
Etomidate	0.2–0.3 mg/kg	5–7.5 mg	2 mg/mL	2.5–3.75 mL
Ketamine#	1–2 mg/kg	25–50 mg	50 mg/mL	0.5–1 mL
Paralysis				
Rocuronium	0.6–1.2 mg/kg	15–30 mg	10 mg/mL	1.5–3 mL
Succinylcholine§	1–2 mg/kg	25–50 mg	20 mg/mL	1.25–2.5 mL

Contraindications: *Glaucoma, thyrotoxicosis; #elevated intracranial pressure; §burn or crush injury, glaucoma, neuromuscular disease, malignant hyperthermia
[†]Minimum dose: 0.1 mg

Table 19.14C   Cardiopulmonary Resuscitation Medications: 25 kg

Drug	Dosing	Dose	Concentration	Volume
Epinephrine 1:10,000	0.01 mg/kg	0.25 mg	0.1 mg/mL	2.5 mL
Epinephrine 1:1000	0.1 mg/kg	2.5 mg	1 mg/mL	2.5 mL
Atropine	0.02 mg/kg	0.5 mg	0.1 mg/mL	5 mL
Calcium chloride 10%	20 mg/kg	500 mg	100 mg/mL	5 mL
Sodium bicarbonate 8.4%	1 mEq/kg	25 mEq	1 mEq/mL	25 mL

Table 19.14D   Defibrillation and Cardioversion: 25 kg

Defibrillation	50 J (2 J/kg), then 100 J (4 J/kg); max 250 J (10 J/kg)
Cardioversion	10 J (½ J/kg), then 20 J (1 J/kg); max 50 J (2 J/kg)

Table 19.14E   Other Emergency Medications: 25 kg

Drug	Dosing	Dose	Concentration	Volume
Adenosine	0.1–0.2 mg/kg	2.5–5 mg	3 mg/mL	0.83–1.67 mL
Amiodarone	5 mg/kg/dose	125 mg	50 mg/mL	2.5 mL
Benadryl	1–2 mg/kg	25–50 mg	50 mg/mL	0.5–1 mL
Glucose (D_{50}W)	0.5–1 g/kg	12.5–25 g	0.5 g/mL	Dilute 25–50 mL 1:1 with sterile water

(Continued)

Table 19.14E   Other Emergency Medications: 25 kg *(Continued)*

Drug	Dosing	Dose	Concentration	Volume
Flumazenil	0.01 mg/kg	0.2 mg (max)	0.1 mg/mL	2 mL
Hydrocortisone	1–5 mg/kg	25–125 mg	50 mg/mL	0.5–2.5 mL
Lidocaine	1 mg/kg	25 mg	20 mg/mL	1.25 mL/dose
Lorazepam	0.05–0.1 mg/kg	1.25–2.5 mg	2 mg/mL	0.63–1.25 mL
Magnesium	25–50 mg/kg/dose	625–1250 mg	500 mg/mL	1.25–2.5 mL
Naloxone	0.1 mg/kg	2 mg (max)	1 mg/mL	2 mL

EMERGENCY DRUG QUICK REFERENCE: 30 kg

TABLE 19.15A   Resuscitation Equipment: 30 kg

Item	Size	Other
Endotracheal tube (ETT) (16 + age (yr) / 4)	5.5–6.5 cuffed	O_2 mask: Small
		Oral airway: Medium
Laryngoscope blade	2	Foley: 10- to 12-Fr
		Self-inflating bag: Child
ETT depth of insertion (cm) (3 × internal diameter of tube)	17–20 cm	Femoral line: 5- to 7-Fr
		Chest tube: 28- to 32-Fr

Table 19.15B   Rapid-Sequence Intubation (RSI) (see section on RSI for details): 30 kg

	Dosing	Dose	Concentration	Volume
Premedication				
Atropine*	0.01–0.02 mg/kg[†]	0.3–0.5 mg	0.1 mg/mL	3–5 mL
Lidocaine	1–2 mg/kg	30–60 mg	20 mg/mL	1.5–3 mL
Sedation				
Midazolam	0.05–0.1 mg/kg	1.5–3 mg	1 mg/mL	1.5–3 mL
Etomidate	0.2–0.3 mg/kg	6–9 mg	2 mg/mL	3–4.5 mL
Ketamine#	1–2 mg/kg	30–60 mg	50 mg/mL	0.6–1.2 mL
Paralysis				
Rocuronium	0.6–1.2 mg/kg	18–36 mg	10 mg/mL	1.8–3.6 mL
Succinylcholine§	1–2 mg/kg	30–60 mg	20 mg/mL	1.5–3 mL

Contraindications: *Glaucoma, thyrotoxicosis; #elevated intracranial pressure; §burn or crush injury, glaucoma, neuromuscular disease, malignant hyperthermia
[†]Minimum dose: 0.1 mg

Table 19.15C   Cardiopulmonary Resuscitation Medications: 30 kg

Drug	Dosing	Dose	Concentration	Volume
Epinephrine 1:10,000	0.01 mg/kg	0.3 mg	0.1 mg/mL	3 mL
Epinephrine 1:1000	0.1 mg/kg	3 mg	1 mg/mL	3 mL
Atropine (bradycardia)	0.02 mg/kg	0.5 mg	0.1 mg/mL	5 mL (max dose)
Calcium chloride 10%	20 mg/kg	600 mg	100 mg/mL	6 mL
Sodium bicarbonate 8.4%	1 mEq/kg	30 mEq	1 mEq/mL	30 mL

TABLE 19.15D   Defibrillation and Cardioversion: 30 kg

Defibrillation	50 J (2 J/kg), then 100 J (4 J/kg); max 300 J (10 J/kg)
Cardioversion	10 J (½ J/kg), then 30 J (1 J/kg); max 60 J (2 J/kg)

Table 19.15E   Other Emergency Medications: 30 kg

Drug	Dosing	Dose	Concentration	Volume
Adenosine	0.1–0.2 mg/kg	3–6 mg	3 mg/mL	1–2 mL
Amiodarone	5 mg/kg/dose	150 mg	50 mg/mL	3 mL
Benadryl	1–2 mg/kg	25–50 mg	50 mg/mL	0.5–1 mL
Glucose ($D_{50}W$)	0.5–1 g/kg	15–30 g	0.5 g/mL	Dilute 30–60 mL 1:1 with sterile water
Flumazenil	0.01 mg/kg	0.2 mg (max)	0.1 mg/mL	2 mL
Hydrocortisone	1–5 mg/kg	30–150 mg	50 mg/mL	0.6–3 mL
Lidocaine	1 mg/kg	30 mg	20 mg/mL	1.5 mL/dose
Lorazepam	0.05–0.1 mg/kg	1.5–2 mg	2 mg/mL	0.75–1 mL
Magnesium	25–50 mg/kg/dose	750–1500 mg	500 mg/mL	1.5–3 mL
Naloxone	0.1 mg/kg	2 mg (max)	1 mg/mL	2 mL

EMERGENCY DRUG QUICK REFERENCE: 35 kg

Table 19.16A   Resuscitation Equipment: 35 kg

Item	Size	Other
Endotracheal tube (ETT) (16 + age (yr) / 4)	6.5 cuffed	O₂ mask: Small / adult
		Oral airway: Medium
Laryngoscope blade	2–3	Foley: 10- to 12-Fr
		Self-inflating bag: Child
ETT depth of insertion (cm) (3 × internal diameter of tube)	20 cm	Femoral line: 5- to 7-Fr
		Chest tube: 28- to 32-Fr

Table 19.16B   Rapid Sequence Intubation (RSI) (see section on RSI for details): 35 kg

	Dosing	Dose	Concentration	Volume
Premedication				
Atropine*	0.01–0.02 mg/kg†	0.35–0.5 mg	0.1 mg/mL	3.5–5 mL
Lidocaine	1–2 mg/kg	35–70 mg	20 mg/mL	1.75–3.5 mL
Sedation				
Midazolam	0.05–0.1 mg/kg	1.75–3.5 mg	1 mg/mL	1.75–3.5 mL
Etomidate	0.2–0.3 mg/kg	7–10.5 mg	2 mg/mL	3.5–5.25 mL
Ketamine#	1–2 mg/kg	35–70 mg	50 mg/mL	0.7–1.4 mL
Paralysis				
Rocuronium	0.6–1.2 mg/kg	21–42 mg	10 mg/mL	2.1–4.2 mL
Succinylcholine§	1–2 mg/kg	35–70 mg	20 mg/mL	1.75–3.5 mL

Contraindications: *Glaucoma, thyrotoxicosis; #elevated intracranial pressure; §burn or crush injury, glaucoma, neuromuscular disease, malignant hyperthermia
†Minimum dose: 0.1 mg

Table 19.16C   Cardiopulmonary Resuscitation Medications: 35 kg

Drug	Dosing	Dose	Concentration	Volume
Epinephrine 1:10,000	0.01 mg/kg	0.35 mg	0.1 mg/mL	3 mL
Epinephrine 1:1000	0.1 mg/kg	3.5 mg	1 mg/mL	3 mL
Atropine (bradycardia)	0.02 mg/kg	0.5 mg	0.1 mg/mL	5 mL (max dose)
Calcium chloride 10%	20 mg/kg	700 mg	100 mg/mL	7 mL
Sodium bicarbonate 8.4%	1 mEq/kg	35 mEq	1 mEq/mL	35 mL

Table 19.16D   Defibrillation and Cardioversion: 35 kg

Defibrillation	50 J (2 J/kg), then 100 J (4 J/kg); max 300 J (10 J/kg)
Cardioversion	10 J (½ J/kg), then 30 J (1 J/kg); max 70 J (2 J/kg)

Table 19.16E   Other Emergency Medications: 35 kg

Drug	Dosing	Dose	Concentration	Volume
Adenosine	0.1–0.2 mg/kg	3.5–7 mg	3 mg/mL	1.17–2.33 mL
Amiodarone	5 mg/kg/dose	175 mg	50 mg/mL	3.5 mL
Benadryl	1–2 mg/kg	25–50 mg	50 mg/mL	0.5–1 mL
Glucose ($D_{50}W$)	0.5–1 g/kg	17.5–35 g	0.5 g/mL	Dilute 35–70 mL 1:1 with sterile water
Flumazenil	0.01 mg/kg	0.2 mg (max)	0.1 mg/mL	2 mL

(Continued)

Table 19.16E   Other Emergency Medications: 35 kg *(Continued)*

Drug	Dosing	Dose	Concentration	Volume
Hydrocortisone	1–5 mg/kg	35–175 mg	50 mg/mL	0.7–3.5 mL
Lidocaine	1 mg/kg	35 mg	20 mg/mL	1.75 mL/dose
Lorazepam	0.05–0.1 mg/kg	1.75–2 mg	2 mg/mL	0.88–1 mL
Magnesium	25–50 mg/kg/dose	875–1750 mg	500 mg/mL	1.75–3.5 mL
Naloxone	0.1 mg/kg	2 mg (max)	1 mg/mL	2 mL

EMERGENCY DRUG QUICK REFERENCE: 40 kg

Table 19.17A   Resuscitation Equipment: 40 kg

Item	Size	Other
Endotracheal tube (ETT) (16 + age (yr) / 4)	7 cuffed	O_2 mask: Adult
		Oral airway: Medium
Laryngoscope blade	3 Mac	Foley: 12-Fr
		Self-inflating bag: Child or adult
ETT depth of insertion (cm) (3 × internal diameter of tube)	21 cm	Femoral line: 6- or 7-Fr
		Chest tube: 28- to 38-Fr

Table 19.17B   Rapid-Sequence Intubation (RSI) (see section on RSI for details): 40 kg

	Dosing	Dose	Concentration	Volume
Premedication				
Atropine*	0.01–0.02 mg/kg[†]	0.4–0.5 mg	0.1 mg/mL	4–5 mL
Lidocaine	1–2 mg/kg	40–80 mg	20 mg/mL	2–4 mL
Sedation				
Midazolam	0.05–0.1 mg/kg	2–4 mg	1 mg/mL	2–4 mL
Etomidate	0.2–0.3 mg/kg	8–12 mg	2 mg/mL	4–6 mL
Ketamine#	1–2 mg/kg	40–80 mg	50 mg/mL	0.8–1.6 mL
Paralysis				
Rocuronium	0.6–1.2 mg/kg	24–48 mg	10 mg/mL	2.4–4.8 mL
Succinylcholine§	1–2 mg/kg	40–80 mg	20 mg/mL	2–4 mL

Contraindications: *Glaucoma, thyrotoxicosis; #elevated intracranial pressure; §burn or crush injury, glaucoma, neuromuscular disease, malignant hyperthermia
[†]Minimum dose: 0.1 mg

Table 19.17C   Cardiopulmonary Resuscitation Medications: 40 kg

Drug	Dosing	Dose	Concentration	Volume
Epinephrine 1:10,000	0.01 mg/kg	0.4 mg	0.1 mg/mL	4 mL
Epinephrine 1:1000	0.1 mg/kg	4 mg	1 mg/mL	4 mL

(Continued)

Table 19.17C   Cardiopulmonary Resuscitation Medications: 40 kg *(Continued)*

Drug	Dosing	Dose	Concentration	Volume
Atropine (bradycardia)	0.02 mg/kg	0.8 mg	0.1 mg/mL	8 mL
Calcium chloride 10%	20 mg/kg	800 mg	100 mg/mL	8 mL
Sodium bicarbonate 8.4%	1 mEq/kg	40 mEq	1 mEq/mL	40 mL

Table 19.17D   Defibrillation and Cardioversion: 40 kg

Defibrillation	100 J (2 J/kg), then 150 J (4 J/kg); max 360 J (adult max)
Cardioversion	20 J (½ J/kg), then 40 J (1 J/kg); max 80 J (2 J/kg)

Table 19.17E   Other Emergency Medications: 40 kg

Drug	Dosing	Dose	Concentration	Volume
Adenosine	0.1–0.2 mg/kg	4–8 mg	3 mg/mL	1.33–2.67 mL
Amiodarone	5 mg/kg/dose	200 mg	50 mg/mL	4 mL
Benadryl	1–2 mg/kg	50 mg	50 mg/mL	1 mL
Glucose ($D_{50}W$)	0.5–1 g/kg	20–40 g	0.5 g/mL	Dilute 40–80 mL 1:1 with sterile water
Flumazenil	0.01 mg/kg	0.2 mg (max)	0.1 mg/mL	2 mL
Hydrocortisone	1–5 mg/kg	40–200 mg	50 mg/mL	0.8–4 mL
Lidocaine	1 mg/kg	40 mg	20 mg/mL	2 mL/dose
Lorazepam	0.05–0.1 mg/kg	2 mg	2 mg/mL	1 mL
Magnesium	25–50 mg/kg/dose	1–2 g	500 mg/mL	2–4 mL
Naloxone	0.1 mg/kg	2 mg (max)	1 mg/mL	2 mL

EMERGENCY DRUG QUICK REFERENCE: 50 kg

Table 19.18A   Resuscitation Equipment: 50 kg

Item	Size	Other
Endotracheal tube (ETT) (16 + age (yr) / 4)	7–8 cuffed	O_2 mask: Adult
		Oral airway: Medium
Laryngoscope blade	3 Mac	Foley: 12-Fr
		Self-inflating bag: Child or adult
ETT depth of insertion (cm) (3 × internal diameter of tube)	21–24 cm	Femoral line: 7-Fr
		Chest tube: 32- to 42-Fr

Table 19.18B   Rapid-Sequence Intubation (RSI) (see section on RSI for details): 50 kg

	Dosing	Dose	Concentration	Volume
Premedication				
Atropine*	0.01–0.02 mg/kg†	0.5–1 mg	0.1 mg/mL	5–10 mL
Lidocaine	1–2 mg/kg	50–100 mg	20 mg/mL	2.5–5 mL
Sedation				
Midazolam	0.05–0.1 mg/kg	2.5–5 mg	1 mg/mL	2.5–5 mL
Etomidate	0.2–0.3 mg/kg	10–15 mg	2 mg/mL	5–7.5 mL
Ketamine#	1–2 mg/kg	50–100 mg	50 mg/mL	1–2 mL
Paralysis				
Rocuronium	0.6–1.2 mg/kg	30–60 mg	10 mg/mL	3–6 mL
Succinylcholine§	1–2 mg/kg	50–100 mg	20 mg/mL	2.5–5 mL

Contraindications: *Glaucoma, thyrotoxicosis; #elevated intracranial pressure; §burn or crush injury, glaucoma, neuromuscular disease, malignant hyperthermia
†Minimum dose: 0.1 mg

Table 19.18C   Cardiopulmonary Resuscitation Medications: 50 kg

Drug	Dosing	Dose	Concentration	Volume
Epinephrine 1:10,000	0.01 mg/kg	0.5 mg	0.1 mg/mL	5 mL
Epinephrine 1:1000	0.1 mg/kg	5 mg	1 mg/mL	5 mL
Atropine (bradycardia)	0.02 mg/kg	1 mg	0.1 mg/mL	10 mL
Calcium chloride 10%	20 mg/kg	1000 mg	100 mg/mL	10 mL
Sodium bicarbonate 8.4%	1 mEq/kg	50 mEq	1 mEq/mL	50 mL

Table 19.18D   Defibrillation and Cardioversion: 50 kg

Defibrillation	100 J 2 (J/kg), then 200 J (4 J/kg); max 360 J (adult max)
Cardioversion	20 J (½ J/kg), then 50 J (1 J/kg); max 100 J (2 J/kg)

Table 19.18E   Other Emergency Medications: 50 kg

Drug	Dosing	Dose	Concentration	Volume
Adenosine	0.1–0.2 mg/kg	5–10 mg	3 mg/mL	1.67–3.33 mL
Amiodarone	5 mg/kg/dose	250 mg	50 mg/mL	5 mL
Benadryl	1–2 mg/kg	50 mg	50 mg/mL	1 mL

(Continued)

Table 19.18E Other Emergency Medications: 50 kg *(Continued)*

Drug	Dosing	Dose	Concentration	Volume
Glucose ($D_{50}W$)	0.5–1 g/kg	25–50 g	0.5 g/mL	Dilute 50–100 mL 1:1 with sterile water
Flumazenil	0.01 mg/kg	0.2 mg (max)	0.1 mg/mL	2 mL
Hydrocortisone	1–5 mg/kg	50–250 mg	50 mg/mL	1–5 mL
Lidocaine	1 mg/kg	50 mg	20 mg/mL	2.5 mL/dose
Lorazepam	0.05–0.1 mg/kg	2 mg	2 mg/mL	1 mL
Magnesium	25–50 mg/kg/dose	1.25–2 g	500 mg/mL	2.5–4 mL
Naloxone	0.1 mg/kg	2 mg (max)	1 mg/mL	2 mL

EMERGENCY DRUG QUICK REFERENCE: 60 kg

Table 19.19A   Resuscitation Equipment: 60 kg

Item	Size	Other
Endotracheal tube (ETT) (16 + age (yr) / 4)	7–8 cuffed	O_2 mask: Adult
		Oral airway: Adult
Laryngoscope blade	3 Mac	Foley: 12-Fr
		Self-inflating Bag: Adult
ETT depth of insertion (cm) (3 × internal diameter of tube)	21–24 cm	Femoral line: 7-Fr
		Chest tube: 32- to 42-Fr

Table 19.19B   Rapid-Sequence Intubation (RSI) (see section on RSI for details): 60 kg

	Dosing	Dose	Concentration	Volume
Premedication				
Atropine*	0.01–0.02 mg/kg[†]	0.6–1 mg	0.1 mg/mL	6–10 mL
Lidocaine	1–2 mg/kg	60–120 mg	20 mg/mL	3–6 mL
Sedation				
Midazolam	0.05–0.1 mg/kg	3–5 mg	1 mg/mL	3–5 mL
Etomidate	0.2–0.3 mg/kg	12–18 mg	2 mg/mL	6–9 mL
Ketamine#	1–2 mg/kg	60–120 mg	50 mg/mL	1.2–2.4 mL
Paralysis				
Rocuronium	0.6–1.2 mg/kg	36–72 mg	10 mg/mL	3.6–7.2 mL
Succinylcholine[§]	1–2 mg/kg	60–120 mg	20 mg/mL	3–6 mL

Contraindications: *Glaucoma, thyrotoxicosis; #elevated intracranial pressure; §burn or crush injury, glaucoma, neuromuscular disease, malignant hyperthermia
[†]Minimum dose: 0.1 mg

Table 19.19C   Cardiopulmonary Resuscitation Medications: 60 kg

Drug	Dosing	Dose	Concentration	Volume
Epinephrine 1:10,000	0.01 mg/kg	0.6 mg	0.1 mg/mL	6 mL
Epinephrine 1:1000	0.1 mg/kg	6 mg	1 mg/mL	6 mL
Atropine (bradycardia)	0.02 mg/kg	1 mg	0.1 mg/mL	10 mL
Calcium chloride 10%	20 mg/kg	1000 mg	100 mg/mL	10 mL
Sodium bicarbonate 8.4%	1 mEq/kg	50 mEq	1 mEq/mL	50 mL

Table 19.19D   Defibrillation and Cardioversion: 60 kg

Defibrillation	100 J (2 J/kg), then 200 J (4 J/kg); max 360 J (Adult max)
Cardioversion	30 J (½ J/kg), then 50 J (1 J/kg); max 100 J (2 J/kg)

Table 19.19E   Other Emergency Medications: 60 kg

Drug	Dosing	Dose	Concentration	Volume
Adenosine	0.1–0.2 mg/kg	6–12 mg	3 mg/mL	2–4 mL
Amiodarone	5 mg/kg/dose	300 mg	50 mg/mL	6 mL rapid IV bolus
Benadryl	1–2 mg/kg	50 mg	50 mg/mL	1 mL
Glucose ($D_{50}W$)	0.5–1 g/kg	30–60 g	0.5 g/mL	Dilute 60–120 mL 1:1 with sterile water
Flumazenil	0.01 mg/kg	0.2 mg (max)	0.1 mg/mL	2 mL
Hydrocortisone	1–5 mg/kg	60–250 mg	50 mg/mL	1.2–5 mL
Lidocaine	1 mg/kg	60 mg	20 mg/mL	3 mL/dose
Lorazepam	0.05–0.1 mg/kg	2 mg	2 mg/mL	1 mL
Magnesium	25–50 mg/kg/dose	1.5–2 g	500 mg/mL	3–4 mL
Naloxone	0.1 mg/kg	2 mg (max)	1 mg/mL	2 mL

RAPID SEQUENCE INTUBATION

RAPID-SEQUENCE INTUBATION

- Rapid-sequence intubation (RSI) describes preparation, sedation, and subsequent paralysis to facilitate safe and controlled airway management
- Preferred method of endotracheal intubation in emergency department (ED) and in any patient with a potentially full stomach
- Not necessary in comatose children or children in cardiac arrest

PREPARATION

- Preoxygenate immediately at highest O_2 concentration available (15 liters/min with non-rebreather mask)
- Assemble equipment and personnel necessary (see weight-based emergency drug sheets)
- Identify any conditions that might make intubation or bag-valve-mask ventilation (BVM) difficult
- Avoid BVM prior to intubation if possible to avoid overinflating stomach
- Insert nasogastric or orogastric tube to decompress stomach if time available

MEDICATIONS SEQUENCE FOR RAPID-SEQUENCE INTUBATION

- Premedicate as per table below with atropine or lidocaine as indicated:
  - Atropine for: All children ≤ 1 year old, children < 5 years old receiving succinylcholine, or any child receiving second-dose succinylcholine
  - Lidocaine indicated if concern for elevated intracranial pressure (ICP)
    - Give 2–3 minutes prior to intubation
- Sedation: Onset generally 1–3 minutes after infusion
- Paralysis as per Table 19.20

INTUBATION

- Position patient
  - Cervical spine immobilization if possible cervical spine injury
  - "Sniffing position" if no concern for cervical spine injury
- Cricoid pressure
  - Apply to unconscious child
  - Can be released if creates difficulty passing endotracheal tube

POST-INTUBATION

- Confirm tracheal intubation with end-tidal CO_2 detection or colorimetric device (changes from purple → yellow with proper placement)
  - An alternate method, a "bulb detector," can falsely indicate esophageal intubation in pliable pediatric airways
  - Chest radiograph to document proper endotracheal tube position
  - Ongoing sedation and analgesia as needed

Table 19.20 Medications for Rapid-Sequence Intubation

	Dose	Uses	
Premedications			
Atropine	0.01–0.02 mg/kg	Min 0.1 mg, max 0.5 mg/dose; can cause paradoxical bradycardia, ↑ secretions	
Lidocaine	1–2 mg/kg	Blunts ICP spike	
Glycopyrrolate	0.005–0.01 mg/kg	Antisialagogue, inhibits bradycardia	
Sedatives			
Midazolam	0.05–0.1 mg/kg	↓ BP, HR; max single dose 10 mg	
Fentanyl	1–3 mcg/kg	Rigid chest (treatment: naloxone, paralyze)	
Etomidate	0.3 mg/kg	Myoclonus	
Ketamine	1–2 mg/kg	↑ ICP, ↑ BP, ↑ HR; laryngospasm, secretions	
Thiopental	0.5–4 mg/kg	↓ BP, bronchospasm	
Paralytics		**Onset**	**Duration**
Rocuronium	0.6–1.2 mg/kg	45–60 sec	30–45 min
Vecuronium	0.1–0.2 mg/kg	70–120 sec	30–90 min
Succinylcholine	1–2 mg/kg	30–60 sec	3–10 min

*Succinylcholine is contraindicated in patients with neuromuscular disease, muscular dystrophy, severe burns, hyperkalemia, rhabdomyolysis, or family history of malignant hyperthermia.

POISONINGS

For expert advice: in United States, call Poison Control a 1-800-222-1222; if outside United States, see www.who.int/gho/phe/chemical_safety/poisons_centres/en/index.html

EPIDEMIOLOGY

- Accidental: More common in toddlers/young children; nonpharmaceutical (cleaning products, plants, etc.) > pharmaceutical (acetaminophen, iron, over-the-counter cough and cold meds, vitamins), boys > girls
- Intentional: More common in adolescent girls, intentional, pharmaceuticals > nonpharmaceuticals
- General principles
  - Activated charcoal
    - Give within 1 hour of ingestion for optimal effect
    - Contraindicated if altered mental status, unprotected/tenuous airway, corrosive ingestion, ileus, bowel obstruction
    - Not effective for alkali substances, arsenic, bromide, camphor, cyanide, ethanol, hydrocarbons, iron, lithium, methanol, organic solvents, phosphorus
  - Bowel decontamination with whole-bowel irrigation (WBI)
    - Theoretic value in potentially toxic ingestions of enteric-coated/sustained-release medications, lithium, metals (iron, zinc)
    - Contraindicated in presence of gastrointestinal bleed, ileus, perforation, obstruction, or CNS depression/altered mental status
    - Polyethylene glycol (*Go-Lytely*®): 25 mL/kg/hour PO/NG
      - Stop when rectal effluent clear and without tablets/pills
  - Rarely recommended:
    - Ipecac: Only for iron ingestion within the last hour
      - Contraindicated: Corrosive or hydrocarbon ingestion, altered mental status, hematemesis
    - Gastric lavage: Only for severe ingestions within the last 30–60 minutes
      - Contraindicated: Infants and young children (ineffective due to small tube size), caustic and hydrocarbon ingestion
    - Cathartics: Occasionally used with activated charcoal. No evidence for efficacy. Not to be used as only method of treatment for ingestion
      - Contraindicated: Caustic and hydrocarbon ingestion, ileus

Table 19.21   Causes of Common Physical Exam Findings in Ingestions

Eye Findings	Mydriasis	Sympathomimetics, anticholinergics, antidepressants, antihistamines
	Miosis	Cholinergics, opiates, barbiturates, clonidine, organophosphates
Skin Findings	Diaphoresis	Sympathomimetics, anticholinergics (organophosphates), aspirin
	Red skin	Carbon monoxide, boric acid
	Blue skin	Methemoglobinemia
Cardiac	Bradycardia	Organophosphates, beta-blockers, calcium channel blockers, clonidine, opiates, digoxin
	Tachycardia	Sympathomimetics, levothyroxine, tricyclic antidepressants (TCAs), anticholinergics, caffeine, antihistamines
Respiration	Bradypnea	Opiates, barbiturates, benzodiazepines, ethanol
	Tachypnea	Salicylates, sympathomimetics, methanol, ethylene glycol

TOXIDROMES
- Sympathomimetics (cocaine, methamphetamine, caffeine)
  - Symptoms: Mydriasis, tachycardia, sweating, fever, irritability, hypertension
  - Treatment: Supportive care, continuous cardiopulmonary monitoring, benzodiazepines (agitation)
- Anticholinergic
  - Symptoms: Hyperpyrexia, urinary retention, constipation, altered mental status, delirium, mydriasis, tachycardia, hypertension, ataxia, seizures
  - Treatment: Physostigmine (controversial)
    - 0.02 mg/kg IM/IV, may repeat q 15–20 min if severe or persistent sx and cholinergic sx absent (have atropine ready; see dosing below)
    - Max dose 0.5 mg/dose; 2 mg total
- Cholinergic (organophosphates nerve agent insecticides)
  - Diarrhea, salivation, lacrimation, emesis, bradycardia, hypotension, polyuria, miosis, bronchospasm
  - Atropine: Treat until muscarinic symptoms abated
    - < 2 years old: 0.05 mg/kg IV/IM (mild sx), or 0.1 mg/kg IV/IM (severe sx) q 10–20 min prn
    - 2–10 years old: 1 mg IV/IM q 5–10 min prn (mild/moderate sx), or 2 mg IV/IM q 5–10 min prn (severe sx), or 1 mg IV q 5–10 min prn
    - > 10 years old: 2 mg IM q 5–10 min prn (mild/moderate sx), or 4 mg IM q 5–10 min prn (severe sx), or 2 mg IV q 5–10 min prn
  - Pralidoxime (2-*PAM*®, *Protopam*®):
    - Pretreat with atropine
    - IV: 20–50 mg/kg × 1 (max 2 g/dose). May repeat in 1 hour and q 10–12 hour if remains symptomatic (muscle weakness). Consider q 3–8 hour dosing if ingested
    - IM (< 40 kg, mild symptoms): 15 mg/kg × 1 (max 600 mg/dose). Repeat × 2 doses q 15 min if mild symptoms persist (max total dose 45 mg/kg)
    - IM (< 40 kg, severe symptoms): 15 mg/kg × 3 successive doses in rapid succession (max 600 mg/dose, 45 mg/kg/series of 3 doses). May repeat 3-dose course in 1 hour if severe symptoms persist
    - IM (> 40 kg, mild symptoms): 600 mg/dose × 1. Repeat × 2 doses q 15 min if mild symptoms persist (max 1800 mg/series of 3 doses)
    - IM (> 40 kg, severe symptoms): 600 mg/dose × 3 successive doses in rapid succession. May repeat 3-dose course in 1 hour if severe symptoms persist

SALICYLATE
- Peak concentration after ingestion
  - Regular aspirin tables: 15–60 minutes
  - Enteric coated: 4–14 hours
- Clinical/laboratory manifestations
  - Mild ingestion (< 300 mg/kg), serum level < 30 mg/dL: hyperpyrexia, nausea, vomiting, tinnitus, diarrhea
  - Moderate–severe ingestion (300–500 mg/kg), serum level > 30–40 mg/dL: Tachypnea, tachycardia, altered mental status, seizures, coma, anion gap metabolic acidosis, hypoglycemia, shock
  - Potentially fatal ingestion (> 500 mg/kg), serum level > 100 mg/dL
- Treatment
  - Dextrose-containing (D5 ½NS or D10 ½NS) IVF to prevent neuroglycopenia
  - Decontamination with activate charcoal: For single-dose treatment needs to be given within 1 hour of ingestion
    - < 1 year old: Single-dose: 0.5–1 g/kg PO or 10–25 g PO × 1
      - Multiple dose: 1–2 g/kg PO q 2–4 hrs prn
    - 1–12 years old: Single-dose: 0.5–1 g/kg PO or 25–50 g PO × 1
      - Multiple dose: 1–2 g/kg PO q 2–4 hrs prn

-     – > 12 years old: Single-dose: 25–100 g PO × 1
  - Multiple dose: 12.5 g PO q 1 hour prn
  - Consider WBI for enteric-coated tablets
    - Polyethylene glycol (*Go-Lytely®*): 25 mL/kg/hour PO/NG
- ○ Alkalization: Add 100–150 mEq NaHCO$_3$ (2–3 vials 8.4% NaHCO$_3$) to 1 liter D$_5$W to infuse at 1.5–2 × maintenance rate
  - Add KCl (20–40 mEq/L) once urine output assured
  - Goal urine pH > 7.5
- ○ Hemodialysis for renal failure, pulmonary edema, CHF, persistent altered mental status, hypotension, uncorrecting acidosis, or electrolyte disturbances. Consider hemodialysis if salicylate level > 100 mg/dL

ACETAMINOPHEN

- Symptoms: Contact poison control and treat any ingestion ≥ 150 mg/kg
  - ○ 0–24 hrs: Nausea, vomiting with normal LFTs
  - ○ 24–48 hrs: Asymptomatic (possible RUQ pain, LFTs may increase)
  - ○ 48–96 hrs: Hepatocellular death leads to coagulopathy, jaundice, encephalopathy; AST most sensitive marker of hepatic injury
  - ○ 4–14 days: Recovery or death
- Draw level 4 hours post-ingestion
- Rumack-Matthew nomogram can help to guide intervention (accessible at http://www.ars-informatica.ca/toxicity_nomogram.php?calc=acetamin or http://en.wikipedia.org/wiki/Rumack-Matthew_nomogram)

Table 19.22   Single Acute Acetaminophen Overdose and Blood Levels for Starting N-Acetylcysteine Treatment

Approximate Hours Postingestion	Consider Treatment with N-acetylcysteine If Plasma Acetaminophen Level Greater or Equal to Approximately:
4 hours	150 mcg/mL
5 hours	125 mcg/mL
6 hours	110 mcg/mL
7 hours	89 mcg/mL
8 hours	75 mcg/mL
9 hours	63 mcg/mL
10 hours	54 mcg/mL
11 hours	45 mcg/mL
12 hours	37 mcg/mL
13 hours	32 mcg/mL
14 hours	27 mcg/mL
15 hours	22 mcg/mL
16 hours	19 mcg/mL
17 hours	16 mcg/mL
18 hours	15 mcg/mL
19 hours	11 mcg/mL

(Continued)

Table 19.22   Single Acute Acetaminophen Overdose and Blood Levels for Starting N-Acetylcysteine Treatment *(Continued)*

Approximate Hours Postingestion	Consider Treatment with N-acetylcysteine If Plasma Acetaminophen Level Greater or Equal to Approximately:
20 hours	9 mcg/mL
21 hours	8 mcg/mL
22 hours	6.5 mcg/mL
23 hours	5.5 mcg/mL
24 hours	4.75 mcg/mL

- Treatment of acetaminophen toxicity/overdose:
  - N-Acetylcysteine (*Mucomyst®*): Begin immediately (do not wait for levels)
    - PO/NG: 140 mg/kg × 1, then 70 mg/kg q 4 hours × 17 doses
      - Repeat dose if emesis within 1 hour of dose
    - IV (*Acetadote®*): 150 mg/kg × 1 over 60 min, then 50 mg/kg (max 5 g) IV × 1 over 4 hours, then 100 mg/kg (max 10 g) IV × 1 over 16 hours. May continue treatment × 48–72 hours if LFTs continue to rise
  - Lactulose (10 g/15 mL): Used for hepatic encephalopathy
    - Dose: 40–90 mL/day PO divided tid–qid. Goal 2–3 soft stools/day
  - Refer to tertiary care/organ transplant center for hepatic failure

BENZODIAZEPINES
- Symptoms: Ataxia, altered mental status, lethargy, coma, hypopnea, apnea, cardiac depression
- Treatment: flumazenil (*Romazicon®*). IV push over 30 seconds
  - > 1 year old: 0.01 mg/kg IV q 1 min prn (max single dose 0.2 mg; total dose 1 mg)

OPIATES
- Symptoms: Altered mental status, slurred speech, lethargy, hypopnea/apnea, coma, miosis, ileus
- Treatment of opiate ingestion/severe toxicity: Naloxone (*Narcan®*)
  - < 1 month old: 0.1 mg/kg IV q 2–3 min or 0.1 mg/kg IM q 3–8 min
  - > 1 month (< 20 kg): 0.1 mg/kg IV (max 0.4 mg) q 2–3 min or 0.1 mg/kg IM/IO/SQ/ETT q 3–8 min (max single dose: 0.4 mg)
  - > 1 month (> 20 kg): 0.4–2 mg IV q 2–3 min
- Treatment of mild/moderate opiate toxicity/effect: Naloxone (*Narcan®*):
  - < 20 kg: 0.001–0.01 mg/kg IV q 2–3 min or 0.001–0.01 mg/kg IM/SQ q 3–8 min
  - > 20 kg: 0.1–0.2 mg IV q 2–3 min or 0.1–0.2 mg IM/SQ q 3–8 min

NEUROMUSCULAR BLOCKADE REVERSAL
- Neostigmine 0.025–0.08 mg/kg/dose slow IV push; use w/ atropine or glycopyrrolate
- Pyridostigmine 0.1–0.25 mg/kg/dose IV; use w/ atropine or glycopyrrolate
- Secretion prevention:
  - Glycopyrrolate 0.2 mg IV for each 1 mg neostigmine or 5 mg pyridostigmine

DIGOXIN
- Symptoms: Nausea, vomiting, diarrhea, headache, confusion, SVT, AV block, bradycardia, hyperkalemia (inhibition of Na^+/K^+ ATP pump)
- Treatment:
  - Digoxin immune Fab (*DigiFab®*); 40/vial; IV. Dose varies based on following formulas. Give as single infusion over 30 minutes

- Chronic intoxication: Number of vials = [digoxin level (ng/mL) × weight (kg)] / 100.
  - In patient < 20 kg, may give 1 vial IV × 1 if digoxin ingestion suspected and level not yet available
- Acute intoxication: Number of vials = total digoxin ingested (mg) / 0.5
  - Alternative: 10 vials IV × 1 for each 25 tabs/caps ingested
○ Multidose charcoal as outlined in salicylate section
○ Atropine for bradycardia
○ Treat hyperkalemia in standard fashion (*except no calcium)

AMPHETAMINE

- Symptoms: Sympathomimetic toxicity
  ○ Children may also have unsteady gait, hyperactive reflexes, talkativeness, nausea, vomiting, abdominal pain
  ○ Infants may present with inconsolability, seizures, altered mental status, or even coma
- Treatment
  ○ Manage symptomatically

METHANOL

- Found in washer fluid, fuel additives
- Metabolite (formic acid) inhibits mitochondrial respiration and leads to acidosis
- Symptoms:
  ○ Initial: Headache, abdominal pain, nausea, vomiting, malaise
  ○ > 24 hours post-ingestion: Blurred vision, photophobia, altered mental status, severe anion-gap acidosis
- Treatment:
  ○ GI decontamination not effective
  ○ Sodium bicarbonate: 1–2 mEq/kg IV if pH < 7.3. If still acidotic, initiate $NaHCO_3$ via continuous infusion by adding 2–3 ampules (50 mEq/amp) to 1000 mL dextrose 5% at 1–2 × maintenance until pH > 7.35
  ○ Alcohol dehydrogenase inhibition: Prefer fomepizole over ethanol infusion
    - Fomepizole (4-methylpyrazole, *Antizol*®): 15 mg/kg IV × 1, followed by 10 mg/kg IV q 12 hours × 4 doses; then 15 mg/kg q 12 hours until methanol level < 20 mg/dL
      - Give q 4 hours if undergoing hemodialysis
    - IV ethanol 600–800 mg/kg of 10% solution in dextrose 5% (D5W)
      - Goal blood ethanol concentration > 100 mg/dL
      - Monitor in ICU setting given cardiac and respiratory risks
  ○ Hemodialysis if large anion gap acidosis or end-organ damage (see above)

References: *J Toxicol Clin Toxicol.* 2002;40(4):415; *Pediatrics.* 2001;108(4): e77.

LEAD

- Symptoms of lead encephalopathy: Coma, seizures, bizarre behavior, ataxia, apathy, incoordination, vomiting, alteration in the state of consciousness, and subtle loss of recently acquired skills
- Symptoms of lead toxicity: Decrease in activity, lethargy, anorexia, sporadic vomiting, intermittent abdominal pain, and constipation
- Lead level > 5 mcg/dL is considered a call for investigation
- If level ≥ 70 mcg/dL on repeat venous sample, hospitalize for IV chelation therapy
  ○ Dimercaprol (BAL): 4 mg/kg/dose 75 mg/m²/dose IM q 4 hrs × 3–7 days
    - First dose should precede $CaNa_2$ ethylenediaminetetraacetic acid (EDTA) by at least 4 hours
    - 30–50% patients have side effects: fever, vomiting, headache, elevated transaminases. Avoid in patients with G6PD deficiency

- CaNa$_2$ EDTA 1500 mg/m^2/day via continuous IV infusion × 5 days
  - Dilute in dextrose 5% or 0.9% saline
  - Concentration of CaNa$_2$ EDTA not to exceed 0.5%
  - Monitor urine output, urine sediment, BUN, creatinine, transaminases daily. Life-threatening renal failure can occur
- Consider chelation when blood lead 45–69 mcg/dL as follows:
  - If *symptomatic*: CaNa$_2$ EDTA + dimercaprol (BAL) treatment as above
  - If asymptomatic: CaNa$_2$ EDTA 1000 mg/m^2/day via continuous IV infusion × 5 days. Second course may be necessary if lead level rebounds in 7–14 days
  - Oral succimer 350 mg/m^2/dose PO q 8 hours × 5 days, then q 12 hours × 14 days; repeat courses may be necessary. Experience limited in children
- Blood lead level 25–40 mcg/dL
  - If asymptomatic, options include oral succimer, D-penicillamine (not FDA approved). See cdc.gov for latest recommendations

IRON

- Identify when, what type, and how much (mg/kg) elemental iron was ingested
  - Elemental iron (% eFe) varies per preparation: Ferrous sulfate (20% eFe), ferrous gluconate (12% eFe), ferrous fumarate (33% eFe), prenatal vitamins (60–65 mg eFe/pill), MVI (15–18 mg eFe/pill)
  - Toxic dose (of elemental iron): < 20 mg/kg generally asymptomatic, 20–60 mg/kg variable symptoms, > 60 mg/kg can cause severe toxicity, lethal dose ranges from 60–300 mg/kg
- Multiphase presentation (overlap of phases occurs regularly)
  - Gastrointestinal (GI) phase (30 min–6 hours): emesis, diarrhea, abdominal pain, hematemesis, melena, metabolic acidosis, lethargy, shock
  - Latent (6–24 hours): Tachypnea, tachycardia, improvement in GI symptoms
  - Shock/acidosis (4 hours–4 days): CNS, renal, pulmonary, and cardiac dysfunction leads to severe shock and metabolic acidosis
  - Hepatotoxicity (first 2 days): coagulopathy, hyperbilirubinemia, coma
  - Bowel obstruction (2–4 weeks): emesis, abdominal pain, gastric outlet obstruction
- Management:
  - Aggressive volume repletion with isotonic fluids (NS or LR)
  - WBI (as above) if radiograph shows presence of iron in stomach or small bowel
    - Activated charcoal binds Fe poorly; not useful
  - Deferoxamine infusion: 15 mg/kg/hour IV (max 6000 mg/day)
    - Infuse for minimum 24 hours. Consult medical toxicologist
    - Alternate: 90 mg/kg/dose IM q 8 hrs (max 6000 mg/day)
    - Side effects: ARDS, hypotension (with rapid infusion)
    - Used for altered mental status, shock, severe acidosis, iron level > 500 mcg/dL, significant retained iron in bowel noted on radiograph

Reference: *Curr Opin Pediatr.* 2006;18(2):174.

HYDROCARBON (KEROSENE, GASOLINE, TURPENTINE)

- Large-volume ingestion rare in young children as foul-tasting
- Observe for systemic toxicity (arrhythmia, CNS depression) and aspiration
- If asymptomatic, with normal oximetry and CXR 6 hours post-ingestion → discharge
- Admit for symptoms, hypoxia, or abnormal CXR. Supportive care. Decontaminate patient (remove clothing, bathe). Oxygen, bronchodilators. Do not induce emesis or give charcoal

Reference: *Clin Toxicol.* 2010;48(10):979.

TRICYCLIC ANTIDEPRESSANTS (TCA)

- Signs/symptoms: Sedation, confusion, arrhythmias, hypotension, anticholinergic
- ECG: May show widened QRS (> 100 msec) or prolonged PR and QT intervals
- Treatment
  ○ Activated charcoal: 1 g/kg PO/NG if < 2 hours post-ingestion
  ○ Sodium bicarbonate 2 mEq/kg IV for ECG abnormalities (widened QRS)
  ○ Seizures: Lorazepam 0.1 mg/kg IV × 1. **Avoid phenytoin**

Reference: *Clin Toxicol (Phila).* 2007;45(3):203–233.

SELECTIVE SEROTONIN REUPTAKE INHIBITORS (SSRI)

- Observation for mild symptoms: Vomiting, somnolence, mydriasis, or diaphoresis
- More severe symptoms include seizures, hyperthermia, and serotonin syndrome (AMS, myoclonus, ocular clonus, hypertonia, shivering, diaphoresis, diarrhea, agitation, ataxia, hyperthermia, tremors, ankle clonus)
- Admit for observation. Intubate if obtunded. ECG on admission to evaluate QTc. Depending on size of ingestion and QTc, may need repeat ECG every 1–2 hours
- Treatment
  ○ Activated charcoal 1 g/kg PO/NG × 1 if < 2 hours post-ingestion
  ○ Seizures: Lorazepam 0.1 mg/kg IV × 1
  ○ Hyperthermia/serotonin syndrome: Cooling measures. Consider intubation and paralysis. Consider cyproheptadine (serotonin antagonist) 0.25 mg/kg/day (max 12 mg) IV divided bid–tid
  ○ Prolonged QTc: Consider magnesium 25–50 mg/kg if QTc > 560 msec, bradycardia, or frequent premature ventricular beats

References: *Clin Toxicol (Phila).* 2007;45(4):315–332; *Pediatr Emerg Care.* 1999;15(5):325–327.

ORAL HYPOGLYCEMIC AGENTS (SULFONYLUREAS)

- Single tablets, in small children, can lead to significant hypoglycemia and even death
- If < 2 hours postingestion, give activated charcoal 1–2 g/kg (max 100 grams)
- Observe for a minimum of 8 hours postingestion (peak effect meds at 4–6 hours)
- If BG < 70 mg/dL, admit for treatment and observation
  ○ Give D25W 2–4 mL/kg or D10W 5–10 mL/kg → check BG in 15 minutes
  ○ Initiate dextrose 10% infusion at 1.2–3 mL/kg/hr = 2–5 mg/kg/min
  ○ Recheck BG every 15–60 minutes until stabilized > 70 mg/dL
  ○ Consider octreotide (suppresses insulin release) 1 mcg/kg/dose SQ every 6–12 hours. Generally do not need therapy > 24–36 hours, unless large ingestion

Reference: *Pediatr Emerg Care.* 2013;29(3):292–295.

VALPROIC ACID

- Signs/symptoms of toxicity: CNS depression, electrolyte disturbances, transaminitis, hyperammonemia, hepatotoxicity, metabolic acidosis, hypotension
- Patients with > 50 mg/kg ingestion should be observed for signs/symptoms of toxicity
  ○ Immediate-release preparation: Observe minimum 6 hours post-ingestion
  ○ Delayed-release preparation: Observer minimum 12 hours post-ingestion
- Administer activated charcoal if < 1 hour since ingestion
  ○ Immediate-release: Single dose 1 g/kg PO/NG
  ○ Delayed-release: Consider 0.5 g/kg q 6 hours × 4 doses
- If significant CNS depression, consider naloxone 0.1 mg/kg (max 2 mg) IV × 1
- Hyperammonemia or liver toxicity, give carnitine 50 mg/kg/day PO/IV divided tid

Reference: *Clin Toxicol (Phila).* 2008 Aug;46(7):661–676.

Abbreviations: AC: Activated charcoal; AMS: Altered mental status; ARDS: Acute respiratory distress syndrome; BAL: Dimercaprol; bid: Twice daily; BUN: Blood urea nitrogen; CNS: Central nervous system; CXR: Chest radiograph; D10W: dextrose 10%; D25W: dextrose 25%; ECG: Electrocardiogram; eFe: Elemental iron; FDA: Federal Drug Administration; Fe: Iron; LR: Lactated Ringer's solution; NG: Nasogastric; NS: 0.9% Normal saline; OTC: Over-the-counter; PO: oral; QTc: Corrected QT interval; SSRI: Selective serotonin reuptake inhibitor; SQ: Subcutaneous; TCA: Tricyclic antidepressant; tid: Three times daily; WBI: Whole-bowel irrigation

THORACOSTOMY TUBE MANAGEMENT

INDICATION FOR PLACEMENT AND CHOICE OF THORACOSTOMY TUBE

- Moderate–large pneumothorax (spontaneous, post-central line placement):
  - Small-bore thoracostomy or pigtail catheter may be sufficient
- Tension pneumothorax
- Hemothorax (post-traumatic or postoperative) or pleural effusion:
  - Larger-bore thoracostomy tube to prevent obstruction

THORACOSTOMY TUBE ATTACHMENT OPTIONS

- Water-seal devices (Pleur-Evac®, Atrium Ocean®) have 3 chambers
  - Accumulation chamber
    - Collects air, fluid, and blood from thorax
  - Water seal chamber
    - Prevents back flow of air from the drainage system
    - Air bubbling in this chamber represents "air leak"
  - Suction regulation chamber
    - Height of fluid dictates degree of negative pressure
      - Typically: 15–20 cm H_2O in children
    - Wall suction turned on until constant low bubbling of suction chamber
    - Goal is minimum suction needed to maintain full lung expansion
- One-way valve (Heimlich valve)
  - Useful for pneumothorax only
  - Allows for patient ambulation
- Other devices
  - "Dry" and "wet-dry" systems use either exclusive mechanical valve/regulator suction control or a combination of mechanical regulator and water-seal
  - Benefit: No spillage if collection system tips over

THORACOSTOMY TUBE REMOVAL

- Criteria for tube removal
  - Lung fully expanded
  - No air leak
  - < 1 mL/kg/day fluid drainage
- Remove wall suction and leave "water sealed" for desired period of time
  - Generally 4–24 hours
  - If asymptomatic, likely no reaccumulation of air or fluid
  - Most check radiograph to document no reaccumulation of air or fluid
- Removal
  - Take down occlusive dressing, clip any retaining sutures, hold "purse string" sutures, clamp tube
  - Have patient take breath and hold
    - Remove tube while breath is being held

○ Tie purse string sutures if present
○ Reapply dressing
- Consider recheck radiograph after removal to look for reaccumulation of air

TROUBLESHOOTING THORACOSTOMY TUBES

- Do not "clamp" thoracostomy tube except during insertion, removal, changing of full collection chamber, or troubleshooting
- Do not "strip" chest tube
  ○ Can increase intrapleural pressures and cause significant patient pain
- Persistent air leak
  ○ Make sure occlusive dressing is intact at chest wall
  ○ Take down dressing to make sure tube has not migrated out of pleural space
- Shortness of breath or chest pain
  ○ Can indicate lumen obstruction or tube dislodgment
  ○ Determine patency of tube via patient cough/air bubbling in water seal chamber
  ○ Consider replacing tube if still deemed a necessity, as "repair" options often have greater risk than benefit
    – Do not open system to flush tube as this breaks sterility of system
    – Sterile management options can be undertaken or use "closed" tube clearing systems commercially available
    – Consider alteplase (tPA) instillation into thoracostomy tube

DRIPS

CALCULATION OF DRIP RATES

- Drips run at a dose/kg/hour or dose/kg/minute
- Be sure to convert to appropriate dosing units (mg or mcg) and time (per hour or per minute)
- 1 mg = 1000 mcg; 1 hour = 60 minutes
- Infusion rate (mL/hr)= [(Drip dose in mcg/kg/min) × (weight in kg) × 60 minutes] / (drug concentration in mcg/250 mL)
- Example: 5-kg child, want to run dopamine at 5 mcg/kg/min, and you ask the pharmacy to mix dopamine 400 mg / 250 mL NS
  ○ [5 mcg/kg/min × 5 kg × 60 min] / 1600 mcg/mL = 0.94 mL/ hr infusion rate

Table 19.23   Drips Commonly Used in Pediatrics*

Drug	Dosing	Other
Aminophylline (asthma, apnea; max concentration = 25 mg/mL)	6 wks to 6 mo: 0.5 mg/kg/hr >6 mo: 0.6–1 mg/kg/hr after loading dose of 6 mg/kg	Monitor levels: for asthma goal levels 10–20 mcg/mL; Neonatal apnea: 6–13 mcg/mL
Amiodarone (antiarrhythmic; max concentration in central line 6 mg/mL in D5W)	5 mg/kg (max 300 mg) IV over 30 minutes (can be given rapid IV bolus for pulseless VT of VF) then 5–15 mcg/kg/min (max 15 mg/kg/day)	Usually 2–3 mg/mL concentration in peripheral line; avoid in iodine allergy; monitor ECG; Phlebitis with peripheral infusion; watch for ↓ HR, ↓ BP, corneal deposits, tremor

(Continued)

Table 19.23   Drips Commonly Used in Pediatrics* *(Continued)*

Drug	Dosing	Other
Alprostadil (prostaglandin PGE 1; max concentration = 20 mcg/mL)	0.05–0.1 mcg/kg/min (max 0.4 mcg/kg/min)	Used for temporary maintenance of patent PDA. Beware of apnea (~10% neonates), ↓ BP, ↓ HR, flushing
Cisatracurium (max concentration = 0.4 mg/mL)	0.1–0.15 mg/kg over 5–10 seconds then 1 mcg/kg/min	↓ BP, ↓ HR, bronchospasm. Myopathy with prolonged use
Dobutamine (max concentration = 6 mg/mL *or* 6000 mcg/mL)	5–20 mcg/kg/min (max 40 mcg/kg/min)	Side effects ↓ K+, ↑ BP, chest pain, headache, arrhythmias
Dopamine (max concentration = 6400 mcg/mL)	2–20 mcg/kg/min, may ↑ by 5 mcg/kg min q 15 minutes to desired effect, MAX 50 mcg/kg/min If > 20 mcg/kg/min needed consider adding other adrenergic support (epi, norepi)	Beware ventricular arrhythmias, widened QRS, anxiety. Headache; DO NOT infuse in umbilical artery catheter
Epinephrine (max concentration = 64 mcg/mL)	Continuous infusion: 0.01–1 mcg/kg/min; start low and titrate to desired effect	Beware arrhythmias, anxiety, dizziness, diaphoresis
Fentanyl (max concentration = 50 mcg/mL)	1–2 mcg/kg bolus then 1–2 mcg/kg/hr continuous infusion	Beware chest wall rigidity (reverse with naloxone); ↓ BP, ↓ HR, urinary retention, apnea
Furosemide (max concentration = 10 mg/mL)	0.05 mg/kg/hr to start; titrate to effect, max of 0.4 mg/kg/hr (max 10 mg/kg/day)	Beware ototoxicity, bowel changes, dizziness, rash, electrolyte changes, may affect hepatic and renal dysfunction, ↓ BP
Heparin (max concentration = 100 units/mL)	< 1 yr old: load with 50–75 units/kg over 10 min then 25–28 units/kg/hr, titrate to desired aPTT > 1 yr old: load with 50–75 units/kg then 20 units/kg/hr and adjust to desired aPTT	Check aPTT, platelets, Hb, watch for signs of bleeding; monitor for heparin-induced thrombocytopenia (HIT); watch for signs of ↑ LFTs and ↑ K+
Regular insulin (usually mixed 1 unit/mL)	0.05–0.2 units/kg/hr depending on glucose response, goal glucose ↓ 80–100 mg/dL/hr	Closely monitor serum glucose, potassium, pH, serum, HCO₃, and urine ketones
Lidocaine	Mix 4 g in 500 mL D5W = 8 mg/mL; 20–50 mcg/kg/min	↓ Dose in liver failure
Midazolam (max concentration = 5 mg/mL)	Status epilepticus: 0.05–0.1 mg/kg loading dose, then 1–2 mcg/kg/min; may ↑ by 1 mcg/kg/min every 5–30 min to desired effect	Respiratory and cardiac depression; may require mechanical ventilation; extra caution when used with opioid or rapid administration
Milrinone (1 mg/mL)	50 mcg/kg load, then 0.25–075 mcg/kg/min	↓ BP, arrhythmia

(Continued)

Table 19.23   Drips Commonly Used in Pediatrics* *(Continued)*

Drug	Dosing	Other
Morphine (max concentration = 4 mg/mL)	0.05–0.1 mg/kg/dose max 15 mg IV q 2–4 hr (max 15 mg q 2–4hr), or 10–150 mcg/kg/hr continuous infusion	↓ BP, ↓ respiratory drive (naloxone 0.1 mg/kg [repeat q 2–3 min prn] will reverse)
Nicardipine (max concentration = 0.5 mg/mL)	Start at 0.5 mcg/kg/min, max 3 mcg/kg/min; titrate to effect	Monitor BP and HR; use central IV if possible
Nitroprusside (max concentration = 200 mcg/mL)	Start 0.3–0.5 mcg/kg/min for severe hypertension	Thiocyanate levels if > 3 days, renal impairment, high dose; 1 g sodium thiosulfate per 100 mg nitroprusside in drip to neutralize cyanide
Norepinephrine (max concentration = 64 mcg/mL)	0.05 mcg/kg/min, titrate to max 2 mcg/kg/min	↑ BP, ↑ HR, watch peripheral perfusion and UOP. Useful in "warm shock"
Pancuronium (max concentration = 1 mg/mL)	Infants/teens: 0.02–0.04 mg/kg/hr Child: 0.03–0.1 mg/kg/hr	↑ BP, rash, salivation, bronchospasm, burning sensation
Propofol (max concentration = 10 mg/mL)	Sedation: 1–2 mg/kg IV then 100–150 mcg/kg/min × 3–5 min then DECREASE to 25–75 mcg/kg/min	↓ RR, ↓ HR, ↓ BP; not recommended for prolonged use
Vasopressin (max concentration = 1 unit/mL)	Bleeding esophageal varices 0.002–0.005 units/kg/min, max 0.01 units/kg/min Hypotension: 0.0002–0.002 units/kg/min; max 0.04 units/min	↑ BP, ↓ HR, vasoconstriction, ischemia
Vecuronium (max concentration = 1 mg/mL)	0.1 mg/kg bolus, verify spontaneous recovery from bolus dose, then 0.05–0.15 mg/kg/hr infusion	Bronchospasm, ↑ HR, ↑ or ↓ BP

BP: Blood pressure; Hb: Hemoglobin; HR: Heart rate; RR: Respiratory rate; UOP: Urine output

*Not all FDA-approved for use in children. For more information, refer to www.fda.gov or *Tarascon Pharmacopoeia*.

Data from University of Kentucky Intensive Care Unit Nurse's Guide IV drip list, 2005; *Tarascon Pocket Pharmacopoeia* electronic version accessed 1/18/2013.

TRAUMATIC BRAIN INJURY

SEVERE TRAUMATIC BRAIN INJURY (GCS 3–8) IN CHILDREN

Table 19.24   Pediatric Coma Score

	Points	Glasgow Coma Scale	Modified Infant Coma Score
Eye Opening	4	Spontaneous	Spontaneous
	3	To voice	To voice
	2	To pain	To pain
	1	None	None

(Continued)

Table 19.24   Pediatric Coma Score *(Continued)*

	Points	Glasgow Coma Scale	Modified Infant Coma Score
Verbal Response	5	Oriented	Coos, babbles
	4	Confused	Irritable cry, consolable
	3	Inappropriate	Cries to pain
	2	Garbled	Moans to pain
	1	None	None
Motor Response	6	Obeys commands	Normal movements
	5	Localizes pain	Withdraws to touch
	4	Withdraws to pain	Withdraws to pain
	3	Flexion posturing	Flexion posturing
	2	Extension posturing	Extension posturing
	1	No Movement	No movement

PREHOSPITAL/PRE-ICU MANAGEMENT OF TRAUMATIC BRAIN INJURY

(1) **Fluid resuscitation**

Use isotonic crystalloid solutions (normal saline or lactated Ringer's solution) via large-bore peripheral IV, 20 mL/kg. Repeat as necessary to stabilize vital signs

Do not use hypotonic solutions

(2) **Avoid hypoxemia**

Deliver oxygen via non-rebreather mask

(3) **Bag-valve-mask** often preferred over endotracheal intubation in field

Generally BVM is sufficient to provide oxygenation and ventilation until reaching hospital ED

(4) **C-spine precautions**

(5) **Hypoglycemia**

4 mL/kg of D10W or 2 mL/kg of D25W for symptomatic hypoglycemia

BASIC INTENSIVE CARE MANAGEMENT OF INTRACRANIAL INJURY

(1) Priority is adequate cardiac output by maintaining ***PRELOAD***

Keep CVP > 5 mm H_2O; do not fluid restrict unless SIADH

(2) Place **ICP monitor/ventriculostomy** with drain capability (preferred)

(3) **Cerebral perfusion pressure** (CPP = MAP − ICP) goal 50–70 children, > 70 adults. Catecholamines to increase MAP: phenylephrine, norepinephrine, dopamine

(4) **Sedation:** Options include: Fentanyl, benzodiazepines, etomidate, pentobarbital

Propofol: Decreases cerebral metabolic rate, theoretically decreasing CPP

Adverse reactions include metabolic acidosis, arrhythmias (bundle branch block, junctional)

(5) **Paralysis:** If necessary to prevent agitation/ICP spikes: Vecuronium

(6) **Prevent hyperglycemia:** Associated with pro-inflammatory state. Titrate insulin and glucose infusions with goal serum glucose 80–150 mg/dL

(7) **Phenytoin:** Prophylaxis for seizures. Alternate: Levetiracetam

(8) Elevate head of bed 30° (via reverse Trendelenberg if spine is not cleared)

ACUTE MANAGEMENT OF ELEVATED INTRACRANIAL PRESSURE

First Line: ***Mild* Hyperventilation**: Goal pCO_2 30–35 mmHg

                CSF drainage via ventriculostomy

                Mannitol: 0.25–1 g/kg/dose, *or*

                Hypertonic saline: Infuse 3% saline 0.1–1 mL/kg/hr goal Na^+ 150–155 with maximum serum osmolality 360 (better evidence than for mannitol)

Second Line: **Hypothermia**: Goal 32–36° Celsius via external cooling blankets

                Hyperventilation: pCO_2 25–30 mmHg (should monitor CBF, jugular venous saturation, or tissue O_2 tension)

                Barbiturate coma: Needs continuous EEG monitoring

                Craniotomy, craniectomy, temporal lobe resection

INDEX

Note: Page numbers followed by *f* and *t* refer to figures and tables respectively.